Computed Tomography of CNS Disease: A Teaching File

Computed Tomography of CNS Disease: A Teaching File

Douglas H. Yock, Jr., M.D.

Departments of Radiology
Metropolitan Medical Center
Hennepin County Medical Center
Minneapolis, Minnesota

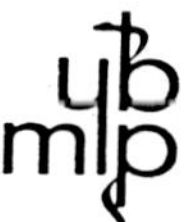

YEAR BOOK MEDICAL PUBLISHERS, INC.
CHICAGO • LONDON • BOCA RATON

4567890Y898887

Library of Congress Cataloging in Publication Data

Yock, Douglas H.
Computer tomography of CNS disease.

Includes bibliographies and index.
1. Central nervous system—Diseases—Diagnosis.
2. Central nervous system—Radiography.
3. Tomography. I. Title. II. Title: Computed tomography of C.N.S. disease. [DNLM: 1. Central Nervous System Diseases— diagnosis. 2. Tomography, X-Ray Computed. WL 141 Y54c] RC361.Y63 1984
616.8'047572 84–19646
ISBN 0–8151–9814–0

Sponsoring editor: James D. Ryan
Editing supervisor: Frances M. Perveiler
Production project manager: Sharon W. Pepping
Proofroom supervisor: Shirley E. Taylor

FOREWORD

THE REAL NEED for a teaching text in craniospinal CT has now been met. In this unique and wonderful book, Dr. Yock succeeds in teaching and delighting his readers simultaneously. The format is beautiful in its simplicity. On facing pages Dr. Yock provides 4 CT images that illustrate the key features of a common diagnosis or a common differential diagnosis. The patient's age, sex, and chief complaint are printed above each image, so they are known before the image is viewed. Detailed captions are printed below each image to explain what the image shows and how to use it to arrive at the correct diagnosis. By this method the reader is first invited to try his skill in interpreting the scan and history in exactly the fashion required in practice. Thereafter, he or she is gently guided to the correct interpretation of the case by the caption beneath. Often the captions conclude with "pearls" of knowledge or just those statistics the physician must know to function effectively.

As in the best teaching conferences, the companion images are carefully selected to complement each other by illustrating, for example, typical and atypical appearances of the same disease or the strikingly-similar appearances of different disease states. Since the complexity of cases and number of possible diagnoses increase from chapter to chapter, Dr. Yock has carefully interwoven special pages, entitled "Differential Diagnosis," that pair diagnoses from different chapters to help the reader review previous material. Throughout the volume, extensive cross references within the captions lead the reader to page back and forth among the cases to glean additional correlations and insights. By this technique, Dr. Yock expands the reader's appreciation of the range of pathology one must consider in each context, and provides a very close approximation to "instant experience." Selected modern references permit especially interested readers to pursue any particular topic easily.

In a book like this, image quality is paramount. Realizing this, Dr. Yock retrieved all the cases illustrated from the archives of magnetic tape and made new hard copies that accentuate the diagnostic features desired. The final results merit this enormous effort.

This book works very well. By painstaking effort and complete control of organization, Dr. Yock has created a teaching tool which combines the best features of first rate teaching conferences and home study. He has eliminated paragraphs of verbiage and replaced them with concise captions which distill for the readers his broad experience and acumen. This excellent volume will be highly useful to all medical students, to all residents in radiology, neurology, neurosurgery, general surgery and medicine, to all attendings who face increasing numbers of CT scans in their daily practice, and to all those knowledgeable physicians who seek to refresh and extend their understanding of this modality. It properly belongs in the departmental and institutional libraries of all hospitals and medical schools and in the personal libraries of those who practice the neurosciences. Unlike compendiums and reference texts, this book is one to enjoy cover to cover.

THOMAS P. NAIDICH, M.D.
Professor of Radiology
Northwestern University Medical School
Chicago, IL

PREFACE

THE APPLICATION OF computed tomography to the study of CNS disease has matured during the past decade. CT now demonstrates a wide spectrum of neuropathology with a high degree of sensitivity and specificity. The following chapters offer an informal survey of this field.

A broad collection of cases has been carefully arranged, with each page featuring a pair of related scans. The four scans on facing pages often form a group of images developing a common subject or comparing different lesions. The "teaching file" format has been used to most effectively combine the text with the illustrations.

A range of CT findings is demonstrated within each pathologic category. "Classic" patterns are followed by examples with atypical features. The potential resemblance of diverse lesions has also been emphasized, with many such comparisons highlighted throughout the book as "Differential Diagnoses."

The distribution of cases reflects the mixture of lesions encountered in an average practice. A comprehensive atlas was not intended. For example, anatomical variants are included only if they mimic pathology, and ENT disease is largely omitted. The chapters on orbital and spinal lesions are thorough introductions rather than comprehensive summaries.

The text focuses on CT interpretation. Comments on clinical presentation, pathophysiology, and therapy are limited, and case histories are intentionally brief. Repetition has been minimized in favor of extensive cross references and a complete index.

In summary, the book has been organized and edited to provide a concise overview of CT interpretation in CNS disease. We hope the result will be enjoyable and informative.

DOUGLAS H. YOCK, JR., M.D.

Note to readers: unless otherwise specified, scans are displayed with the patient's right on the reader's left.

ACKNOWLEDGMENTS

MOST OF THE SCANS in this collection were performed at Metropolitan Medical Center, Minneapolis, where a skilled group of CT technologists manages to combine high quality and high volume. Additional cases were generously contributed by Drs. Lawrence Gold, Robert McGeachie, Kurt Schellhas, Saul Taylor, and David Tubman of Minneapolis and Dr. Glen Forbes of Rochester, Minnesota. Dr. David Larson shared in the daily supervision of CT procedures and in the selection of teaching material. Drs. Larson and McGeachie reviewed the manuscript and offered constructive suggestions.

Jenny Iverson efficiently rephotographed all cases from archival tapes. Joni Mack cheerfully and expertly managed the printing and reprinting of all illustrations. Outstanding transcription assistance and manuscript preparation were provided by Gisela Sime and Carol Jean Davis.

Jim Ryan, Fran Perveiler, and Sharon Pepping of Year Book Medical Publishers were supportive, responsive, and patient as they guided the development of the manuscript.

Finally, the interns and residents of Hennepin County Medical Center are to be thanked for providing the stimulus and encouragement which led to this project.

DOUGLAS H. YOCK, JR., M.D.

CONTENTS

TABLE OF ILLUSTRATED DIFFERENTIAL DIAGNOSES

Cerebral Hemispheres

Posterior Fossa and Tentorium

Sella, Parasellar, and Suprasellar Regions

Subarachnoid Spaces and Ventricles

Orbits

Spine

CHAPTER 1

METASTASES

Case 1

63-year-old man with metastatic lung carcinoma.

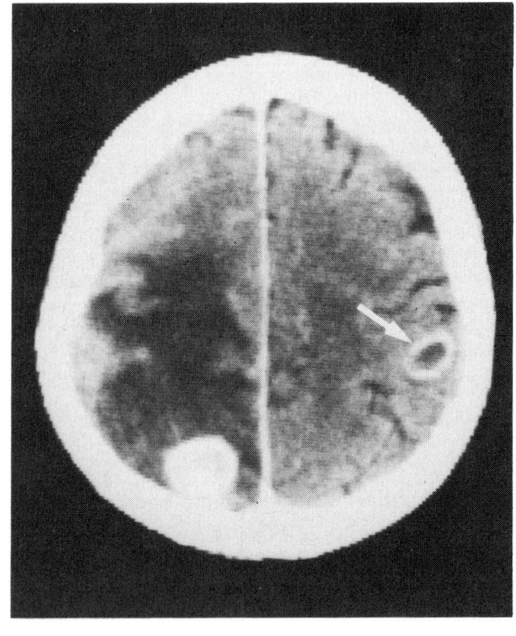

Cerebral metastases are typically found near the junction of gray and white matter. They often provoke cerebral edema, which may be more responsible for symptoms than the tumor itself. Metastases are usually well-defined and are commonly multiple *(arrow)*.

Carcinomas of the breast and lung cause the greatest number of cerebral metastases, although melanoma and hypernephroma metastasize to the brain with higher frequency. An intracranial lesion accounts for the initial presentation of carcinoma in about 10% of cases.

The superficial location of bloodborne metastases reflects the high perfusion of cerebral cortex and is comparable to the distribution of hematogenous cerebral infection (see Case 160).

Case 2

62-year-old woman with metastatic breast carcinoma.

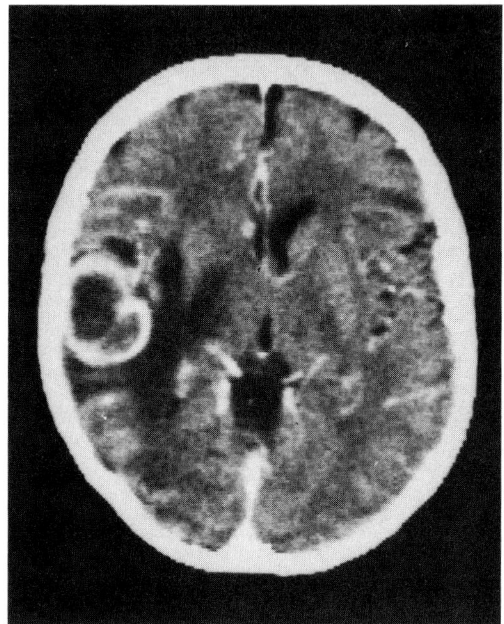

The great majority of cerebral metastases demonstrate abnormal contrast enhancement. The enhancement is homogeneous in small lesions but may be peripheral in larger masses, as is seen in this case. A nonenhancing center within a metastasis (or other tumor) may represent necrosis or a slowly equilibrating compartment that may accumulate contrast on later scans.

Case 3

59-year-old woman with metastatic breast carcinoma.

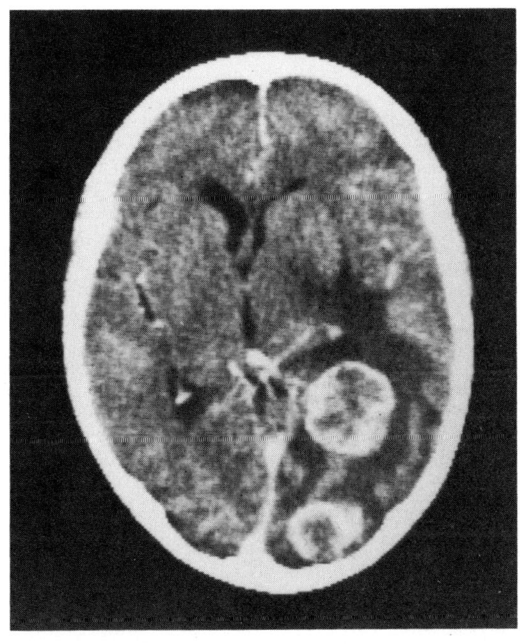

Some metastases are large masses located deep within the cerebral hemispheres. These tumors may mimic primary malignant gliomas (see Cases 48 and 49).

The finding of a second lesion in such cases favors the diagnosis of metastases, and a careful search for distant tumor sites is warranted. Delayed scans and/or increased doses of contrast material may clarify ambiguous lesions by demonstrating additional enhancing masses. However, rare gliomas are multicentric, or may appear so (see Case 43A), so that the demonstration of adjacent masses is not an infallible sign of metastatic disease.

Case 4

52-year-old woman with metastatic hypernephroma.

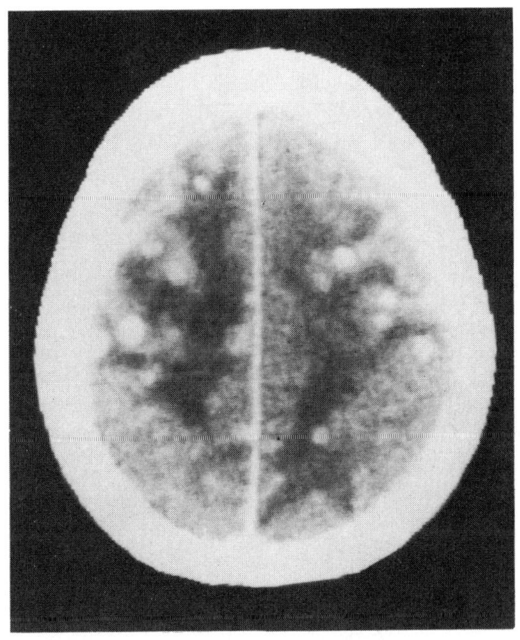

The majority of the small, enhancing nodules in this case are located near the junction of gray and white matter. Edema associated with the multiple lesions coalesces to involve most of the centrum semiovale.

The differential diagnosis of "innumerable" small, enhancing cerebral nodules includes metastases, disseminated infection (e.g., cysticercosis, histoplasmosis, tuberculosis), noninfectious inflammatory processes (e.g., sarcoidosis, multiple sclerosis; see Case 172), primary CNS lymphoma (see Case 138), and subacute multifocal infarction (see Case 236).

CYSTIC METASTASES

Case 5

68-year-old man with metastatic squamous cell carcinoma of the lung.

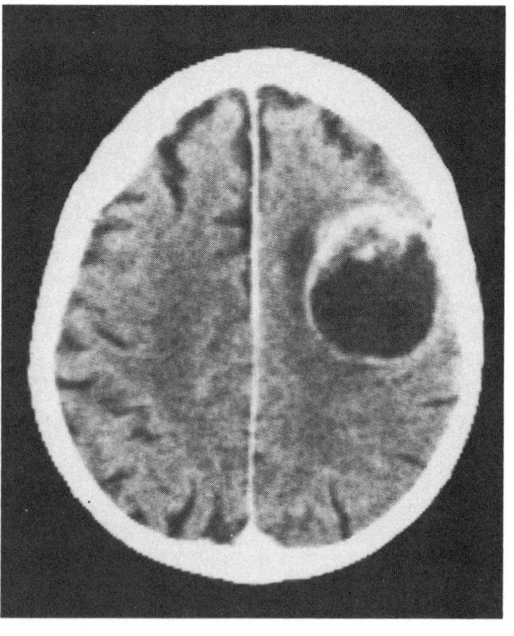

Some cerebral metastases have only a thin rim of tissue surrounding a large central cavity. This appearance is often associated with squamous cell carcinomas but also occurs in adenocarcinomas. Solitary metastases of this type closely resemble malignant gliomas (see Cases 38, 44, and 47), and the two tumors must often be considered together in differential diagnosis.

Up to 50% of cerebral metastases from pulmonary squamous cell tumors are solitary (compared with about 30% of all intracranial metastases).

Case 6

60-year-old woman presenting with confusion. Metastatic adenocarcinoma.

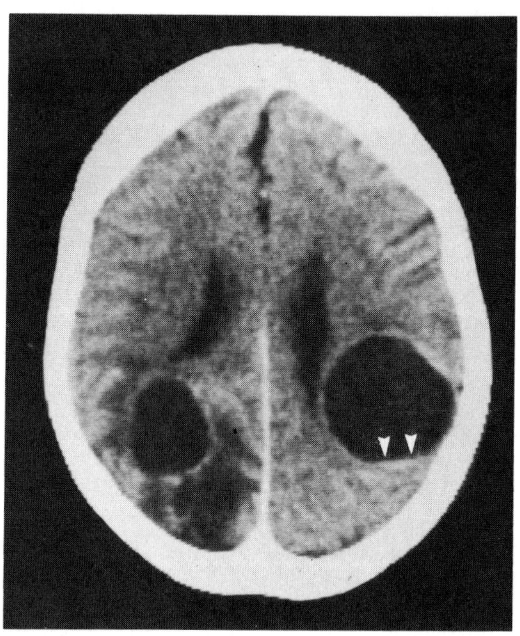

Large, thin-walled cystic-appearing lesions are seen in both hemispheres. The lesion on the left suggests sedimentation of dense material to the dependent portion of the cyst *(arrows)*. Sedimentation is an important finding, since it identifies a homogeneous low-density lesion as a true cyst rather than a region of homogeneous, low-density tissue (see discussion of case 45). In questionable cases, a decubitus scan may demonstrate the appropriate shift of sedimentary material.

HIGH-ATTENUATION METASTASES

Case 7

64-year-old man with metastatic adenocarcinoma of the colon (noncontrast scan).

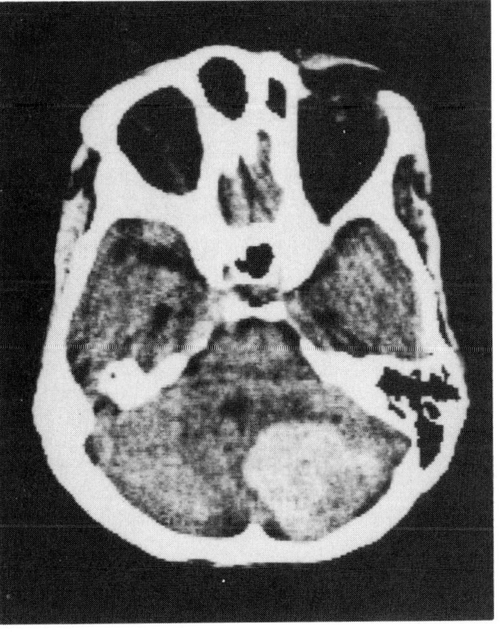

High-attenuation values in a metastasis (or any lesion) may be due to hemorrhage, calcification, and/or dense protein content. Metastases from adenocarcinomas may demonstrate precontrast density in the absence of hemorrhage or macroscopic calcification. The high attenuation is attributable to the tissue density of the tumors and is particularly associated with mucinous carcinomas.

Case 8

58-year-old man with metastatic adenocarcinoma of the colon.

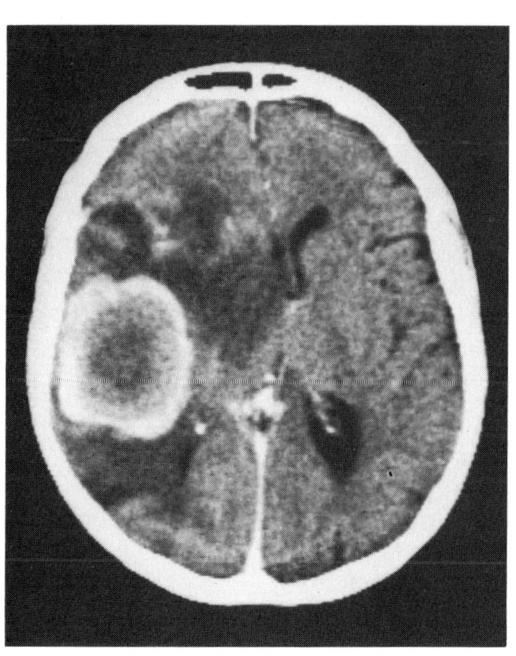

This dense mass was identical in appearance on a precontrast scan. The usually unimpressive contrast enhancement of dense metastases helps to distinguish them from meningiomas (see Cases 21 and 22).

Case 9

67-year-old man with metastatic hypernephroma (noncontrast scan).

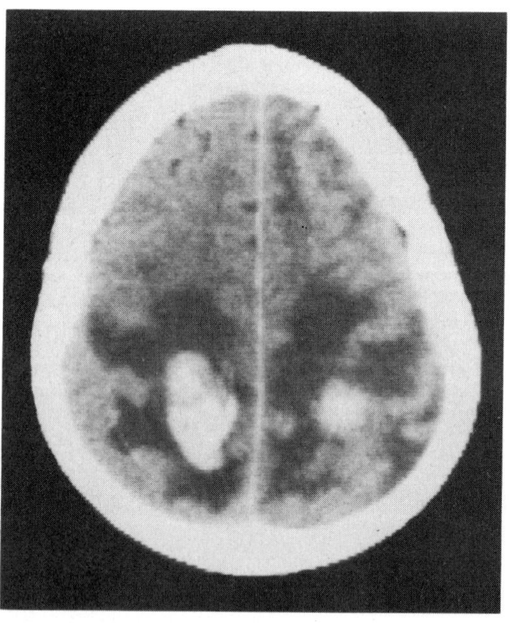

The multiplicity and location of these lesions strongly suggest metastases. The high-attenuation values are more dense than mucinous adenocarcinomas and indicate hemorrhage within the nodules. This feature narrows the likely diagnoses to those primary tumors that cause vascular metastases: melanoma, choriocarcinoma, hypernephroma, bronchogenic carcinoma, and, occasionally, breast carcinoma.

Although hemorrhage into a cerebral metastasis is often the presenting event in metastatic melanoma (see Case 329), a renal or pulmonary neoplasm would be more common in a 67-year-old man. As a result of this scan, a chest roentgenogram and intravenous pyelogram were recommended, and a previously "silent" hypernephroma was discovered.

Case 10

72-year-old woman presenting with a "stroke." Hemorrhage into metastatic ovarian carcinoma.

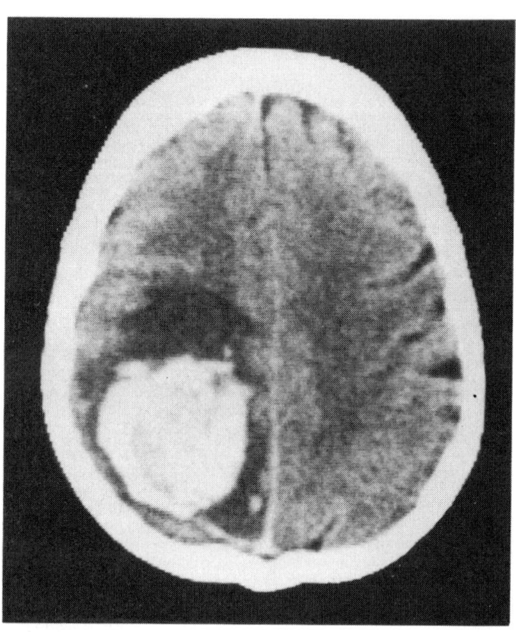

A mass is seen faintly within the large parietal hematoma, suggesting hemorrhage into a preexisting lesion (compare with Case 329). The hematoma was evacuated and metastatic ovarian carcinoma was found.

Hemorrhage into a cerebral neoplasm is one mechanism by which such subacute or chronic lesions may cause acute symptoms ("stroke syndrome"). Other mechanisms include the sudden triggering of reactive cerebral edema (see Case 37), ventricular obstruction causing acute hydrocephalus, and eventual critical vascular compression by an enlarging mass. About 5% of "strokes" are found to be the result of an underlying neoplasm.

METASTATIC INVOLVEMENT OF CEREBROSPINAL FLUID SURFACES

Case 11

76-year-old woman with metastatic breast carcinoma.

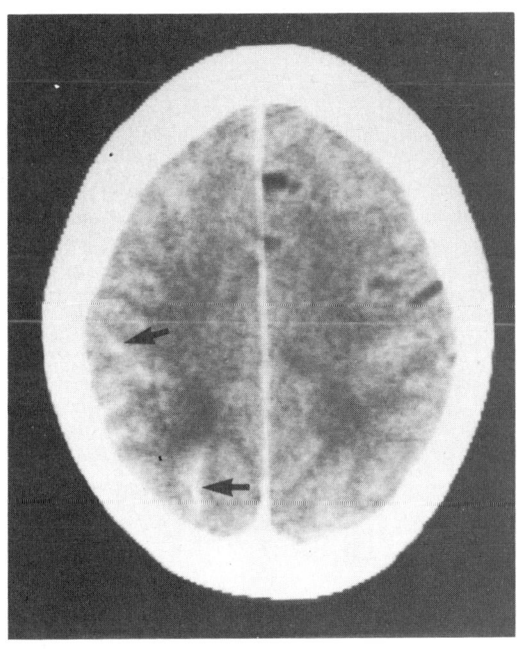

The abnormal contrast enhancement within cortical sulci *(arrows)* represents meningeal carcinomatosis. Meningeal involvement by metastatic solid tumors (especially melanoma and breast carcinoma) is often apparent on CT scans. The detection rate for meningeal lymphoma or leukemia is much lower.

When sulcal enhancement *is* seen, the differential diagnosis includes meningeal tumor (systemic metastasis or seeding of a primary CNS lesion; see Case 301), meningitis (especially granulomatous processes; see Case 162), and the contrast enhancement occurring after subarachnoid hemorrhage (see case 300).

Case 12

62-year-old man with metastatic oat cell carcinoma.

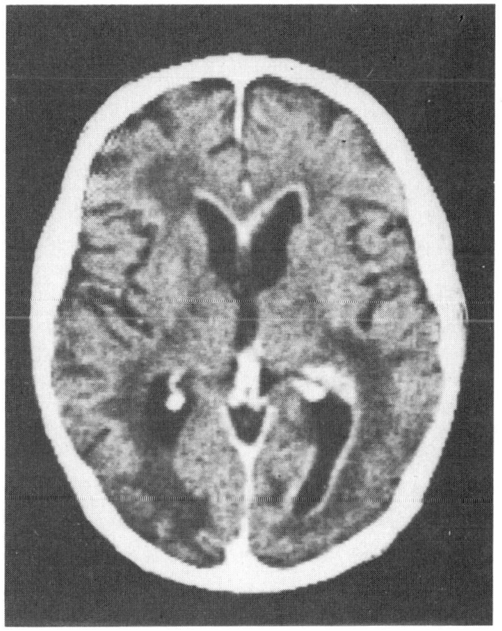

The enhancing ventricular margins in this case represent subependymal spread of metastatic small-cell carcinoma of the lung. This occurrence is less common than meningeal carcinomatosis, but has been observed with several systemic tumors (e.g., melanoma, carcinomas of the lung and breast).

The differential diagnosis of enhancing ventricular margins also includes ependymal seeding or subependymal spread of gliomas and other primary CNS tumors (see Case 54), primary CNS lymphoma, systemic lymphoma (see Case 55), and inflammatory ventriculitis (see Case 163).

REFERENCES

1. Amundsen P., Dugstad G., Syvertsen A.H.: The reliability of computer tomography for the diagnosis and differential diagnosis of meningiomas, gliomas, and brain metastases. *Acta Neurochir. (Wien)* 41:177–190, 1978.
J. Comput. Assist. Tomogr. 4:311–313, 1978.
Demonstration by computed tomography. *A.J.N.R.* 3:527–529, 1982.
3. Brant-Zawadzki M., Enzmann D.R.: Computed tomographic brain scanning in patients with lymphoma. *Radiology* 129:67-71, 1978.
4. Brown S.B., Brant-Zawadzki M., Eifel P., et al.: CT of irradiated solid tumor metastases to the brain. *Neuroradiology* 23:127–131, 1982.
5. Dearnaley D.P., Kingsley D.P., Husband J.E., et al.: The role of CT of the brain in the investigation of breast cancer patients with suspected intracranial metastases. *Clin. Radiol.* 32:375–382, 1981.
6. Deck M.D., Messina A.V., Sackett J.F.: Computed tomography in metastatic disease of the brain. *Radiology* 119:115–120, 1976.
7. Enzmann D.R., Krikorian J., Yorke C., et al.: Computed tomography in leptomeningeal spread of tumor. *J. Comput. Assist. Tomogr.* 2:448–455, 1978.
8. Gildersleeve N., Koo A.H., McDonald C.J.: Metastatic tumor presenting as intracerebral hemorrhage. *Radiology* 124:109–112, 1977.
9. Ginaldi S., Wallace S., Shalen P., et al.: Cranial computed tomography of malignant melanoma. *A.J.N.R.* 1:531–535, 1980.
10. Healy J.F., Marshall W.H., Brahme F.J., White F.: CT of intracranial metastases with skull and scalp involvement. *A.J.N.R.* 2:335–338, 1981.
11. Hilal S.K., Chang C.H.: Specificity of computed tomography in the diagnosis of supratentorial neoplasms. *Neuroradiology* 16:537–539, 1978.
12. Holtas S., Cronquist S.: Cranial computed tomography of patients with malignant melanoma. *Neuroradiology* 22:123–127, 1981.
13. Huckman M.S., Ramsey R.G., Shenk G.I.: CT scanning in patients with suspected cerebral metastases. *J. Comput. Assist. Tomogr.* 2:511–512, 1978.
14. Kingsley D.P., Kendall B.E.: Cranial computed tomography in leukemia. *Neuroradiology* 16:543–546, 1978.
15. Lukin R., Tomsick T.A., Chambers A.A.: Lymphoma and leukemia of the central nervous system. *Semin. Roentgenol.* 15:246, 1980.
16. Naheedy M.H., Kido D.I., O'Reilly G.V., et al.: Computed tomography of subdural and epidural metastases. *J. Comput. Assist. Tomogr.* 4:311–313, 1978.
17. Potts G.D., Abbott G.F., Von Sneidern J.V.: National Cancer Institute study: Evaluation of computed tomography in the diagnosis of intracranial neoplasms. III. Metastatic tumors. *Radiology* 136:657–664, 1980.
18. Rao K.C., Williams J.P.: Intracranial tumors: Metastatic, in Lee S.H., Rao K.C. (eds.): *Cranial Computed Tomography.* New York, McGraw Hill Inc., 1983, pp. 345–369.
19. Voorhies R.M., Sundaresan N., Thaler H.T.: The single supratentorial lesion: An evaluation of preoperative diagnostic tests. *J. Neurosurg.* 53:364–368, 1980.
20. Wendling L.R., Cromwell L.D., Latchaw R.E.: Computed tomography of intracerebral leukemic masses. *A.J.R.* 132:217–220, 1979.
21. Zimmerman R.A., Bilaniuk L.T.: Computed tomography of acute intratumoral hemorrhage. *Radiology* 135: 355–359, 1980.

CHAPTER 2

MENINGIOMAS

Case 13

72-year-old man. Falx meningioma (noncontrast scan).

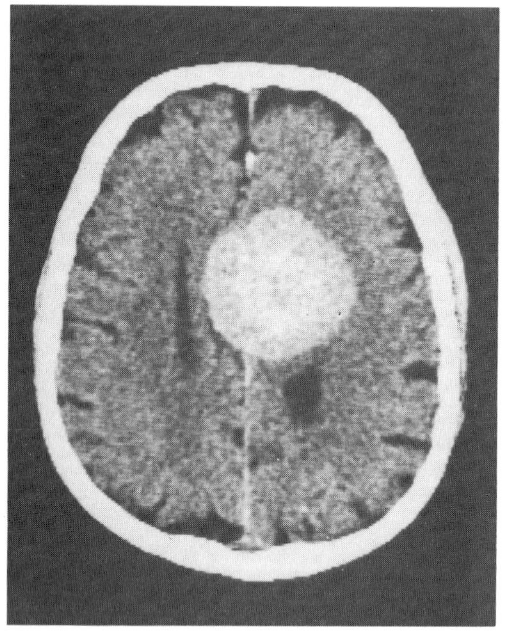

Meningiomas are typically homogeneous, high-attenuation lesions, due to their dense cellularity, fibrous tissue, and/or "psammomatous" calcification. High-resolution scans may show a concentric circular or radial pattern within the tumor, as in this case.

The margins of meningiomas are usually smooth and well-defined. Even large tumors may cause relatively little edema and mass effect. This quiescent appearance implies slow growth, with gradual invagination into adjacent parenchyma.

In this case, the tumor is projecting inferiorly to cross beneath the free margin of the falx, as seen in the coronal section in Case 20.

Meningiomas account for 15% to 20% of intracranial tumors, with a peak age incidence at 45 years and a moderate predominance in women.

Case 14

61-year-old man. Bilateral frontal convexity meningiomas.

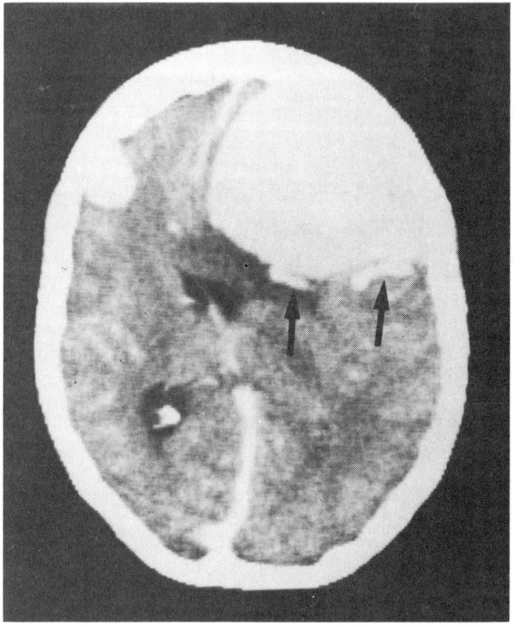

Uniform, intense contrast enhancement is characteristic of meningiomas. The diagnosis of these tumors is based on the combination of homogeneously high precontrast density, uniform contrast enhancement, smooth and well-defined margins, and typical location. (For examples of meningiomas in other common locations, see Cases 79, 83, 135, 295, and 316.)

Other lesions may have similar precontrast and postcontrast features, including aneurysms, pituitary adenomas, germinomas, medulloblastomas, CNS lymphomas, acoustic schwannomas, and, occasionally, craniopharyngiomas and colloid cysts.

It is unusual to identify large draining veins, as are seen in this case along the posterior margin of the larger meningioma *(arrows)*.

ATYPICAL MENINGIOMAS

Case 15

58-year-old man with hemiparesis.

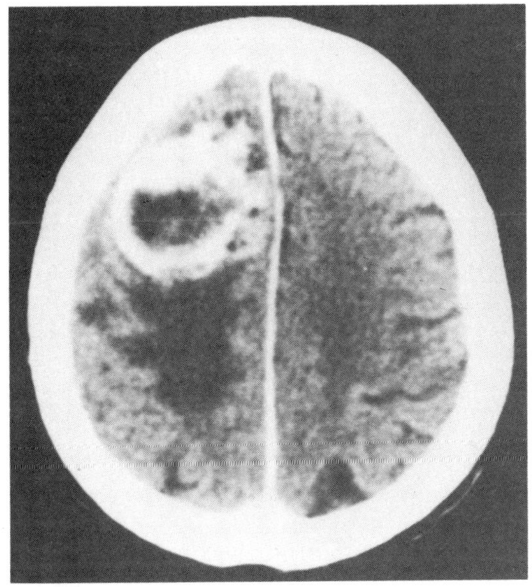

Because the typical appearance of meningiomas is one of the most reliable "stereotypes" on CT, atypical appearances can be confusing. A small number of meningiomas contain or are associated with low-attenuation, nonenhancing areas. These may be due to necrosis, old hemorrhage, cyst formation, or fat within the meningioma tissue.

The diagnosis is not obscured if these atypical regions are small in proportion to the tumor size. If atypical regions predominate, the possibility of other pathologies (e.g., glioma or metastasis) must be considered.

In this case, the thick rim, central low attenuation, irregular margins, and prominent edema mimic a malignant glioma or metastasis (compare with Cases 3 and 38). Coronal scans may contribute to the diagnosis of such lesions by demonstrating that the mass arises from a dural base. However, superficial gliomas may invade the dura, and dural-based metastases are not uncommon (see Cases 23 and 31).

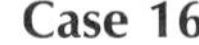

Case 16

44-year-old man.

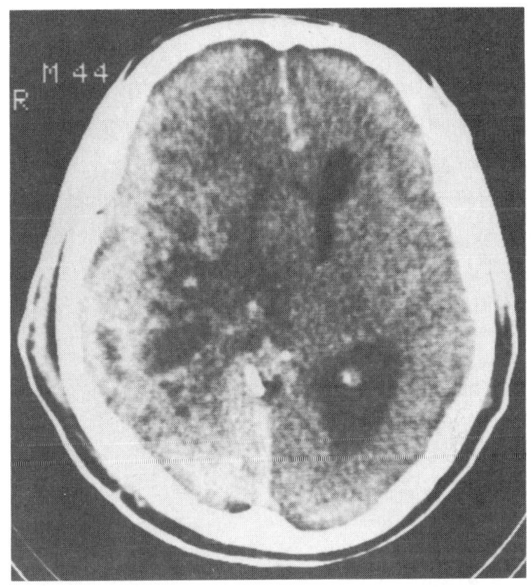

Occasional meningiomas demonstrate aggressive behavior. Sarcomatous transformation may occur in originally benign lesions, and some histologic varieties (e.g., papillary and "angioblastic" meningiomas) are themselves associated with a tendency toward malignant features.

The tumor in this case was recurrent. It had spread over much of the hemisphere and was found to have invaded deeply into cerebral parenchyma at numerous sites. Pathologic examination suggested meningeal sarcoma.

MENINGIOMAS: PLAQUE-LIKE COMPONENTS

Case 17

70-year-old man.

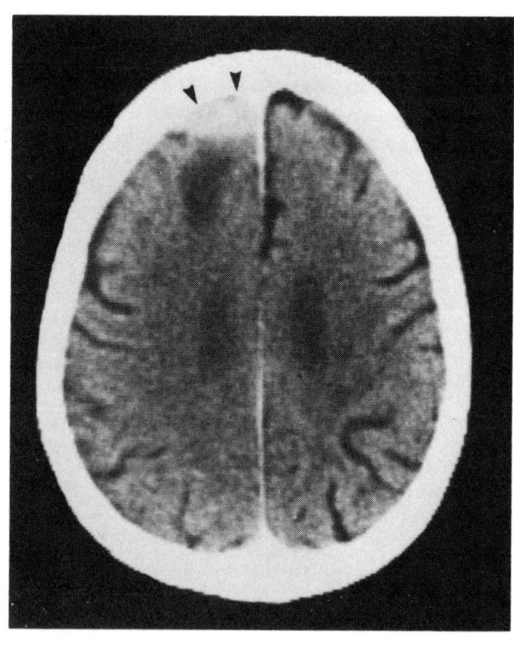

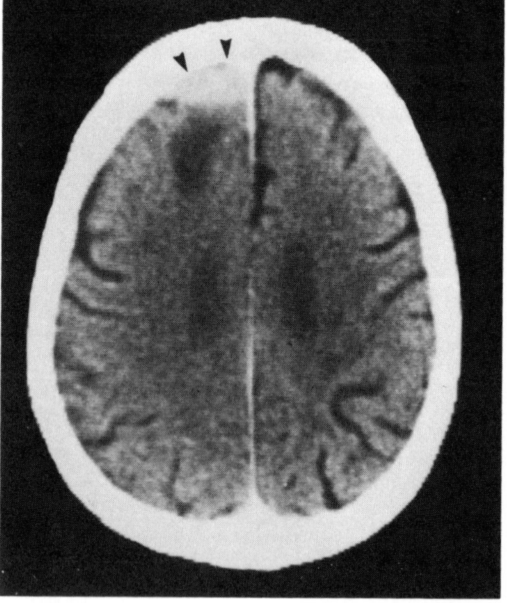

Some meningiomas spread along the inner tables as relatively flat sheets of tissue. This "en plaque" morphology may be seen alone or in association with spherical components. The superficial location, homogeneous density, and intense contrast enhancement remain characteristic.

Case 18

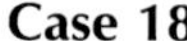

75-year-old man being evaluated for dementia.

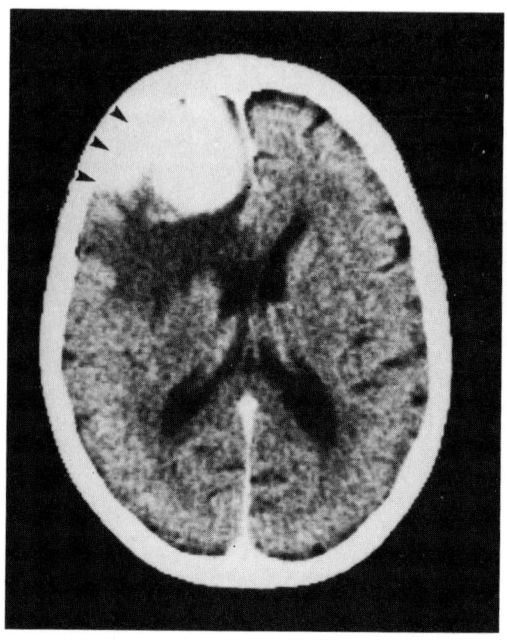

This large frontal meningioma has a "comma" shape due to the combination of spherical and plaque-like components. (Compare this configuration with the comma-shaped masses growing around dural margins in Cases 19 and 20.) Such morphology has been associated with aggressive tumor behavior, a possibility supported here by the extensive reactive edema.

About 20% of patients with dementia are found to have treatable causes for their symptoms. Intracranial masses account for about one fourth of such cases.

MENINGIOMAS: "COMMA" SHAPE

Case 19

52-year-old woman.

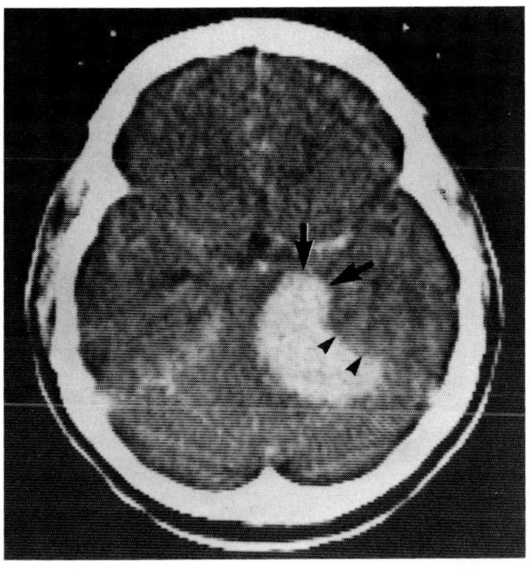

Posterior fossa meningiomas arising from the petrous bone or inferior surface of the tentorium may extend to the incisura. Further growth of the tumor may pass through the tentorial hiatus to accumulate in a parasellar location. While the infratentorial component of the mass retains a straight lateral margin confined by the petrous ridge and tentorium, the middle fossa component is free to assume a spherical shape. The combination of these semilunar and circular components resembles a fat comma.

The lateral tentorial margin similarly shapes the morphology of other adjacent lesions (see Cases 191, 242A, 243, 257, and 258).

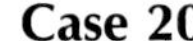

Case 20

72-year-old man (coronal scan; same patient as Case 13).

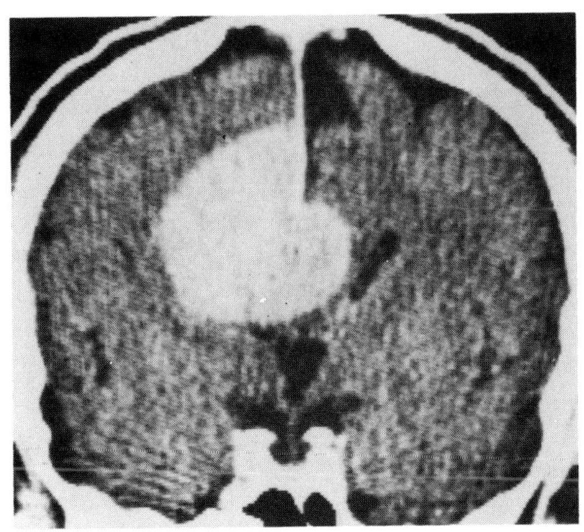

Falx meningiomas may also develop a "comma" shape. A tumor arising along one side of the falx may grow inferiorly to reach the free margin. The mass may then depress the corpus callosum to cross the midline beneath the falx, as seen in this case. Again, the combination of a semilunar component bounded by a dural surface and a spherical component growing beyond the dural margin produces a "comma" shape.

Coronal scans are often useful in the evaluation of falx meningiomas. They may demonstrate (1) the extent of bilateral involvement; (2) the morphology of dependent or exophytic components, as in this case; and (3) possible invasion or compression of the superior sagittal sinus.

DIFFERENTIAL DIAGNOSIS: WELL-DEFINED, SUPERFICIAL, HIGH-ATTENUATION MASS

Case 21

81-year-old woman.

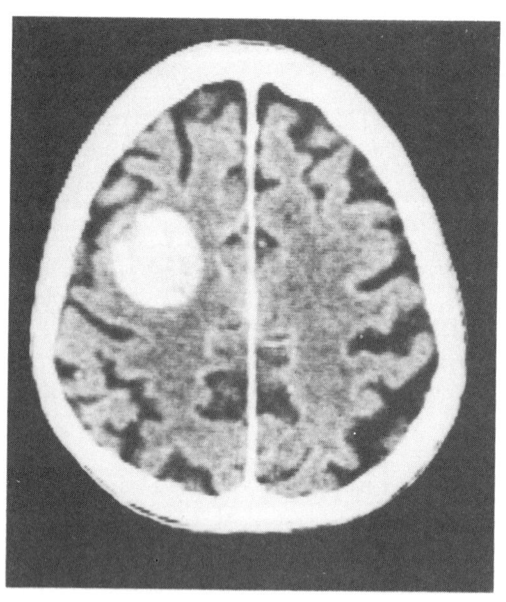

Metastatic Mucinous Adenocarcinoma.

Case 22

80-year-old woman.

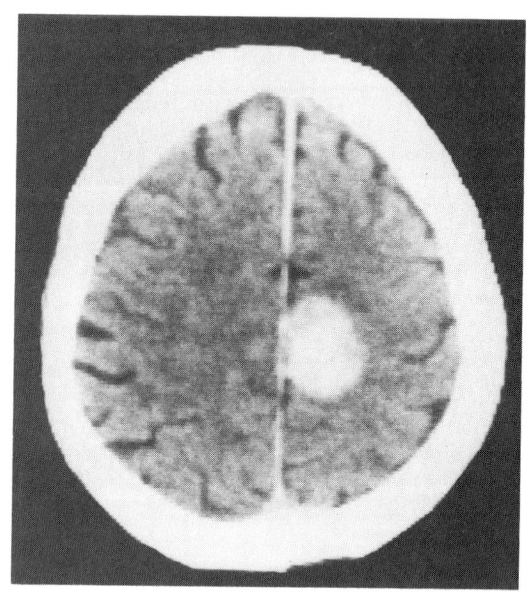

Falx Meningioma.

Some dense metastases may mimic meningiomas because of the shared characteristics of superficial location, well-defined margins, and frequent edema. The correct diagnosis can usually be made by establishing a dural base for a meningioma, vs. an intra-axial location for a metastasis.

The meningioma in Case 22 is clearly attached to the falx. On the other hand, the metastasis in Case 21 is entirely intraparenchymal. (A coronal scan would exclude the possibility that the mass is projecting inferiorly from the calvarial vertex.) Caution: see discussion in Cases 23 and 24 regarding dural-based metastases.

DIFFERENTIAL DIAGNOSIS: DURAL-BASED, INTENSELY ENHANCING, EXTRA-AXIAL MASS

Case 23

75-year-old woman presenting with homonymous hemianopia.

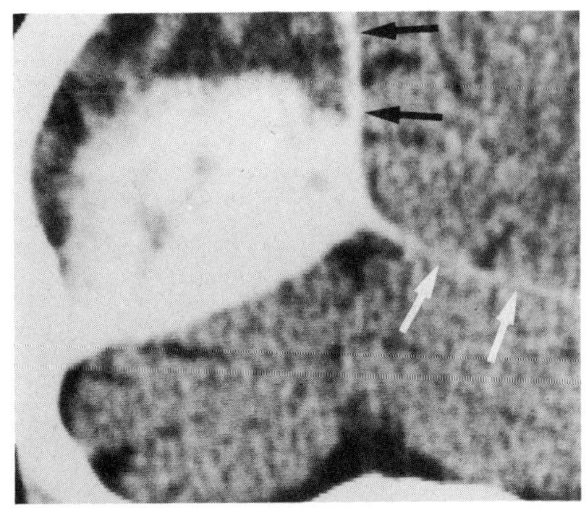

Metastatic Breast Carcinoma (Coronal Scan).

Case 24

83-year-old man presenting with syncope.

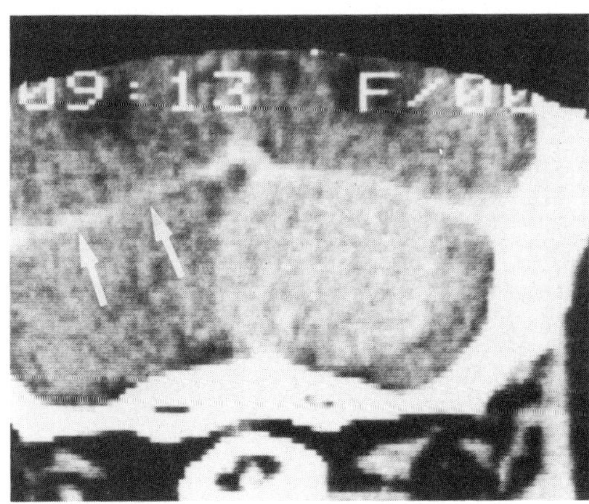

Tentorial Meningioma (Coronal Scan).

Metastases to the skull or dura may produce focal extra-axial masses. Such lesions may closely resemble meningiomas in location, definition, and contrast enhancement. The most common tumor to mimic meningioma in this manner is metastatic prostate carcinoma (see Cases 31 and 32), but melanoma, breast carcinoma, and renal carcinoma may cause similar appearances. Superficial gliomas may also invade the dura and occasionally mimic meningioma in other respects as well (see Case 39).

Coronal scans are helpful in defining the relationship of lesions to the sloping tentorium *(white arrows)* and posterior falx *(black arrows)*. Tentorial meningiomas may thicken the tentorium and/or project from its inferior or superior surfaces. (A thickened tentorium may also be seen in cases of chronic basal meningitis; see Case 162.)

MENINGIOMAS: DENSE TUMOR CALCIFICATION

Case 25

79-year-old woman. Sphenoid wing meningioma (high window level).

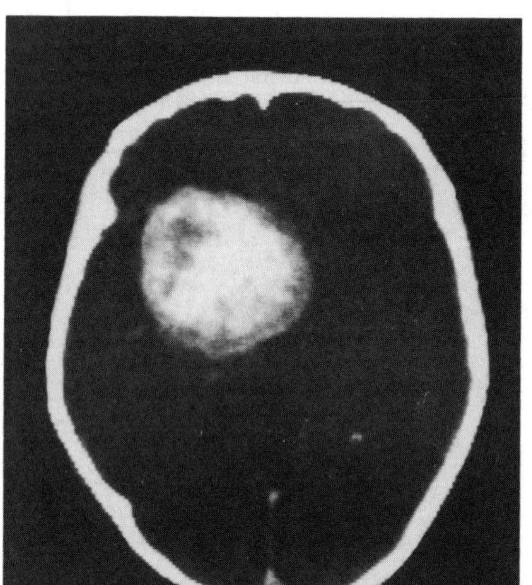

Some meningiomas contain large amounts of dense calcium. Calcification may occupy a portion of the tumor or fill the entire mass, as in this case. Circular and radial components can be seen.

Case 26

63-year-old woman. 'En plaque' convexity meningioma (wide window width, high window level).

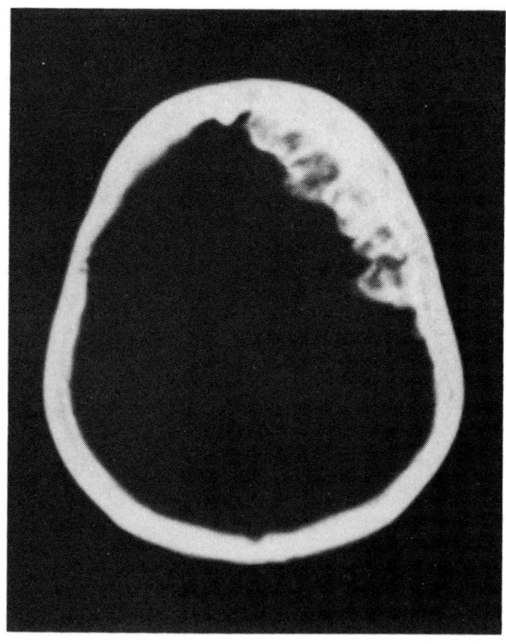

"En plaque" meningiomas may provoke intense calvarial hyperostosis particularly along the skull base. In such cases it is difficult to judge whether the layer of exuberant calcification is within the tumor or represents hyperostosis of the inner table. Often, both components are present.

MENINGIOMAS: ASSOCIATED HYPEROSTOSIS

Case 27

71-year-old woman (coronal scan, wide window width).

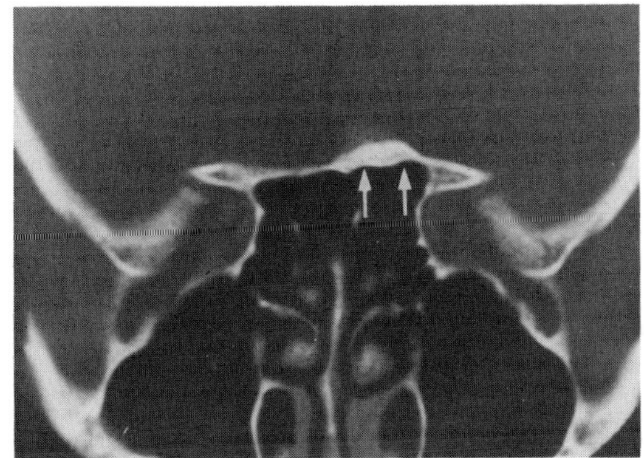

Hyperostosis is frequently seen at the base of meningiomas. This sclerosis may accompany calvarial invasion or be an independent reaction to adjacent tumor.

In this case, the planum sphenoidale is focally thickened *(arrows)* at the attachment of the mass. In addition, tumor-induced remodeling of bone has caused expansion of the sinus toward the meningioma. This "blistering" of the sinus roof is a hallmark of meningiomas arising from the planum sphenoidale or tuberculum sellae.

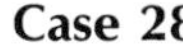

Case 28

75-year-old woman with proptosis (wide window width).

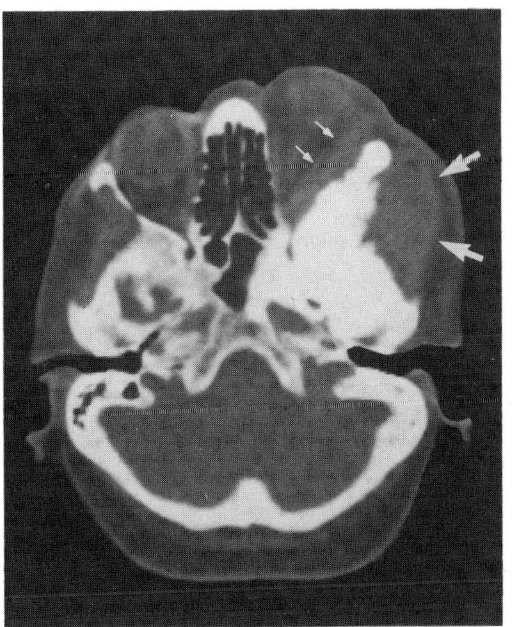

The left sphenoid bone is very dense and greatly thickened due to a meningioma permeating the sphenoid wing ("intraosseous meningioma"). Sphenoid involvement by sclerosing meningioma may have both orbital and cerebral consequences. This scan demonstrates proptosis primarily resulting from bone deformity. Tumor tissue is seen in the lateral aspect of the orbit *(small arrows)* and extracranially in the infratemporal fossa *(large arrows)*.

The major differential diagnosis for this CT appearance would be fibrous dysplasia of bone, which is usually seen in the first decades of life.

DIFFERENTIAL DIAGNOSIS: DENSELY CALCIFIED MASS ADJACENT TO THE INNER TABLE

Case 29

65-year-old woman.

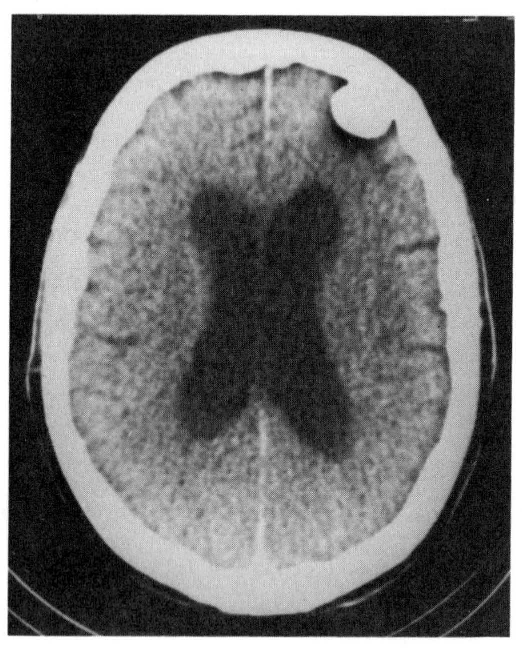

Osteoma.

Case 30

58-year-old woman.

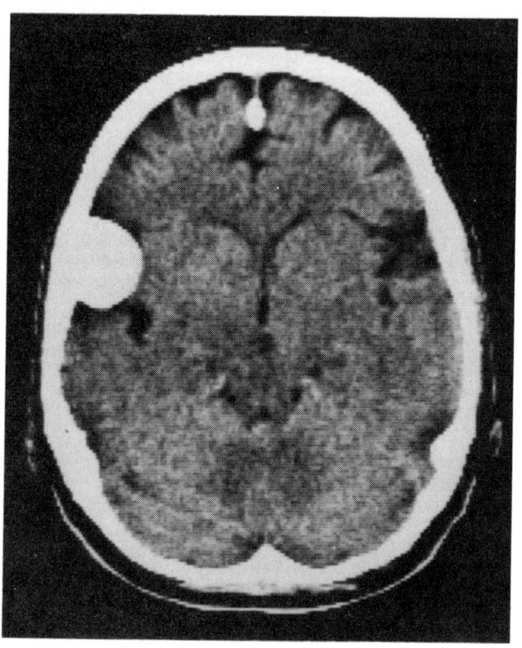

Meningioma.

Densely calcified meningiomas adjacent to the inner table may resemble osteomas. Osteomas are benign bone tumors which may arise from either the inner or outer table of the skull. They typically consist of homogeneous, dense bone with a smooth, hemispheral shape based against the table of origin.

Skull roentgenograms or routine tomograms may be useful in distinguishing the characteristic "ivory" density of an osteoma from the less uniform calcification of a dense meningioma. Examination of CT scans at wide window widths and high window levels may provide similar differentiation.

In many cases, the two lesions are indistinguishable. Both meningiomas and osteomas may be separated from the adjacent inner table by a thin line of relative lucency.

DIFFERENTIAL DIAGNOSIS: INTENSELY ENHANCING, EXTRA-AXIAL MASS ARISING FROM THE SPHENOID WING

Case 31

56-year-old man.

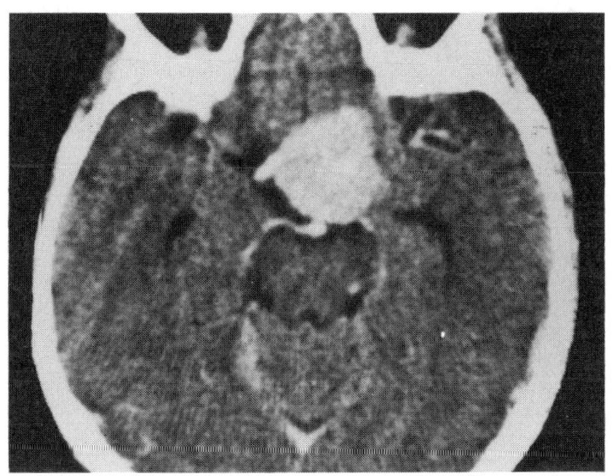

Metastatic Prostate Carcinoma.

Case 32

61-year-old woman.

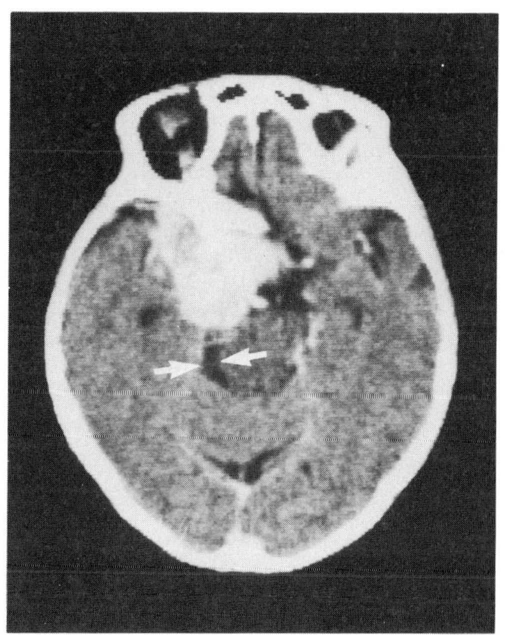

Meningioma.

Metastatic prostate carcinoma involving the skull may be indistinguishable from meningioma on a single scan. (A similar appearance is occasionally caused by epidural melanoma or carcinomas of the breast and kidney.) The two lesions may also be identical on an angiogram, with dural arterial supply and well-defined tumor strains.

Rapid growth of a metastasis or the discovery of systemic lesions usually clarifies initial confusion. The tumor in Case 31 had been found six months earlier, when it was 5 mm in diameter (see Case 111).

The meningioma in Case 32 has displaced the brain stem, causing widening of the adjacent cistern *(arrows)*. This finding is typical of extra-axial masses (see Cases 69 and 74).

REFERENCES

1. Amundsen P., Dugstad G., Syvertsen A.H.: The reliability of computer tomography for the diagnosis and differential diagnosis of meningiomas, gliomas, and brain metastases. *Acta Neurochir. (Wien)* 41:177–190, 1978.
2. Becker D., Norman D., Wilson C.B.: Computerized tomography and pathological correlation in cystic meningiomas. *J. Neurosurg.* 50:103–105, 1979.
3. Claveria L.E., Sutton D., Tress B.M.: The radiological diagnosis of meningiomas: The impact of EMI scanning. *Br. J. Radiol.* 50:15–22, 1977.
4. Dell S., Ganti R., Steinberger A., et al.: Cystic meningiomas: A clinicoradiological study. *J. Neurosurg.* 57:8–13, 1982.
5. Dietemann J.L., Heldt N., Burguet J.L., et al.: CT findings in malignant meningiomas. *Neuroradiology* 23:207–209, 1982.
6. Fine M., Brazis P., Palacios E.: Computed tomography of sphenoid wing meningiomas: Tumor location related to distal edema. *Surg. Neurol.* 13:385–397, 1980.
7. Fornari M., Savoiaro M., Morello G., et al.: Meningiomas of the lateral ventricles. *J. Neurosurg.* 54:64–74, 1981.
8. Kadis G.N., Mount L.A., Ganti S.R.: The importance of early diagnosis and treatment of meningiomas of the planum sphenoidale and tuberculum sellae: A retrospective study of 105 cases. *Surg. Neurol.* 12:367–371, 1979.
9. Kendall B.E., Pullicine P.: Comparison of consistency of meningiomas and computed tomography appearances. *Neuroradiology* 18:173–176, 1979.
10. Nahser H.C., Grote W., Lohr E., et al.: Multiple meningiomas: Clinical and computed tomographic observations. *Neuroradiology* 21:259–263, 1981.
11. New P.F., Aronow S., Hesselink J.: National cancer institute study: Evaluation of computed tomography in the diagnosis of intracranial neoplasms. IV. Meningiomas. *Radiology* 136:665–675, 1980.
12. New P.F., Hesselink J.R., O'Carroll C.P., et al.: Malignant meningiomas: CT and histologic criteria, including a new CT sign. *A.J.N.R.* 3:267–276, 1982.
13. Rozario R., Adelman L., Prager R.J., et al.: Meningiomas of the pineal region and third ventricle. *Neurosurgery* 5:489–495, 1979.
14. Russell E.J., George A.E., Kricheff I.I., et al.: Atypical computed tomographic features of intracranial meningiomas. *Radiology* 135:673–682, 1980.
15. Smith H.P., Challa V.R., Moody D.M., et al.: Biological features of meningiomas that determine the production of cerebral edema. *Neurosurgery* 8:428–433, 1981.
16. Stevens J.M., Ruiz J.S., Kendall B.E.: Observations on peritumoural oedema in meningioma: II. Mechanisms of oedema production. *Neuroradiology* 25:125–131, 1983.
17. Valavanis A., Schubiger D., Hayek J., et al.: CT of meningiomas on the posterior surface of the petrous bone. *Neuroradiology* 22:111–121, 1981.
18. Vassilouthis J., Ambrose J.: Computerized tomography scanning appearances of intracrania meningiomas. An attempt to predict the histological features. *J. Neurosurg.* 50:320–327, 1979.

CHAPTER 3

GLIOMAS

LOW-GRADE GLIOMAS: DEEP LOCATION, LOW ATTENUATION, INDISTINCT MARGINS, AND MINIMAL ENHANCEMENT

Case 33

18-year-old man presenting with seizures.
Grade 1 or 2 astrocytoma.

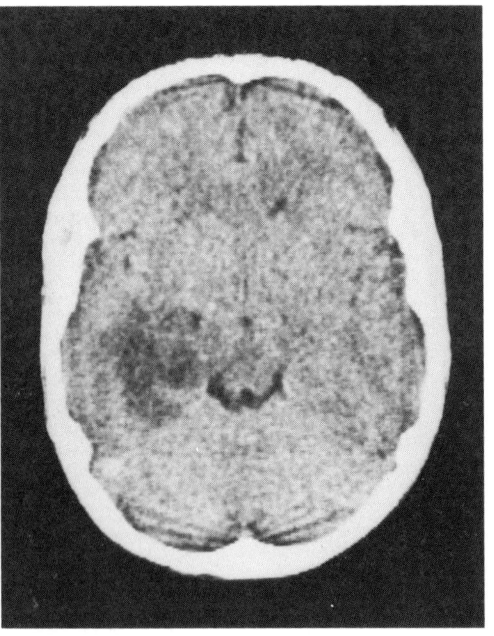

Low-grade gliomas are usually seen as poorly defined areas of low attenuation. Mass effect is variable and contrast enhancement is rarely impressive. The deep temporal lobe is a common location for these lesions in young adults, and the history of seizures is typical for such patients.

Many low-grade gliomas are found in the perisylvian region, where their low density may mimic a recent infarction in the distribution of the middle cerebral artery. The sparing of cortex, indistinct margins, and clinical context of a glioma usually allow distinction from ischemic lesions (see Cases 245, 246, and 262).

Case 34

34-year-old woman presenting with headaches.
Grade 2 astrocytoma.

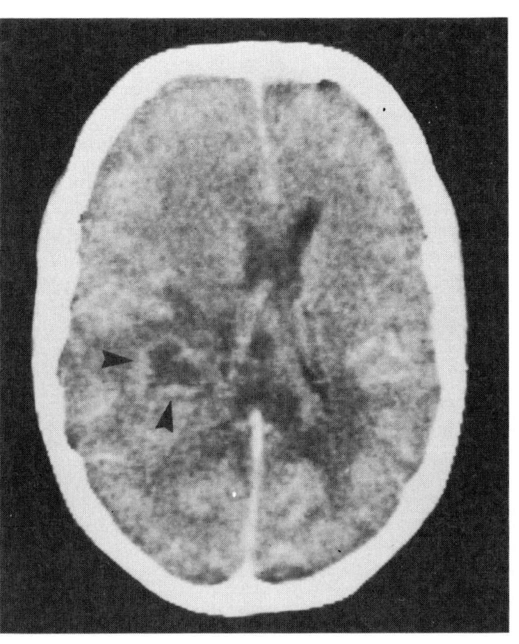

The tumor is seen as a vague area of low attentuation deep within the right cerebral hemisphere. This characteristic deep-hemisphere location of glial tumors contrasts with the metastases and meningiomas illustrated in Chapters 1 and 2.

Minimal contrast enhancement is seen in this lesion *(arrows)*. The more superficial enhancement represents normal vessels within cerebral sulci.

LOW-GRADE GLIOMAS: CALCIFICATION

Case 35

61-year-old woman presenting with seizures.
Low-grade astrocytoma.

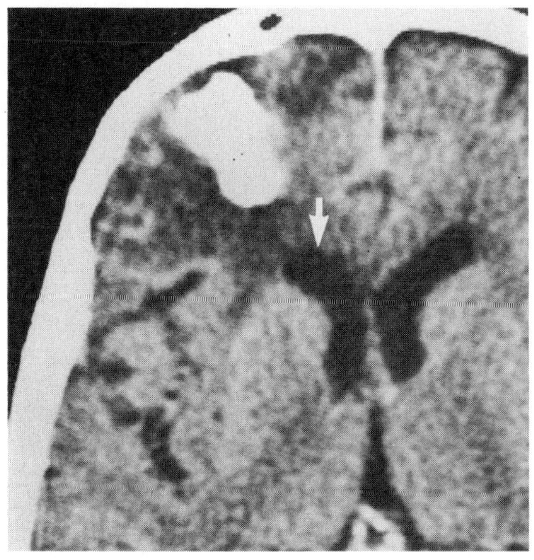

About 10% to 20% of low-grade gliomas contain calcification. The pattern is variable and nonspecific. A large "rock"-like calcification, as in this case, could also be seen as the residual of old injury or inflammation ("brain stone").

Here the adjacent frontal lobe demonstrates intermediate low attenuation and mass effect, with mild displacement of the frontal horn *(arrow)*. These features indicate an active lesion and exclude an old insult (which would be associated with volume loss and lower attenuation values).

Case 36

39-year-old woman presenting with dementia.
Low-grade glioma.

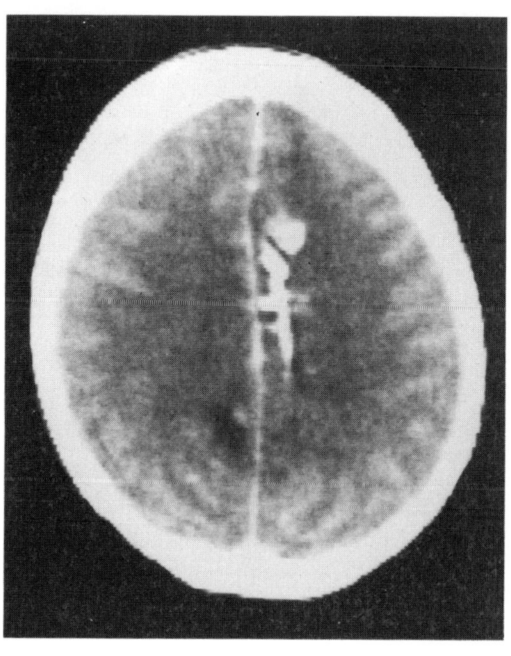

The calcification in this glioma is predominantly linear, following the course of the cingulate gyrus superior to the corpus callosum. Vague, low-attenuation areas are associated anteriorly and posteriorly. (These were better seen at another level, presented as Case 245.)

Low-grade gliomas should be considered in the differential diagnosis of most intracerebral calcifications. (See Cases 42 and 289 for other examples.) Calcification is less common in high-grade gliomas, except for those representing malignant transformation of low-grade tumors.

HIGH-GRADE GLIOMAS: THICK, IRREGULAR RIM ENHANCEMENT

Case 37

60-year-old woman thought to have had a "stroke." Glioblastoma multiforme.

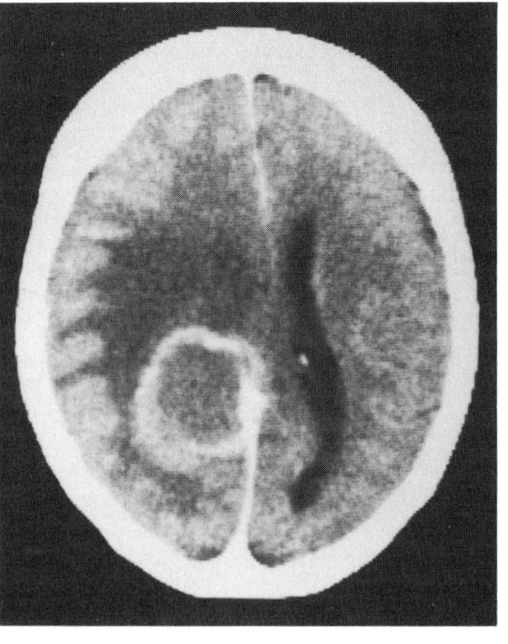

Most high-grade gliomas (grade 3 or 4 astrocytoma, "anaplastic astrocytoma," "glioblastoma multiforme," "malignant glioma") demonstrate definite contrast enhancement. The converse is usually true: extensive contrast enhancement in a glial tumor suggests a high-grade lesion.

The enhancement commonly consists of a thick, nodular rim surrounding a low-attenuation center of necrosis, cyst, or slowly equilibrating tissue. The central, nonenhancing regions may vary widely in size and number.

Prominent edema has contributed to mass effect in this case, compressing the lateral ventricle and effacing cortical sulci. It is possible that a rapid increase in edema caused the patient's apparent "stroke syndrome" (see discussion of Case 10).

Case 38

75-year-old woman with poorly defined symptoms. Glioblastoma multiforme.

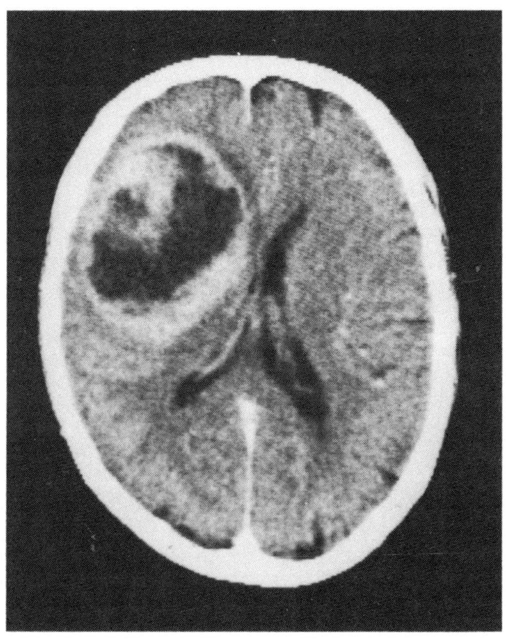

Malignant gliomas may enhance centrally as well as peripherally. The amount of central enhancement may be time-dependent, with the low-attenuation center of the tumor "filling in" with contrast density on delayed scans.

Compare the predominantly peripheral enhancement of this glioblastoma with the metastasis in Case 5.

Case 39

64-year-old woman with repeated transient ischemic attacks. Malignant glioma, grade 4.

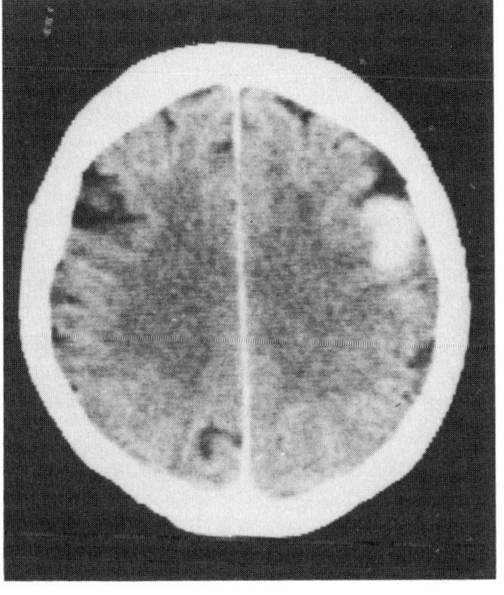

Occasional high-grade gliomas demonstrate homogeneous enhancement and superficial location. This uniformly enhancing lesion resembles a meningioma, but appears to be intra-axial. It had been initially confused with a small, subacute infarction (see chapter 9). The persistent symptoms and CT enlargement warranted a biopsy, which confirmed glioblastoma multiforme.

Case 40

48-year-old man presenting with seizures and hemiparesis. Grade 3 anaplastic astrocytoma (postcontrast scan).

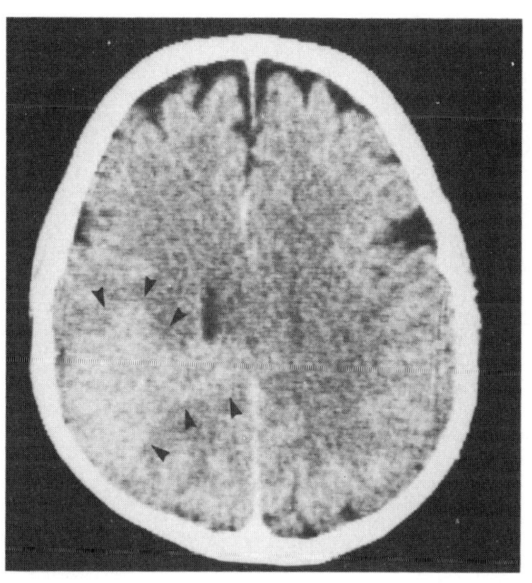

High-grade gliomas may be surprisingly inconspicuous with unusual tissue uniformity. In this case, an area of homogeneous, mildly increased attenuation values is seen in the right parietal lobe *(arrows)*. The lesion extends medially to involve the splenium of the corpus callosum.

GLIOMAS OF THE CORPUS CALLOSUM: GENU

Case 41

74-year-old woman. Glioblastoma multiforme (postcontrast scan).

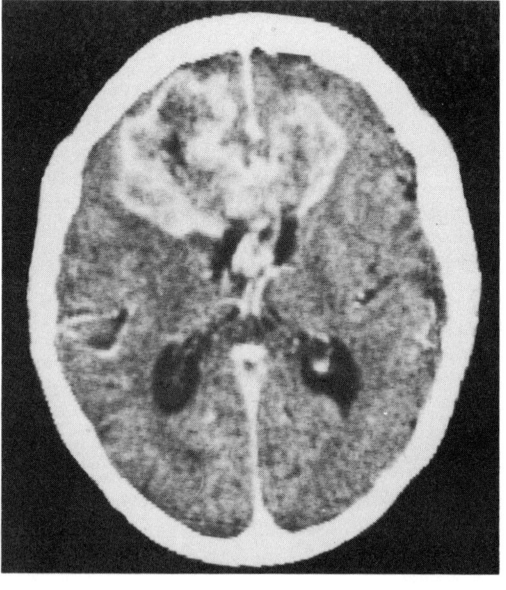

This tumor occupies the genu of the corpus callosum, extending through the minor forceps into both frontal lobes to assume a "butterfly" configuration. The genu of the corpus callosum is thickened, with deformity of the frontal horns and invasion of the septum pellucidum. Septum pellucidum involvement is often a clue to the glial origin of smaller tumors near the forearm of Monro (see Case 115).

Case 42

48-year-old man. Hemorrhage into calcified oligodendroglioma (noncontrast scan).

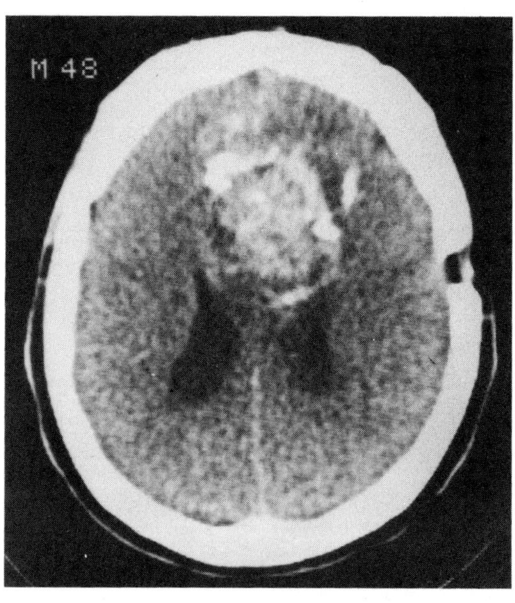

Most oligodendrogliomas are found in the cerebral hemispheres, particularly in the frontal lobes. Although the midline location of this tumor is unusual, its other CT features are characteristic.

Oligodendrogliomas are more frequently calcified than any other glial tumors, with the large majority demonstrating this finding. While hemorrhage into gliomas is relatively uncommon (about 5%), oligodendrogliomas make up a disproportionate share of such cases. Intratumoral hemorrhage is one means by which these slow-growing tumors may come to attention. (Seizures are a more common initial manifestation.)

Case 43A

60-year-old woman. Glioblastoma multiforme.

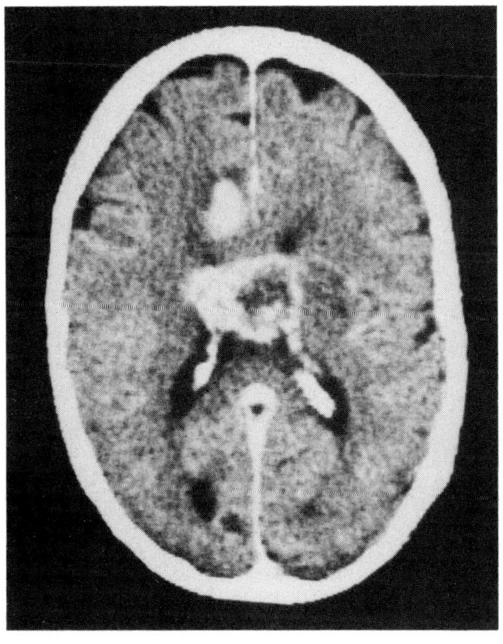

The large tumor in this case has the characteristic features of a malignant glioma. It is centered in the midline, immediately superior to the lateral ventricles. This location places the lesion within the body of the corpus callosum, which forms the ventricular roof.

A smaller nodule, seen more anteriorly, was thought to be part of the same mass. Multicentric origin of gliomas does occur, but connecting strands of nonenhancing tumor frequently join such apparently discrete nodules.

Case 43B

Same patient.

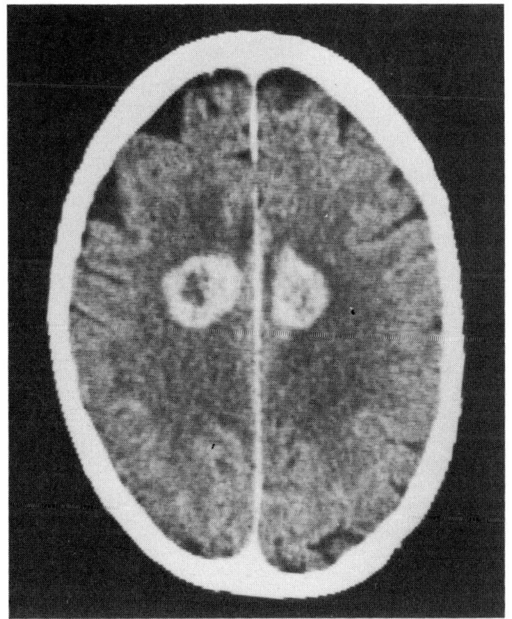

A higher section demonstrates extensions of tumor following callosal radiations into the medial portions of both cerebral hemispheres. The appearance of separate masses at this level reflects a "U"-shaped tumor with an interhemispheric bridge at the ventricular level. Coronal scans are useful for defining the relationship of such masses to the corpus callosum (see Case 20).

Cases 40 and 51 present examples of gliomas involving the splenium of the corpus callosum.

CYSTS WITHIN GLIOMAS

Case 44

68-year-old man. Glioblastoma multiforme.

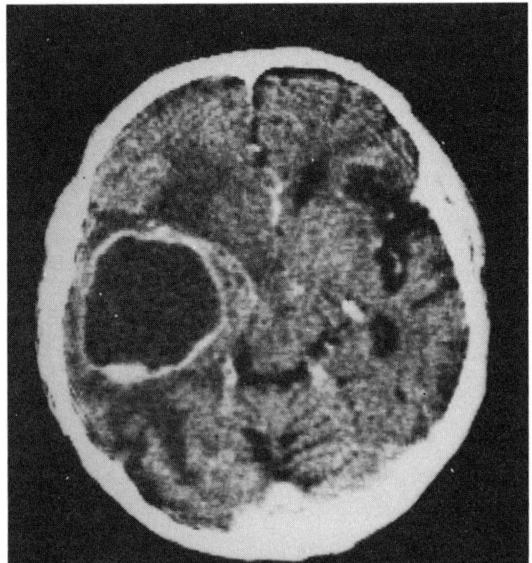

Many low- and high-grade gliomas contain one or more cysts of variable size. When a tumor cyst is large and unilocular, palliative drainage may provide symptomatic improvement by reducing mass effect. Aspiration can often be accomplished under CT guidance. Repeated aspiration or continuous drainage may be necessary due to rapid reaccumulation of fluid.

The large tumor in this case is surrounded by an unusually thin, uniform, rim of enhancement. The resulting appearance resembles that of a cerebral abscess (see Cases 150 and 151). Extensive edema contributes to the prominent mass effect, with the brain stem being flattened and displaced by uncal herniation.

Case 45

31-year-old woman. Cystic cerebellar astrocytoma.

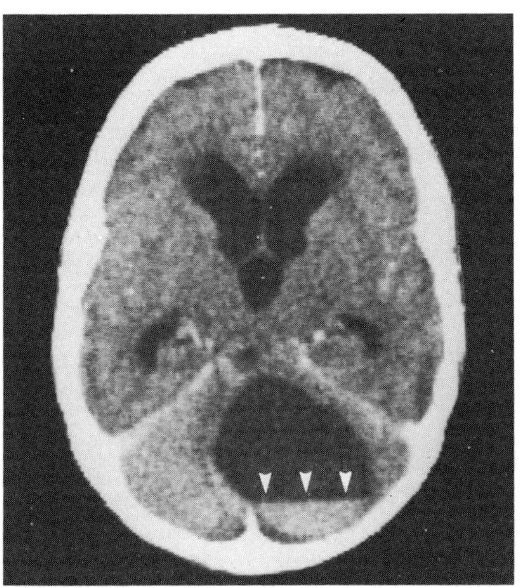

The most reliable CT indication of a truly cystic tumor is the demonstration of a sedimentation level within the lesion *(arrows)*. The dense material settling in the dependent portion of a cyst may be cellular debris, hemorrhage, or accumulated contrast material.

In the absence of a sedimentation level, a cyst may be predicted by the homogeneity of its contents. This uniformity may be demonstrated by an image with a narrow window width or by a histogram of attenuation values within the region of interest.

A coronal scan of this lesion is presented as Case 67.

DIFFERENTIAL DIAGNOSIS: CYSTIC NEOPLASM WITHIN THE TEMPORAL LOBE

Case 46

26-year-old man.

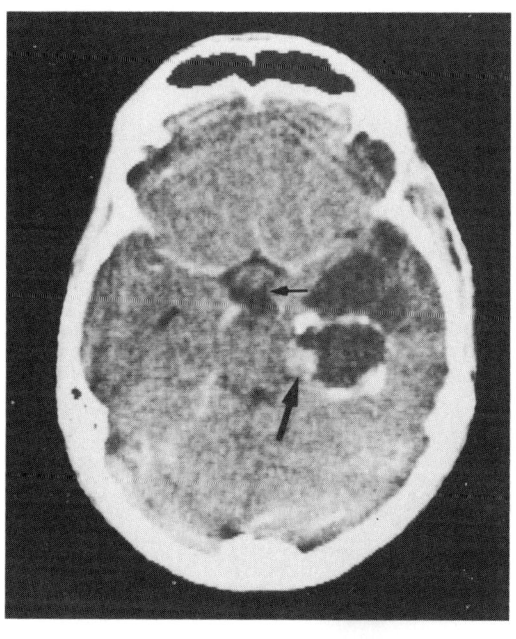

Astrocytoma, Grade 1.

Case 47

69-year-old man.

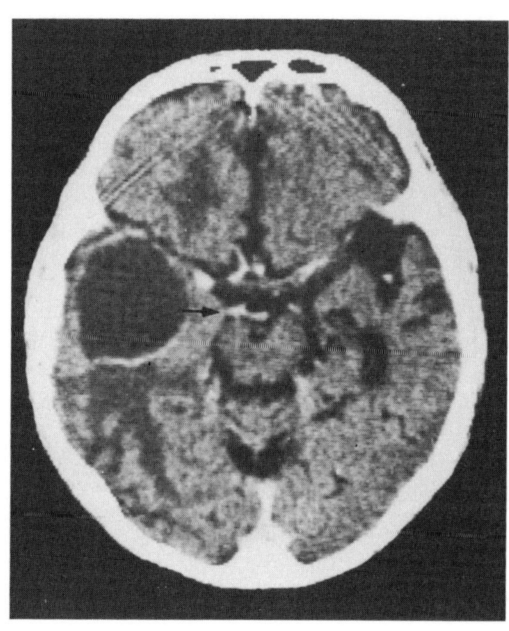

Glioblastoma Multiforme.

The CT features illustrated in Cases 33 to 38 usually allow distinction between low-grade and high-grade glial tumors. However, the CT spectrum of malignant gliomas overlaps that of low-grade neoplasms, and occasional tumors have intermediate characteristics.

In Case 46, the extensive calcification and minimal contrast enhancement favor diagnosis of a long-standing, low-grade neoplasm. However, the possibility of malignant degeneration is raised when areas of thick contrast enhancement *(large arrow)* are superimposed on otherwise benign features.

On the other hand, some high-grade gliomas present deceptively uniform and well-organized appearances. Such well defined lesions may be seen in the form of solid masses (see Cases 39 and 40) or thin-walled cysts (as seen here and in Case 44).

Both of these cases demonstrate medial displacement of the adjacent uncus *(small arrows)*. Both tumors were found to be grossly cystic at surgery.

DIFFERENTIAL DIAGNOSIS: RIM-ENHANCING, DEEP HEMISPHERE MASS WITH EDEMA

Case 48

59-year-old woman.

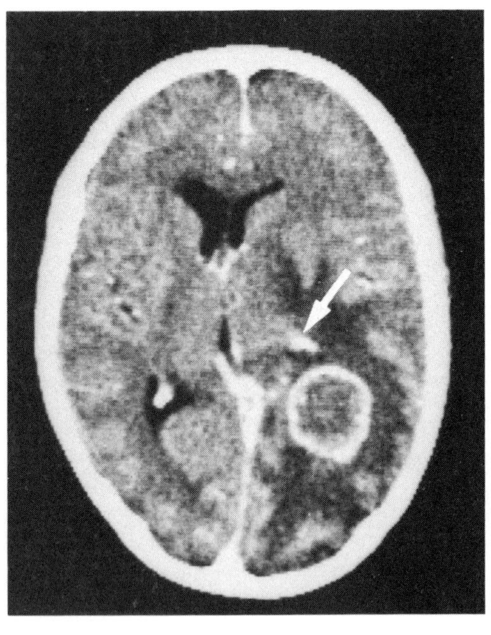

Metastatic Bronchogenic Carcinoma.

Case 49

68-year-old woman.

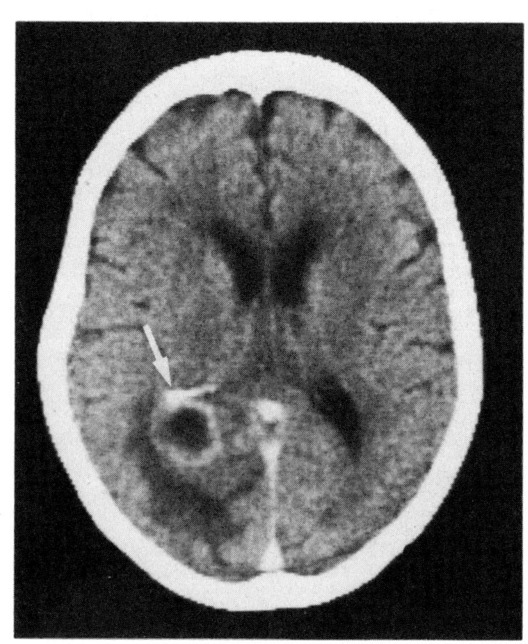

Glioblastoma Multiforme.

The appearance and location of these two lesions are very similar. In each case, the ipsilateral calcified choroid glomus is greatly displaced anteriorly *(arrows)*.

Malignant glioma is the leading possibility when a solitary, peripherally enhancing, deep hemisphere lesion is discovered. However, an unusual metastasis should be included in the differential diagnosis and appropriate evaluation recommended (e.g., chest roentgenogram).

DIFFERENTIAL DIAGNOSIS:
TUMOR INVOLVING THE SPLENIUM OF THE CORPUS CALLOSUM

Case 50

46-year-old woman.

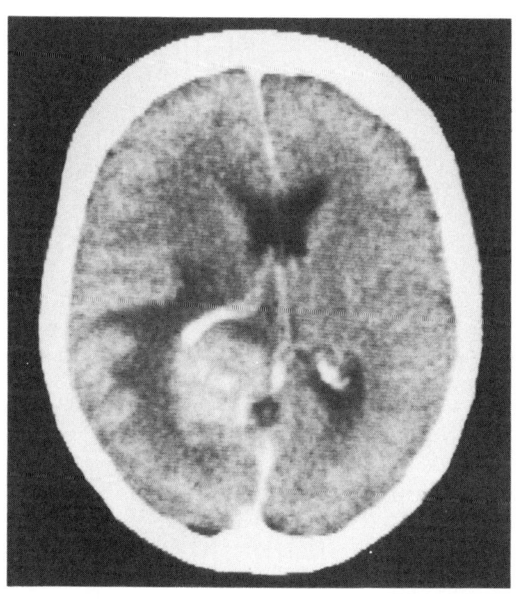

Metastatic Embryonal Cell Carcinoma of the Ovary.

Case 51

87-year-old woman.

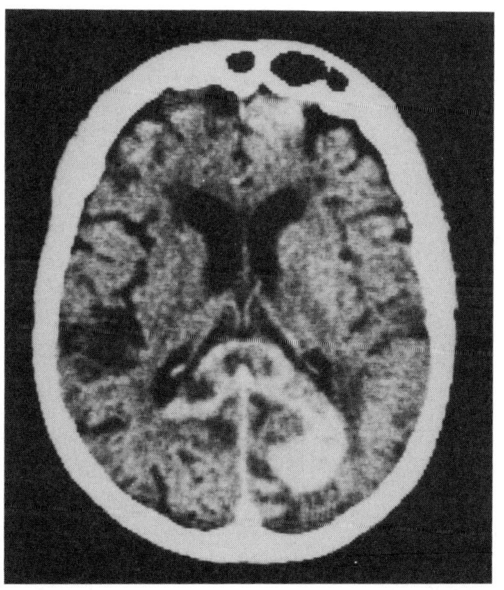

Glioblastoma Multiforme.

Occasional metastases involve the major forceps and splenium of the corpus callosum, strongly resembling a malignant glioma. The tumor in Case 51 crosses the splenium from one hemisphere to the other, and is analogous to a "butterfly" glioma of the genu.

Primary CNS lymphoma ("microglioma" or "reticulum cell sarcoma") is a third tumor type that may involve the corpus callosum and should be included in the differential diagnosis.

DIFFERENTIAL DIAGNOSIS: INTRAVENTRICULAR AND PARAVENTRICULAR RIM-ENHANCING MASS

Case 52

38-year-old man.

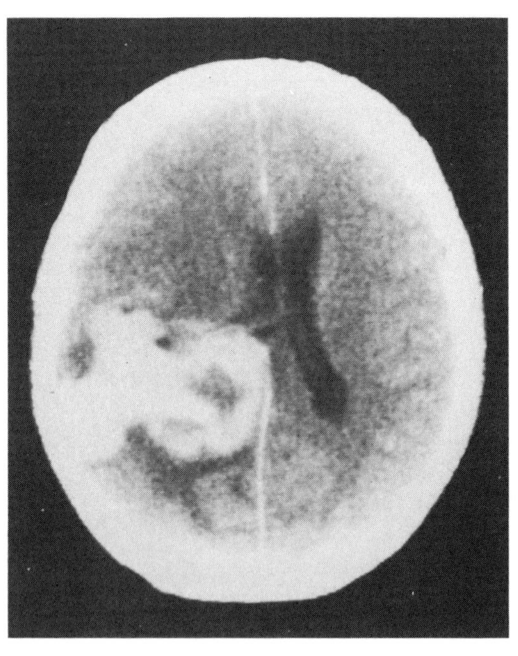

Trigone Meningioma.

Case 53

60-year-old man.

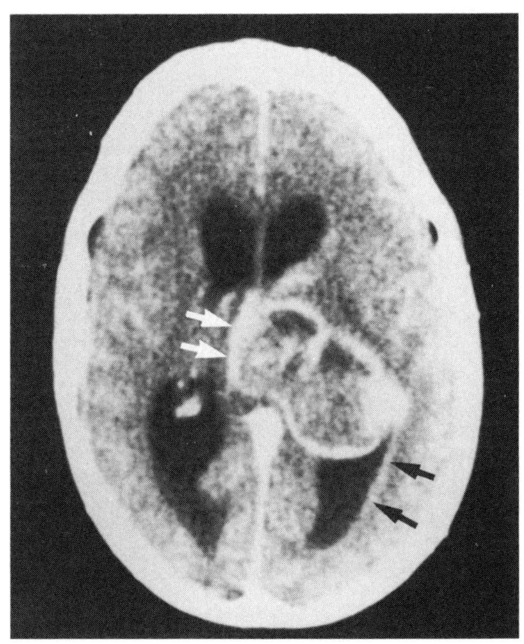

Glioblastoma Multiforme.

In Case 52, the deep hemisphere location, thick-walled contrast enhancement, and occurrence in a young man would make malignant glioma a likely diagnosis. However, the tumor is a meningioma, arising within the trigone of the lateral ventricle and extending into the posterior temporal lobe. One clue to the correct diagnosis is the predominantly smooth, well-defined, intensely enhancing margin of the mass.

Intraventricular meningiomas account for 2% of intracranial meningiomas and most commonly occur within the atrium of the lateral ventricle. The differential diagnosis for an enhancing tumor in this location would include choroid plexus papilloma (see Case 123), ependymoma, metastasis, and vascular malformation.

In both Case 52 and 53 the midline shift is smaller than might be expected because a portion of the tumor bulk has been accommodated within the ventricular chambers. Relatively mild mass effect is characteristic of intraventricular masses, which can enlarge by simply displacing CSF. (See also Case 123.)

The internal cerebral veins are deformed in Case 53 *(white arrows)*. There is a small amount of subependymal tumor extension along the lateral margin of the occipital pole (*black arrows;* see Case 54).

DIFFERENTIAL DIAGNOSIS: SUBEPENDYMAL TUMOR SPREAD

Case 54

64-year-old woman.

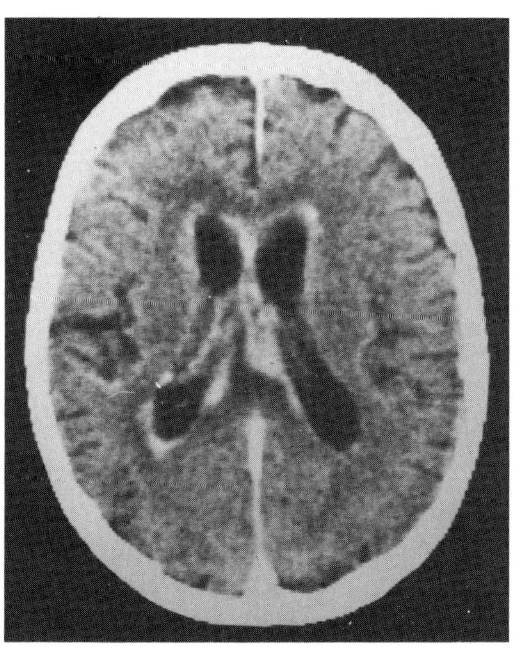

High-Grade Glioma.

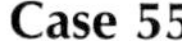

Case 55

77-year-old man.

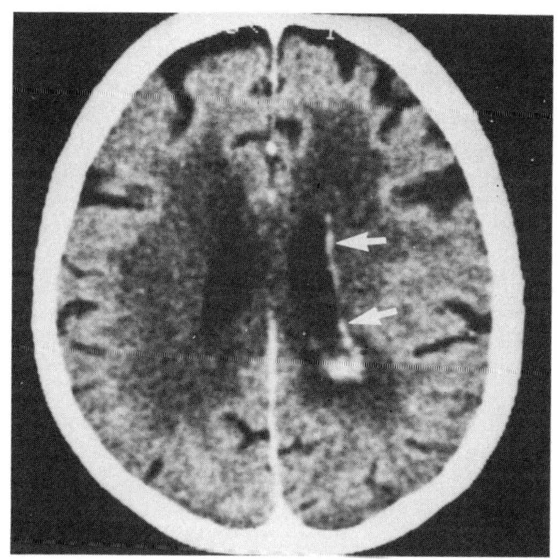

Systemic Lymphoma.

Enhancement along ventricular margins may be due to inflammatory ventriculitis or to subependymal neoplasm. Gliomas and ependymomas are primary considerations in the latter category because of their frequent periventricular location (Case 54; see also Case 53).

Many other tumors can also spread along ventricular surfaces. Metastases from systemic solid tumors (especially oat cell carcinoma of the lung, melanoma, and breast carcinoma; see Case 12), or from other intracranial neoplasms (e.g., medulloblastoma, germinoma) can cause a periventricular "cast" of tumor.

Primary CNS lymphoma or secondary brain involvement by systemic lymphoma (as in Case 55) may present a similar appearance.

REFERENCES

1. Afra D., Norman D., Levin V.A.: Cysts in malignant gliomas: Identification by computerized tomography. *J. Neurosurg.* 53:821–825, 1980.
2. Amundsen P., Dugstad G., Syvertsen A.H.: The reliability of computer tomography for the diagnosis and differential diagnosis of meningiomas, gliomas, and brain metastases. *Acta Neurochir. (Wien)* 41:177–190, 1978.
3. Andreou J., George A.E., Wise A., et al.: CT prognostic criteria of survival after malignant glioma surgery. *A.J.N.R.* 4:488–490, 1983.
4. Belender N., Cromwell L.D., Graves D., et al.: Interval appearance of glioblastomas not evident in previous CT examinations. *J. Comput. Assist. Tomogr.* 7:599–603, 1983.
5. Braun I.F., Chambers E., Leeds N.E., Zimmerman R.D.: The value of unenhanced scans in differentiating lesions producing ring enhancement. *A.J.N.R.* 3:643–647, 1982.
6. Burger P.C., Dubois P.J., Schold S.C., et al.: Computerized tomographic and pathologic studies of the untreated, quiescent, and recurrent glioblastoma multiforme. *J. Neurosurg.* 58:159–169, 1983.
7. Butler A.R., Horri S.C., Kricheff I.I., et al.: Computed tomography in astrocytomas: A statistical analysis of the parameters of malignancy and the positive contrast-enhanced CT scan. *Radiology* 129:433–439, 1978.
8. Butler A.R., Passalaqua A.M., Berenstein A., Kricheff I.I.: Contrast enhanced CT scan and radionuclide brain scan in supratentorial gliomas. *A.J.R.* 132:607–611, 1979.
9. Dubois P.J., Martinez A.J., Myerowitz R.L., et al.: Subependymal and leptomeningeal spread of systemic malignant lymphoma demonstrated by cranial computed tomography. *J. Comput. Assist. Tomogr.* 2:218–221, 1978.
10. Hoffman W.F., Levin V.A., Wilson C.B.: Evaluation of malignant glioma patients during the post-irradiation period. *J. Neurosurg.* 50:624–628, 1979.
11. Jooma R., Kendall B.E.: Intracranial tumours in the first year of life. *Neuroradiology* 23:267–274, 1982.
12. Kendall B.E., Jakubowski J., Pullicino P., et al.: Difficulties in diagnosis of supratentorial gliomas by CAT scan. *J. Neurol. Neurosurg. Psych.* 42:485–492, 1979.
13. Kieffer S.A., Lee S.H.: Intracranial neoplasms, in Haaga J.R., Alfidi R.J. (eds.): *Computed Tomography of the Whole Body.* St. Louis, C.V. Mosby Co., 1983, pp. 64–109.
14. Kieffer S.A., Salibi N.A., Kim R.C., et al.: Multifocal glioblastoma: Diagnostic implications. *Radiology* 143: 709–710, 1982.
15. Lewander R.: Contrast enhancement with time in gliomas. *Acta Radiol. (Diagn)* 20:689–702, 1979.
16. Lilja A., Bergstom K., Spannare B., et al.: Reliability of computed tomography in assessing histopathological features of malignant supratentorial gliomas. *J. Comput. Assist. Tomogr.* 5:625–636, 1981.
17. Marks J.E., Gado M.: Serial computed tomography of primary brain tumors following surgery, irradiation, and chemotherapy. *Radiology* 125:119–125, 1977.
18. McGeachie R.E., Gold L.H., Latchaw R.E.: Periventricular spread of tumor demonstrated by computed tomography. *Radiology* 125:407–410, 1977.
19. Pedersen H., Gjerris F., Klinken L.: Computed tomography of benign supratentorial astrocytomas in infancy and childhood. *Neuroradiology* 21:87–91, 1981.
20. Rao K., Levine H., Itani A., et al.: CT findings in multicentric glioblastoma: Diagnostic-pathologic correlation. *J. Comput. Tomogr.* 4:187–192, 1980.
21. Russell E.J., Naidich T.P.: The enhancing septal alveal wedge: A septal sign of intraaxial mass. *Neuroradiology* 23:33–40, 1982.
22. Saloman M., Levine H., Rao K.: Value of sequential computed tomography in the multimodality treatment of glioblastoma multiforme. *Neurosurgery* 8:15–19, 1981.
23. Steinhoff H., Lanksch W., Kazner E., et al.: Computed tomography in the diagnosis and differential diagnosis of glioblastomas. *Neuroradiology* 14:193–200, 1977.
24. Vonofakos D., Marca H., Hacker H.: Oligodendrogliomas: CT patterns with emphasis on features indicating malignancy. *J. Comput. Assist. Tomogr.* 3:783–788, 1979.

CHAPTER 4

POSTERIOR FOSSA TUMORS

Case 56

7-year-old boy presenting with dizziness and staggering gait.

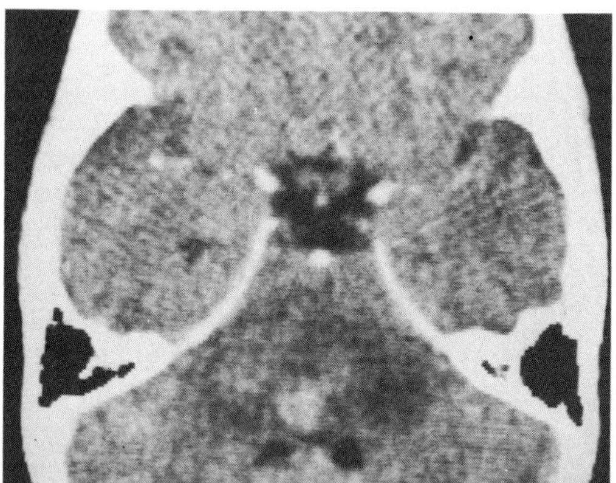

Most brain stem gliomas demonstrate slightly decreased attenuation values. Some tumors are isodense, and a few show increased attenuation or even gross calcification (see Case 120). Mass effect depends on tumor size and may be generalized, as seen here, or focal, as in Case 57. Contrast enhancement may be obvious, minimal, or absent. Cysts may occur, allowing palliative decompression.

In this case, the pons is enlarged by a low-attenuation mass, with obliteration of peripontine cisterns and posterior displacement of the fourth ventricle. A single nodule of contrast enhancement is seen indenting the floor of the fourth ventricle. (The cerebellar vermis causes the normal indentation along the posterior wall or roof of the fourth ventricle.) Cases 59 and 291 present other scans of this patient.

Case 57

42-year-old woman.

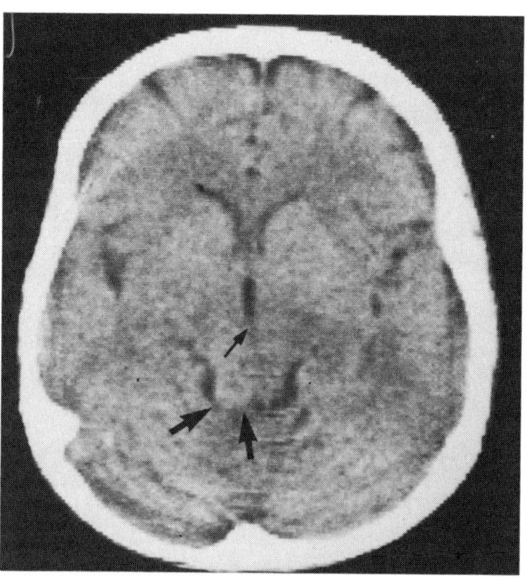

Brain stem gliomas may be relatively inconspicuous lesions on CT scans. They often cause early symptoms that lead to evaluation while the tumor is still small. Diagnostic difficulty is increased by the frequent lack of significant attenuation changes and by the common presence of artifacts on scans of the posterior fossa. Here, a small, isodense midbrain tumor fattens the right superior colliculus *(large arrows)* and displaces the posterior portion of the third ventricle *(small arrow)*.

Subtle abnormalities of brain stem contour may be highlighted by CT scans performed after subarachnoid contrast material has been injected (see Case 130). Magnetic resonance imaging is a sensitive alternative for detecting and assessing brain stem pathology.

DIFFERENTIAL DIAGNOSIS: BRAIN STEM MASS

Case 58

55-year-old woman.

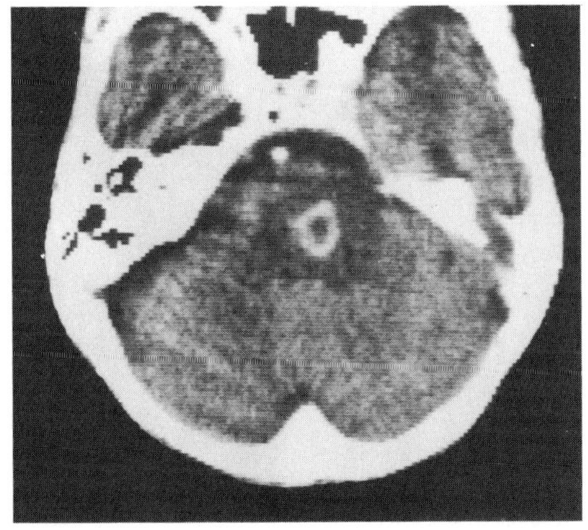

Metastatic Breast Carcinoma.

Case 59

7-year-old boy.

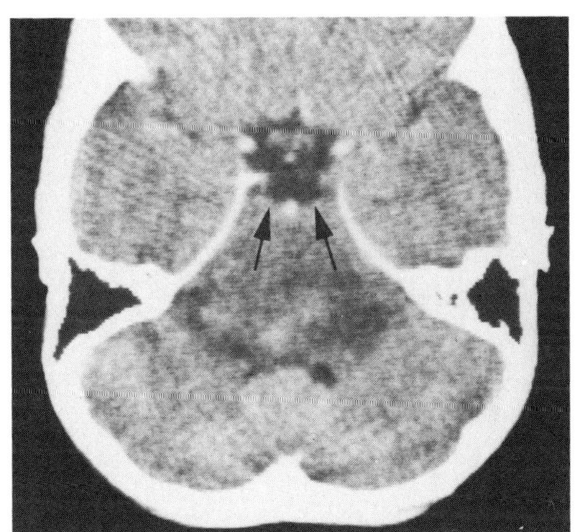

Brain Stem Glioma.

The possibility of metastasis should be considered when brain stem masses are encountered in adults. The well-defined contrast enhancement in Case 58 contrasts with the typically indistinct margins and vague enhancement of most brain stem gliomas.

Case 59 is a second scan of the patient presented in Case 56. The ventral margin of the pons bulges anteriorly on both sides of the basilar artery *(arrows)*. The artery is sometimes encased and posteriorly displaced by an exophytic brain stem neoplasm.

Brain stem infarction or demyelination may cause a combination of low attenuation, mass effect, and vague contrast enhancement resembling a tumor. Clinical information or follow-up scans will usually establish the diagnosis in such cases.

Rarely, a granuloma (e.g., tuberculosis, sarcoidosis) or an abscess may occupy the brain stem and mimic a neoplasm. Diagnosis in these situations may require biopsy.

MEDULLOBLASTOMAS

Case 60A

5-month-old boy presenting with vomiting and ataxia (noncontrast scan).

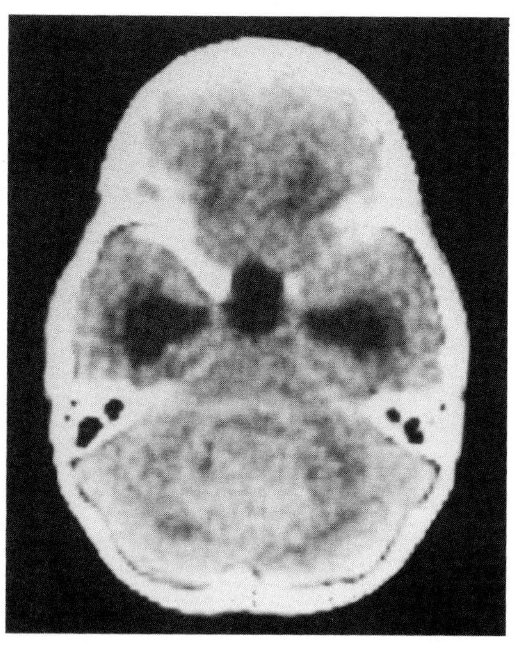

Medulloblastomas are highly cellular tumors arising from primitive cells in the neuroepithelial roof of the fourth ventricle (external granular layer of the inferior medullary velum). They usually present as midline masses with homogeneous, mildly increased attenuation. Calcification and cysts are rare.

Medulloblastomas rank with cerebellar astrocytomas as the most common posterior fossa tumors in children.

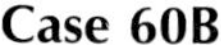

Case 60B

Same patient (postcontrast scan).

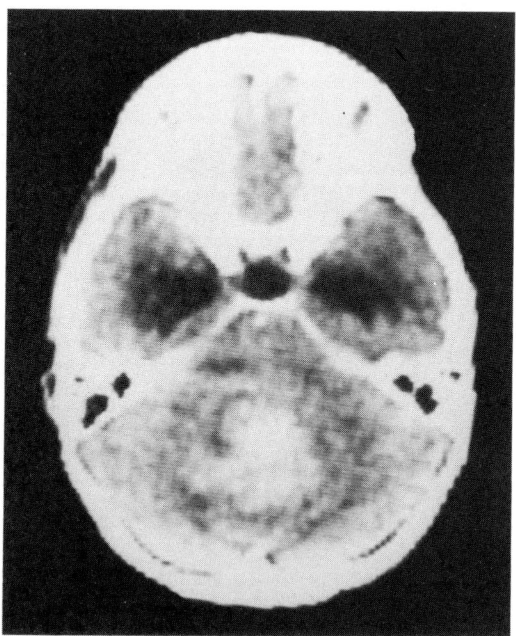

Contrast enhancement in medulloblastomas is typically uniform and intense, as seen here. The posterior fossa is often "tight," with compression of the fourth ventricle causing obstructive hydrocephalus.

Medulloblastomas are among the primary CNS neoplasms commonly associated with seeding of the cerebrospinal fluid. (Others include ependymoma, germinoma, and glioma.) For this reason, isodense or enhancing subarachnoid spaces should be noted on initial and follow-up scans in these patients.

Case 61A

3-year-old boy (noncontrast scan).

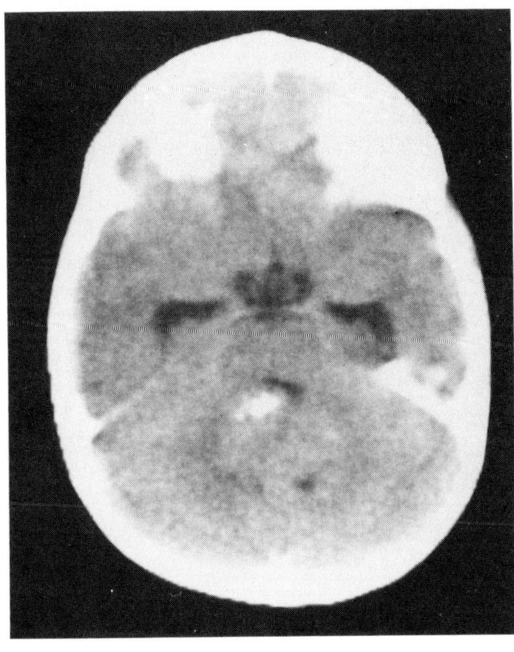

Case 61B

Same patient (postcontrast scan).

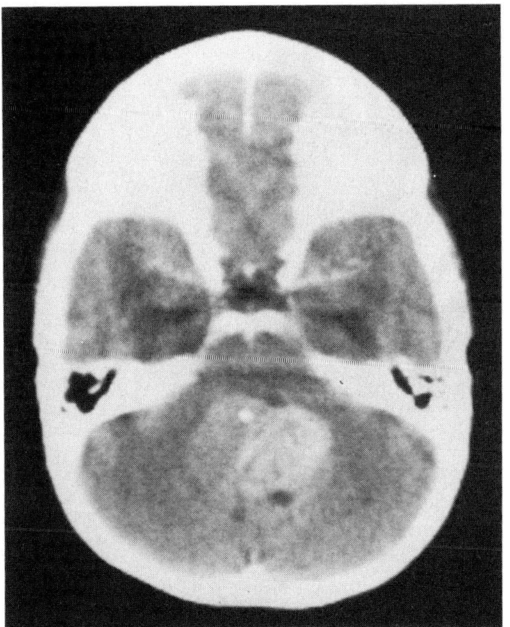

Ependymomas arising from the fourth ventricle are among the posterior fossa masses encountered in children. Their location mimics the more common medulloblastomas, but other CT features usually suggest the correct diagnosis.

Ependymomas are frequently calcified, as seen in this case. They may be inhomogeneous, with mixed attenuation values, sometimes including cysts or hemorrhage. Both calcification and inhomogeneity contrast with the usual appearance of medulloblastomas (see Case 60).

This tumor is relatively isodense. Portions of the expanded fourth ventricle are seen at the margins of the mass anteriorly and possibly posteriorly. The brain stem is anteriorly displaced, and obstructive hydrocephalus is present.

The enhancement pattern of ependymomas is usually less homogeneous and intense than that of medulloblastomas. Tumor margins are often irregular and poorly defined, and multilobulation is frequent.

In this case, the tumor consists of nodules with varying and somewhat inhomogeneous enhancement. The basilar artery and pons are compressed anteriorly against the dorsum sellae and clivus.

Although the characteristics discussed above are useful clues to the diagnosis of ependymoma, some of these tumors demonstrate uniform density and enhancement indistinguishable from medulloblastomas.

Case 62A

29-year-old man. Medullomyoblastoma.

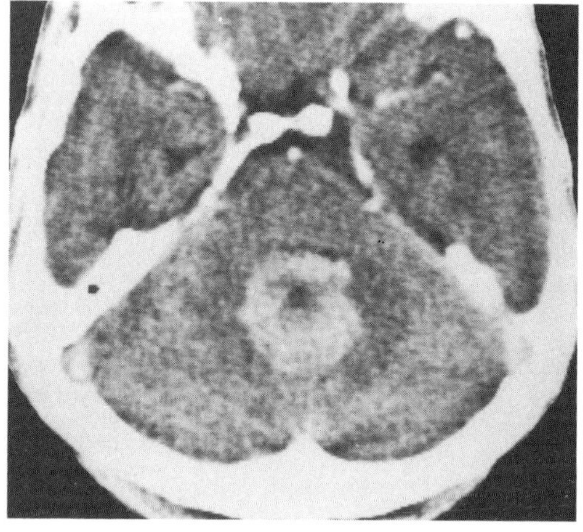

Case 62B

Same patient (coronal scan).

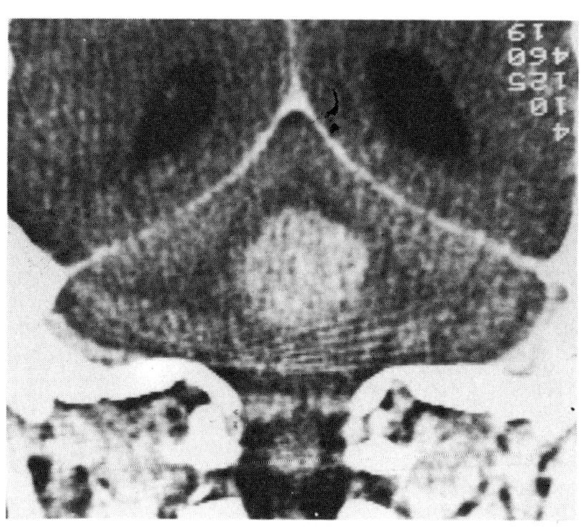

Medulloblastomas and fourth-ventricular ependymomas are much less common in adults than in children.

Medulloblastomas in adolescents and adults may arise laterally in the cerebellar hemisphere. Such "cerebellar sarcomas" often have a fibrotic histologic pattern ("desmoplastic").

In this case, an unusual midline tumor demonstrates inhomogeneous but well-defined enhancement. Surgery disclosed a rare malignant variant of medulloblastoma with differentiation toward muscle cells.

Coronal scans are useful for localizing posterior fossa masses with respect to the fourth ventricle, tentorium, and cerebellopontine angles (see also Cases 23, 24, 67, 68, 70, 79, and 80). Here the enhancing mass occupies the center of the posterior fossa, filling the site of the fourth ventricle.

The differential diagnosis of a fourth-ventricular mass in an adult includes choroid plexus papilloma (see Case 124), ependymoma/glioma, hemangioblastoma, vermian metastasis, arteriovenous malformation, rare epidermoid tumors, and inflammatory mass or cyst.

Case 63

4-year-old girl presenting with nystagmus.

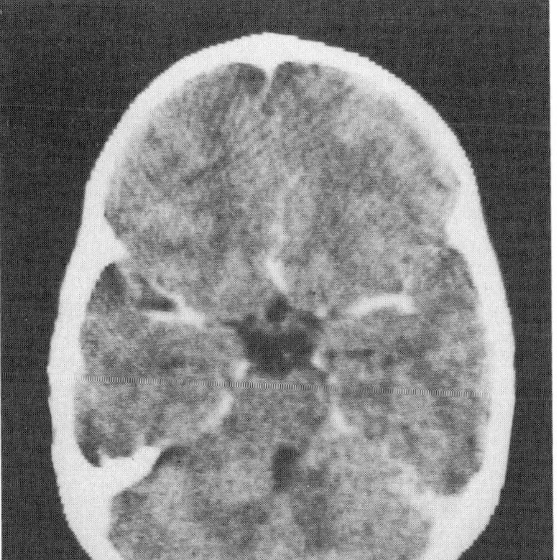

Gliomas of the cerebellum are among the most common posterior fossa tumors in children. These "juvenile cerebellar astrocytomas" often display benign behavior and may carry a relatively good prognosis.

The majority of cerebellar astrocytomas are cystic, but solid masses may be seen, as in this case. Low-attenuation tumors sometimes prove to be solid lesions with microcystic histology.

Contrast enhancement is variable but is usually more prominent than noted here. The lateral compression of the fourth ventricle indicates that the mass has arisen in the brachium pontis or medial cerebellum, contrasting with the midline tumors illustrated in Cases 60 to 62.

Case 64

6-year-old girl.

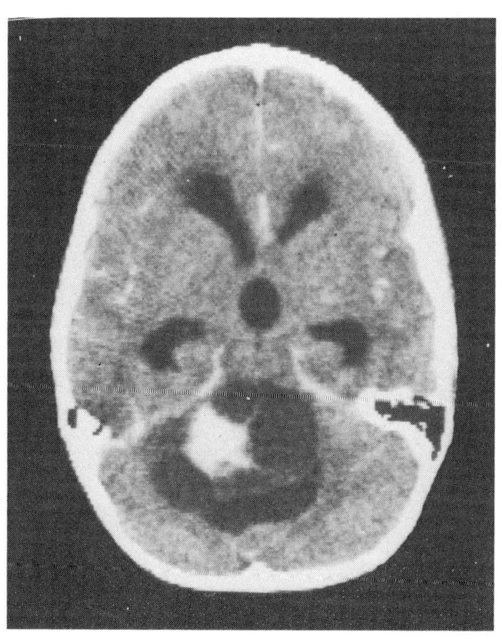

Cystic cerebellar astrocytomas may display an enhancing rim of tissue surrounding the circumference of the cyst. Alternatively, a localized mural nodule may be found along non-enhancing cyst margins, as seen here.

The cyst may be unilocular or multilocular. In this case, septations radiate from the mural nodule.

Severe compression of the brain stem is present and associated with obstructive hydrocephalus. (Compare the anteroposterior diameter of the brain stem with that in Case 56.)

HEMANGIOBLASTOMAS

Case 65

60-year-old man with ataxic gait.

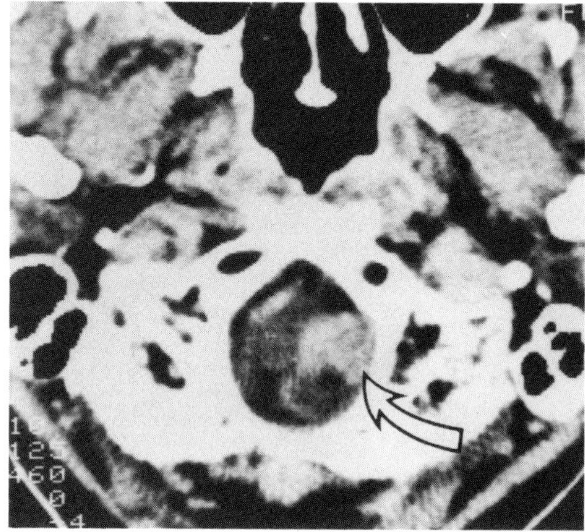

Hemangioblastomas are relatively uncommon tumors of the posterior fossa and spinal cord, usually seen in adults. These masses are often cystic and typically demonstrate an intensely enhancing mural nodule.

Higher scans in this case had disclosed a nonenhancing cerebellar cyst. The associated mural nodule was not apparent until scanning was continued inferiorly through the level of the foramen magnum. The hemangioblastoma nodule *(arrow)* occupies the cerebellar tonsil, displacing the brain stem. (Case 68 presents a coronal scan of this patient.)

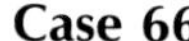

Case 66

45-year-old woman.

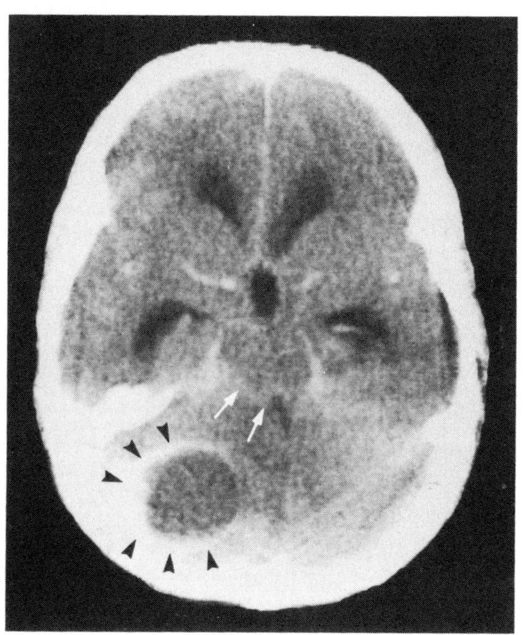

A cystic mass is present in the right cerebellar hemisphere, with a broad crescent of contrast enhancement along the lateral margin *(black arrows)*. The fourth ventricle and brain stem are compressed *(white arrows)*, and obstructive hydrocephalus is present.

The differential diagnosis of this mass in an adult would include hemangioblastoma of unusual morphology, cerebellar astrocytoma, metastasis, and unusual lateral medulloblastoma ("cerebellar sarcoma"). An angiogram showed the lateral cyst wall to be intensely vascular, and a hemangioblastoma was found at surgery.

DIFFERENTIAL DIAGNOSIS: CYSTIC CEREBELLAR TUMOR WITH A MURAL NODULE

Case 67

31-year-old woman with headaches (same patient as Case 45).

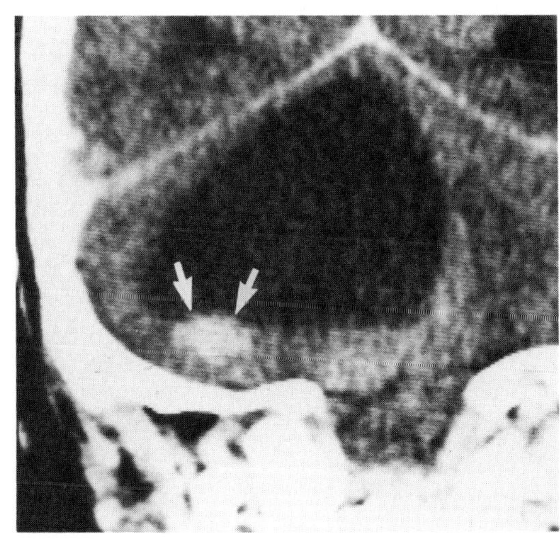

Cystic Cerebellar Astrocytoma (Coronal Scan).

Case 68

60-year-old man (same patient as Case 65).

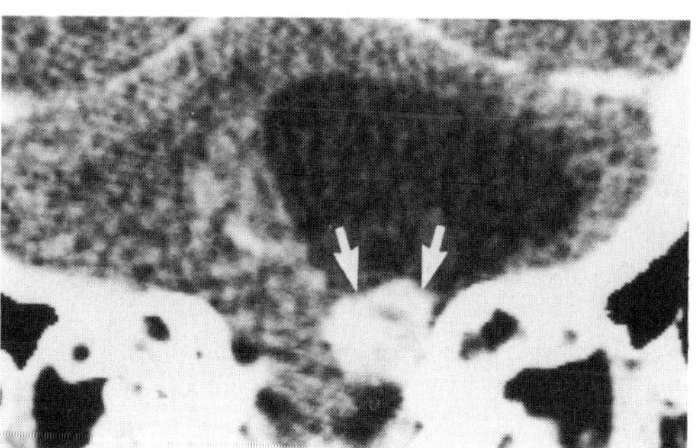

Hemangioblastoma (Coronal Scan).

Coronal scans define the relationship of the cyst to the mural nodule *(arrows)* in each case. Case 67 also demonstrates a sedimentation level, which had been apparent on axial scans (see Case 45).

The CT appearance of these lesions is indistinguishable, and the diagnoses were made angiographically. The angiogram in Case 67 demonstrated an avascular mass, excluding hemangioblastoma. The angiogram in Case 68 showed the mural nodule to be intensely vascular, which is characteristic of hemangioblastoma.

Angiography of hemangioblastomas may demonstrate additional small tumors of the cerebellum or cervical spinal cord inapparent on CT scans.

ACOUSTIC SCHWANNOMAS (NEURINOMAS, "NEUROMAS")

Case 69

75-year-old woman presenting with tinnitus, dizziness, and nausea.

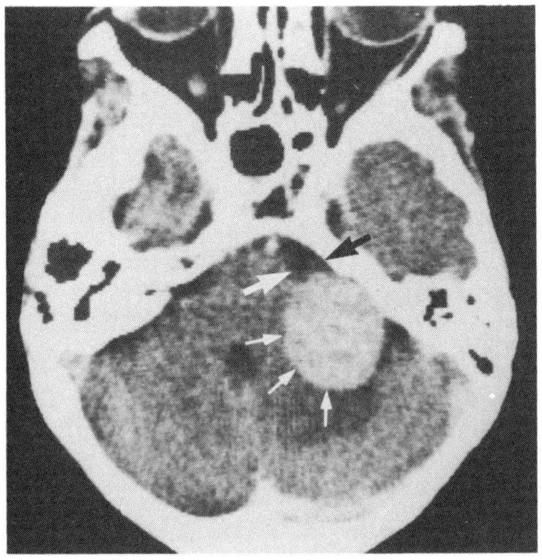

Acoustic schwannomas represent about 10% of primary intracranial tumors and account for the majority of masses in the cerebellopontine angle. They are typically well-defined, uniformly enhancing tumors with smooth, rounded margins. The masses are centered on the midposterior petrous ridge, where they arise at the internal auditory meatus.

Slow growth may allow acoustic schwannomas to gradually invaginate far into the adjacent cerebellum and brain stem *(small arrows)*. However, the extra-axial origin of the mass is usually indicated by contralateral brain stem displacement, causing widening of the ipsilateral cisterns at the margins of the tumor (*large arrows;* see also Cases 72 and 74).

A small amount of cerebellar edema is seen posterior to the schwannoma.

Case 70

24-year-old woman with recent hearing impairment (neurofibromatosis, coronal scan).

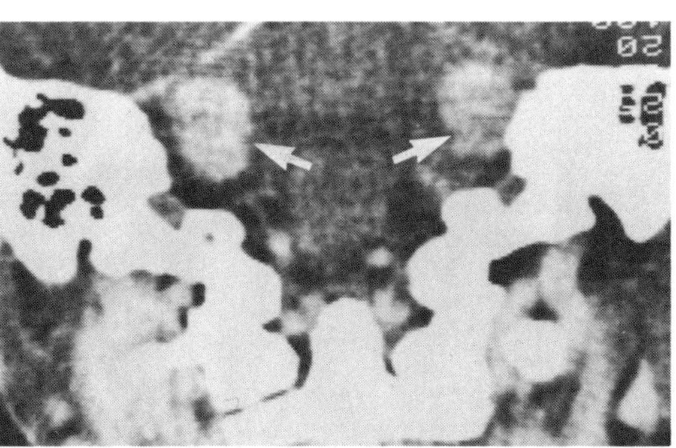

Bilateral acoustic schwannomas suggest neurofibromatosis, even if the diagnosis has not been previously apparent. Here, a coronal scan demonstrates the well-defined, uniformly enhancing masses arising in the cerebellopontine angles along the midposterior surface of the petrous ridges.

Almost all patients who present with acoustic schwannomas have hearing loss, and about three fourths experience dysequilibrium and/or tinnitus. On the other hand, only about 10% of patients with unilateral hearing loss are found to have acoustic schwannomas.

Case 71

74-year-old man.

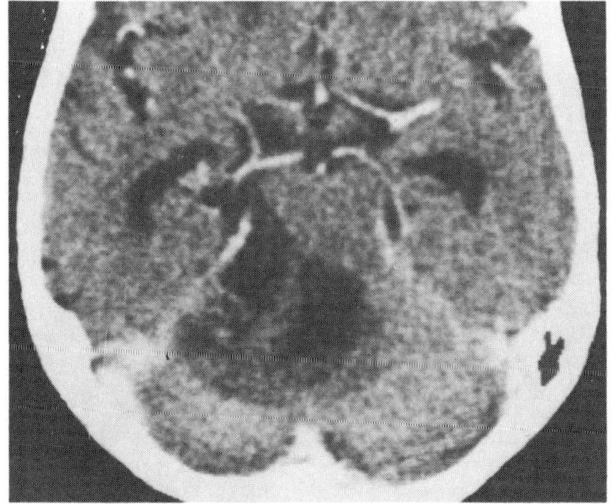

Many acoustic schwannomas have an atypical appearance caused by prominent areas of low attenuation within or adjacent to the tumor. These low-density regions are often cystic, but solid tissue with low attenuation may also occur.

When the bulk of the mass is of low density, as in this case, the lesion may be confused with an intra-axial tumor extending exophytically into the cerebellopontine angle. Alternatively, a low-attenuation acoustic schwannoma may resemble other low-density extra-axial masses (see Cases 131 and 132).

The relationship of the lesion to a widened internal auditory canal may provide the diagnosis. In difficult cases, scans with subarachnoid contrast material will help to separate intra-axial and extra-axial processes.

Case 72

75-year-old woman.

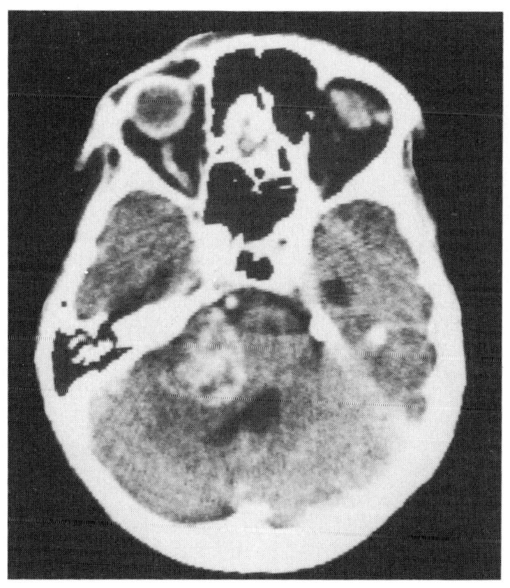

In this case, an inhomogeneous enhancement pattern causes an appearance intermediate between the typical uniform schwannoma (e.g., Case 69) and the low-density lesion in Case 71. Although the tumor has invaginated far into the cerebellum and brain stem, the widening of the ipsilateral cisterns at the margins of the mass suggests an extra-axial origin.

INTERNAL AUDITORY CANAL WIDENING IN ACOUSTIC SCHWANNOMAS

Case 73

19-year-old woman presenting with hearing loss and facial numbness (wide window width).

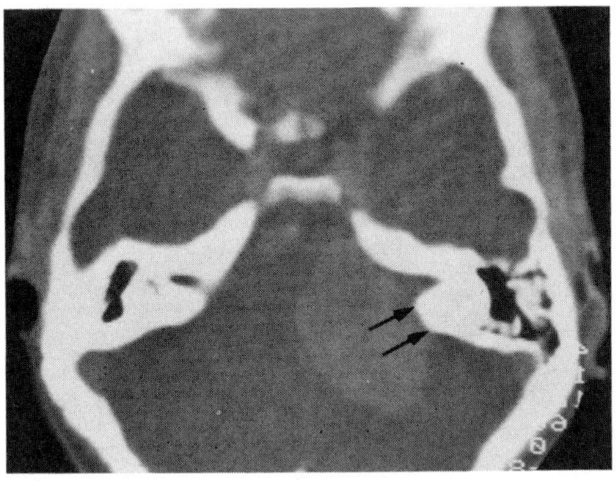

A secondary hallmark of acoustic schwannomas is widening or "flaring" of the internal auditory canal (IAC) from which they arise. The degree of IAC erosion is not necessarily related to the size of the tumor, which may expand exophytically in the adjacent cistern.

In this case, the involved IAC is clearly widened when compared with the contralateral side. The canal is also shortened, due to erosion of the posterior lip of the internal auditory meatus *(arrows)*.

The large cerebellopontine angle mass is faintly seen at this wide window width, and appears centered on the widened internal auditory meatus. This relationship of an enhancing mass to an expanded IAC is useful in distinguishing acoustic schwannomas from meningiomas or aneurysms of the cerebellopontine angle, which rarely cause widening of the canal.

Case 74

57-year-old woman presenting with hearing loss (intermediate window width).

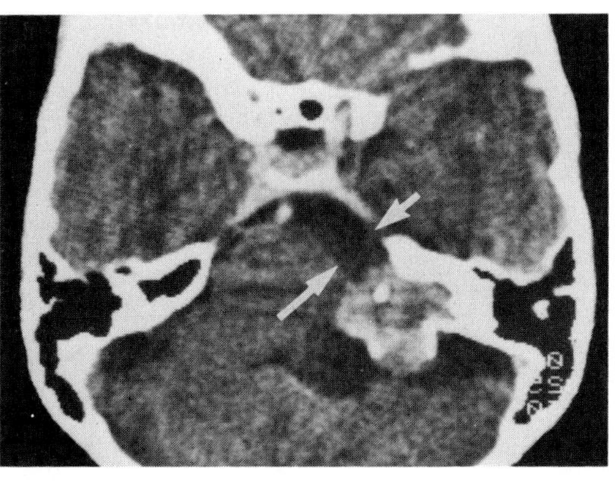

The expansion of the internal auditory canal caused by an acoustic schwannoma may be markedly irregular, as in this case. The lobular tumor has displaced the brain stem, with prominent widening of the ipsilateral cisterns *(arrows)*. An area of low attenuation medial to the enhancing mass may represent edema and/or a low-attenuation component of the tumor.

Case 75

54-year-old woman with hearing loss (decubitus scan with nose to the reader's right).

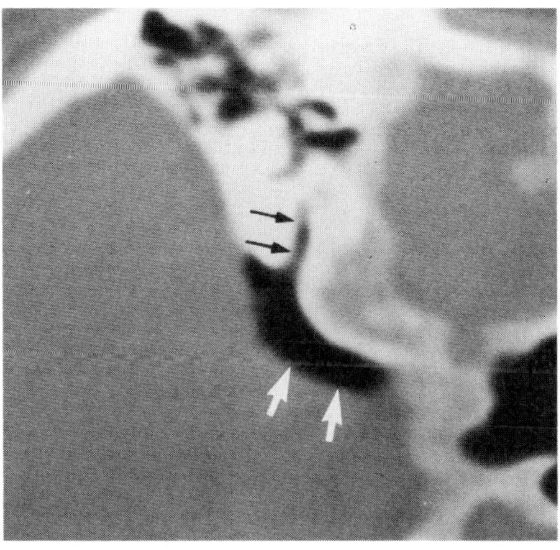

A standard scan may fail to define small acoustic schwannomas, particularly those confined to the internal auditory canal. When initial scans are negative and the clinical suspicion of acoustic schwannoma is strong, the possibility of an intracanalicular tumor is raised.

Such lesions can be better imaged after a few cubic centimeters of gas are injected via a lumbar puncture and maneuvered into the cerebellopontine angle *(white arrows).* The head is turned to a decubitus position, so that gas in the cistern should rise into the adjacent internal auditory canal. Even small canals will normally fill with gas as in this case *(black arrows),* thereby excluding an intracanalicular schwannoma. (It is important to image the middle of the IAC with thin sections to avoid the misleading density of partial volume.)

Case 76

58-year-old man with ten-year history of impaired hearing (decubitus scan with nose to the reader's right).

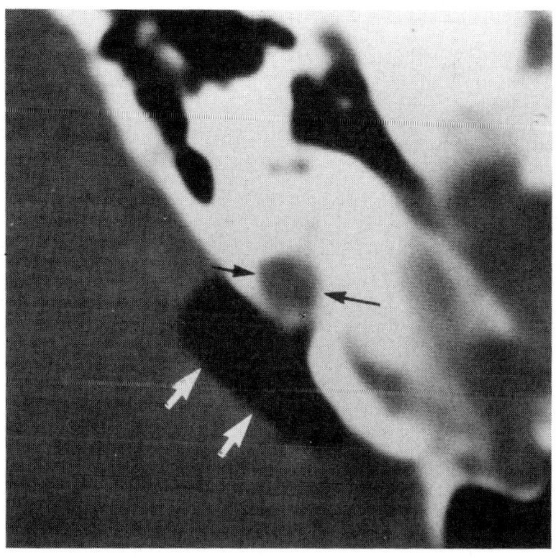

Here, the cerebellopontine angle cistern is filled with gas *(white arrows).* The air fails to enter the widened internal auditory canal *(black arrows)* because it is occupied by a soft-tissue mass. The mass was surgically proved to be a small, intracanalicular acoustic schwannoma.

Such tumors may cause more symptoms due to intracanalicular nerve compression than much larger schwannomas growing freely in the cerebellopontine angle.

DIFFERENTIAL DIAGNOSIS: SMALL, ROUND, DENSE TISSUE IN THE CEREBELLOPONTINE ANGLE

Case 77

76-year-old woman.

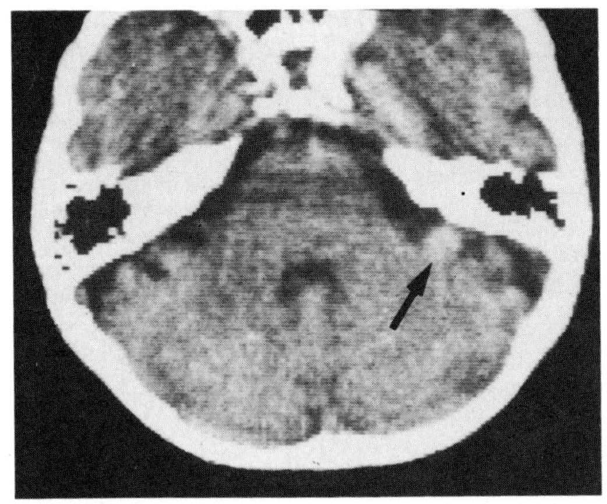

Normal Flocculus (Noncontrast Scan).

Case 78

66-year-old man.

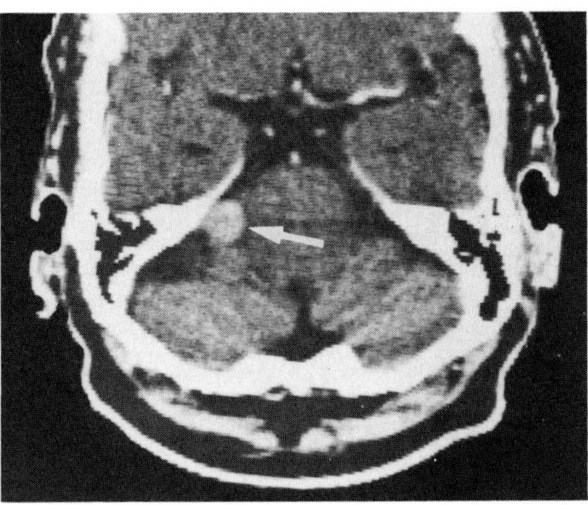

Acoustic Schwannoma (Postcontrast Scan).

The flocculus of the cerebellum forms a nodule along its lateral surface near the IAC. When seen in cross-section on axial scans, this rounded density (*arrow,* Case 77) may mimic a small acoustic schwannoma.

The flocculus does not enhance as prominently as the usual acoustic schwannoma (Case 78), and there is no associated widening of the IAC. In addition, the location of the flocculus is posterior to the IAC.

DIFFERENTIAL DIAGNOSIS: UNIFORMLY ENHANCING, EXTRA-AXIAL POSTERIOR FOSSA MASS

Case 79

76-year-old woman with a four-month history of poor balance.

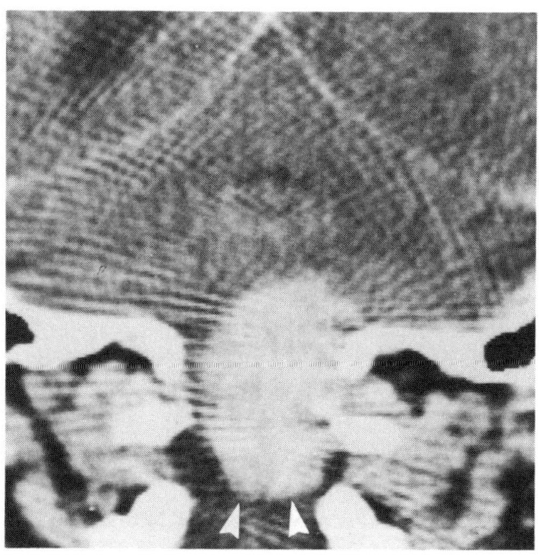

Foramen Magnum Meningioma.

Case 80

75-year-old woman presenting with dizziness and tinnitus.

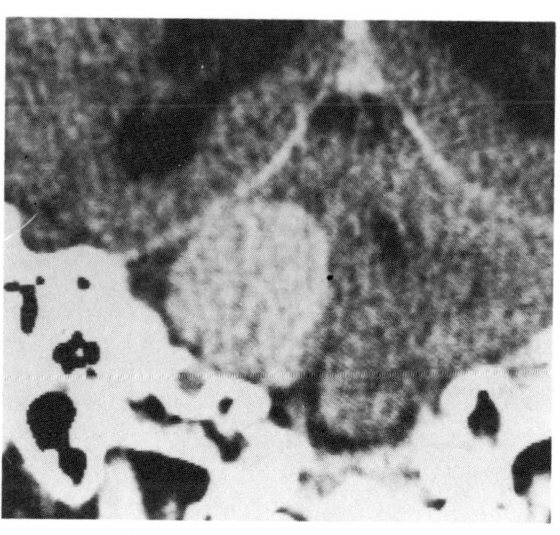

Acoustic Schwannoma.

The CT features of meningiomas and acoustic schwannomas may be very similar. However, most posterior fossa meningiomas are centered above or below the internal auditory meatus, and few are associated with widening of the IAC (or hearing loss).

Coronal views help to define the location of a cerebellopontine angle mass. Coronal scans (and/or sagittal reconstructions of axial scans) are also valuable for evaluating foramen magnum lesions (see also Case 430). In Case 79, the meningioma is seen to extend from the posterior fossa through the plane of C-1 to the level of C-2 *(arrows)*.

Aneurysms of the vertebral or basilar arteries may appear as dense, enhancing extra-axial masses. They should be included in this differential diagnosis (see Cases 310 and 319), along with glomus jugulare tumors (See Case 81) and rare jugular foramen schwannomas and choroid plexus papillomas.

Case 81A

33-year-old woman with tongue weakness (wide window width).

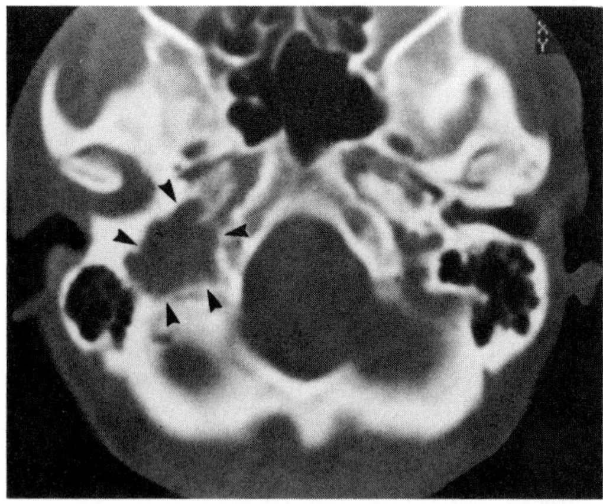

Glomus tumors ("chemodectomas," "paragangliomas") originate from paraganglionic cells in numerous locations, including the carotid sinus ("carotid body tumor"), jugular bulb ("glomus jugulare"), and middle ear ("glomus tympanicum").

Although most of these neoplasms are histologically benign, they may be locally invasive. Associated bone erosion is often irregular and poorly defined, suggesting malignancy. In this case, a large area of bone destruction at the right jugular foramen *(arrows)* demonstrates typically indistinct margins.

Case 81B

Same patient (postcontrast scan).

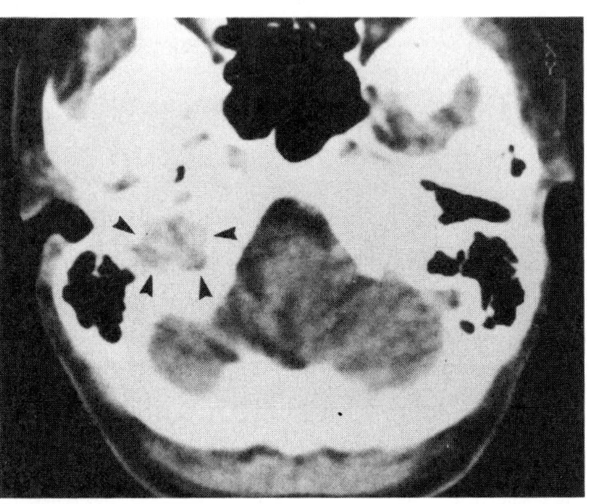

Glomus tumors are highly vascular with prominent contrast enhancement. Here the enhancing mass fills the bone defect demonstrated in Case 81A.

Glomus jugulare tumors may span the skull base, with posterior fossa and extracranial components. Coronal scans provide a useful composite view of these intracranial and extracranial extensions.

A glomus jugulare tumor growing into the cerebellopontine angle may resemble other enhancing extra-axial lesions at this site (e.g., meningioma, acoustic neuroma, aneurysm; see Cases 69, 79, and 80). However, associated erosion of the jugular foramen usually provides the diagnosis.

REFERENCES

1. Bilaniuk L.T., Zimmerman R.A., Littman P., et al.: Computed tomography of brain stem gliomas in children. *Radiology* 134:89–95, 1980.
2. Daniels D.L., Haughton V.M., Williams A.L., et al.: The flocculus in computed tomography. *A.J.N.R.* 2:227–229, 1981.
3. Dubois P.J., Drayer B.P., Bank W.O., et al.: An evaluation of current diagnostic radiologic modalities in the investigation of acoustic neurilemmoma. *Radiology* 126:173– 179, 1978.
4. Duffner P.K., Klein D.M., Cohen M.E.: Calcification in brainstem gliomas. *Neurology* 28:832–834, 1978.
5. Enzmann D.R., Norman D., Levin V., et al.: Computed tomography in the follow-up of medulloblastomas and ependymomas. *Radiology* 128:57–63, 1978.
6. Ganti S.R., Silver A.J., Hilal S.K., et al.: Computed tomography of cerebellar hemangioblastomas. *J. Comput. Assist. Tomogr.* 6:912–919, 1982.
7. Glanz S., Geehr R.B., Duncan C.C., et al.: Metrizamide-enhanced CT for evaluation of brainstem tumors. *A.J.N.R.* 1:31–35, 1980.
8. Johnson D.W.: Air cisternography of the cerebellopontine angle using high resolution computed tomography. *Radiology* 151:401–403, 1984.
9. Mawad M.E., Silver A.J., Hilal S.K., et al.: Computed tomography of the brain stem with intrathecal metrizamide: II. Lesions in and around the brain stem. *A.J.N.R.* 4:13–19, 1983.
10. Möller A., Hatam A., Olivecrona H.: The differential diagnosis of pontine angle meningioma and acoustic neuroma with computed tomography. *Neuroradiology* 17:21–23, 1978.
11. Möller A., Hatam A., Olivecrona H.: Diagnosis of acoustic neuroma with computed tomography. *Neuroradiology* 17:25–30, 1978.
12. Naidich T.P., Lin J.P., Leeds N.E., et al.: Primary tumors and other masses of the cerebellum and fourth ventricle. *Neuroradiology* 14:153–174, 1977.
13. Phelps P.D., Lloyd E.A.: High resolution air CT meatography: The demonstration of normal and abnormal structures in the cerebellopontine cistern and internal auditory meatus. *Br. J. Radiol.* 55:19–22, 1982.
14. Pinto R.S., Kricheff I.I., Bergeron R.T., et al.: Small acoustic neuromas: Detection by high resolution gas CT cisternography. *A.J.N.R.* 3:283–286, 1982.
15. Seeger J.F., Burke D.P., Knake J.E., et al.: Computed tomographic and angiographic evaluation of hemangioblastomas. *Radiology* 138:65–73, 1981.
16. Segall H.D., Zee C.S., Naidich T.P., et al.: Computed tomography in neoplasms of the posterior fossa in children. *Radiol. Clin. North. Am.* 20:237–253, 1982.
17. Shaffer K.A.: Computed tomography of the temporal bone. *Radiographics* 1:62–72, 1981.
18. Solti-Bohman L.G., Magaram D.L., Lo W.W., et al.: Gas-CT cisternography for detection of small acoustic nerve tumors. *Radiology* 150:403–407, 1984.
19. Swartz J.D., Zimmerman R.A., Bilaniuk L.T.: Computed tomography of intracranial ependymomas. *Radiology* 143:97–101, 1982.
20. Taylor S.: The petrous temporal bone (including the cerebellopontine angle). *Radiol. Clin. North. Am.* 20:67–86, 1982.
21. Zee C.S., Segall H.D., Miller C., et al.: Less common CT features of medulloblastoma. *Radiology* 144:97–102, 1982.
22. Zimmerman R.A., Bilaniuk L.T., Bruno L., et al.: Computed tomography of cerebellar astrocytoma. *A.J.R.* 130:929–933, 1980.
23. Zimmerman R.A., Bilaniuk L.T., Pahlajani H.: Spectrum of medulloblastomas demonstrated by computed tomography. *Radiology* 126:137–141, 1978.

CHAPTER 5

PITUITARY AND SUPRASELLAR TUMORS

PITUITARY ADENOMAS: UNIFORM ENHANCEMENT AND SUPRASELLAR EXTENSION

Case 82A

81-year-old man presenting with hypothyroidism.

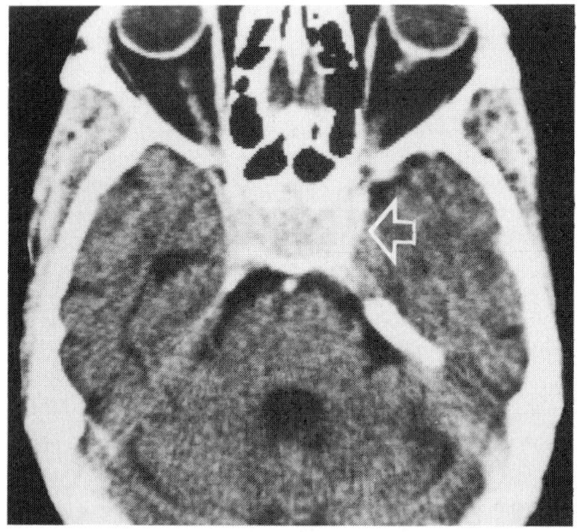

The most reliable CT feature of pituitary adenomas is their origin within the sella turcica. Large adenomas may have confusing suprasellar or parasellar components (see Cases 86 and 90), and enhancement patterns may be variable and nonspecific (see Case 85).

In this case, the sella is moderately enlarged and filled with a uniformly enhancing adenoma. The lateral margins of enhancing tumor merge with contrast density in the cavernous sinuses, which are bowed slightly laterally *(arrow)*.

Pituitary hyperplasia may cause diffuse enlargment of the gland, mimicking an adenoma. This possibility should be considered when a pituitary "mass" is found in appropriate clinical settings (e.g., hypothyroidism, pregnancy).

Case 82B

Same patient.

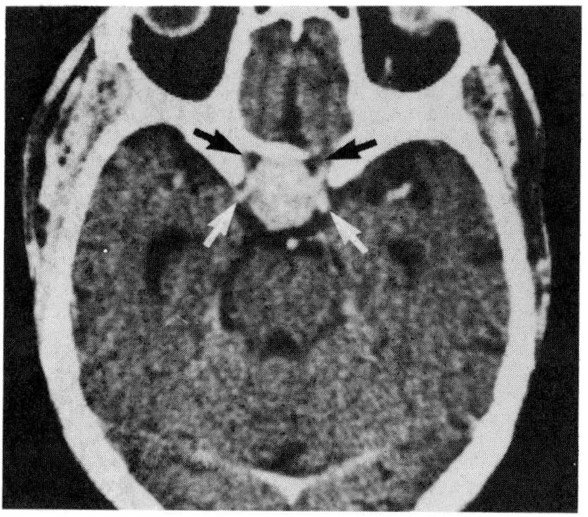

A higher scan demonstrates superior extension of the adenoma into the suprasellar cistern. The tumor is centered in the midline, spanning the distance between the supraclinoid internal carotid arteries *(white arrows)*.

The optic nerves pass between the anterior clinoid process and the tumor *(black arrows)*, so that further tumor growth would lead to increasingly compromised visual acuity. Nerve compression or bitemporal hemianopia (from pressure on the optic chiasm) depend both on the tumor size and on the congenitally variable proximity of the optic chiasm to the optic canals.

The well-defined, uniform enhancement of pituitary adenomas may closely resemble other suprasellar lesions (compare this scan with Cases 83 and 84).

DIFFERENTIAL DIAGNOSIS: INTENSELY ENHANCING, MIDLINE SUPRASELLAR MASS

Case 83

43-year-old woman presenting with decreased visual acuity.

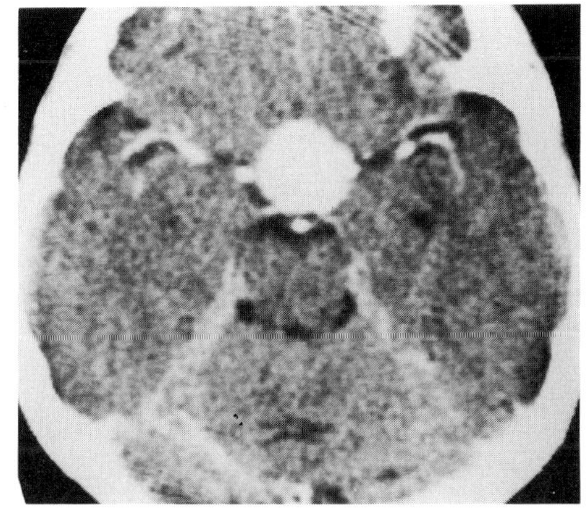

Suprasellar Meningioma.

Case 84

68-year-old man presenting with dementia.

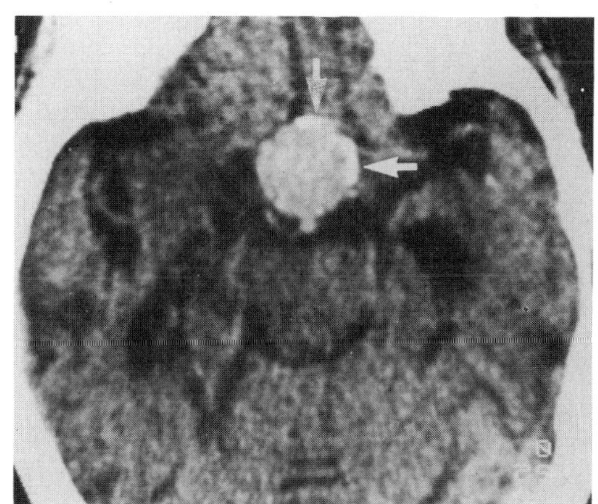

Aneurysm.

Many lesions can present as well-defined, densely enhancing suprasellar masses. In children, chiasmatic-hypothalamic glioma, unusual craniopharyngioma, and rare histiocytosis should be considered when this appearance is encountered (see Cases 95 and 106). In adolescents or young adults, germinomas are included in the differential diagnosis (see Cases 102 and 103). In adults, the most common mass with these features is a pituitary adenoma, but Cases 83 and 84 illustrate the need for caution.

Suprasellar aneurysms may contain characteristic rim calcification *(arrows)* or intraluminal thrombus. They are often located slightly away from the midline. Aneurysms may be readily documented by digital subtraction angiography.

Metastasis to the hypothalamus/infundibulum is another enhancing lesion that may present in the suprasellar region, most often seen with primary tumors of the breast and lung. Large colloid cysts may extend inferiorly into the suprasellar region, usually with little enhancement (see Cases 113 and 114). Suprasellar inflammatory processes (e.g., sarcoidosis) often enhance less intensely than seen here.

As discussed in Cases 103 and 104, expansion of the sella turcica and continuity of suprasellar and intrasellar masses on coronal scans are hallmarks of pituitary adenoma. The absence of these features should suggest an alternative diagnosis.

Case 85A

35-year-old asymptomatic volunteer fireman struck on the head; skull roentgenograms showed a large sella.

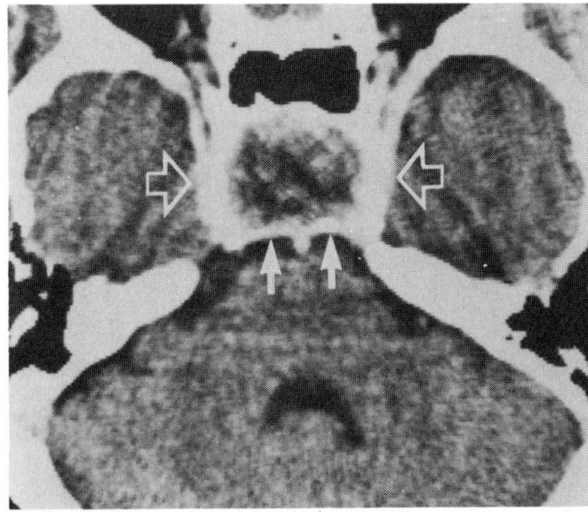

Many pituitary adenomas contain nonenhancing regions representing cysts, necrosis, or inhomogeneous tissue. Sometimes the entire tumor has this appearance, with only a rim of contrast enhancement.

In this case, the sella is enlarged, with the dorsum displaced posteriorly as far as the basilar artery *(solid arrows)*. The lack of central tumor enhancement allows visualization of the cavernous sinuses, which are compressed and bowed laterally *(open arrows)*.

Case 85B

Same patient.

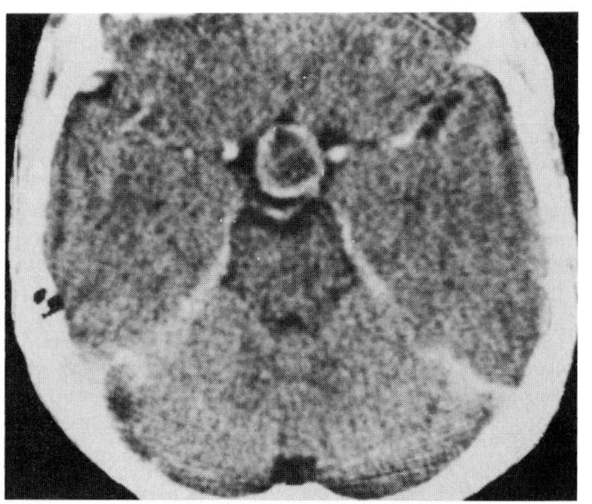

The suprasellar extension of this pituitary adenoma has the same rim-enhancing appearance as the intrasellar component.

Necrosis and hemorrhage are common in pituitary tumors. Acute infarction or hemorrhage may cause rapid swelling of an adenoma, leading to sudden visual and endocrine compromise ("pituitary apoplexy").

Like solid adenomas, rim-enhancing pituitary tumors may resemble other suprasellar lesions (see Cases 100, 101, 313, and 314).

PITUITARY ADENOMAS: CORONAL VIEWS

Case 85C

35-year-old man (same patient as Cases 85A and B).

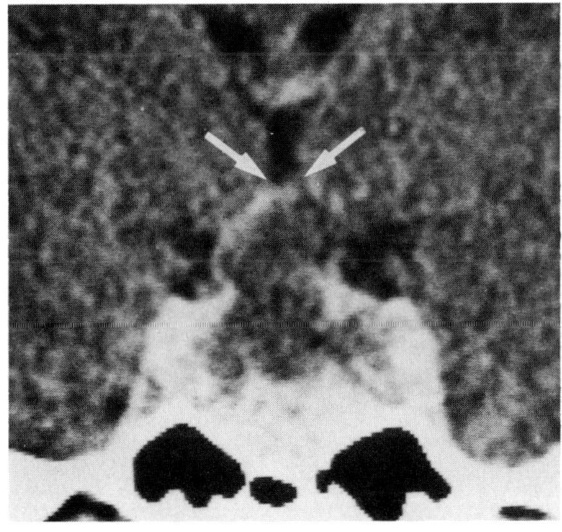

The coronal plane is useful for evaluating infrasellar, suprasellar, and parasellar extension of pituitary adenomas.

Here the suprasellar extension seen axially in Case 85B is defined as a snowman-like nodule arising on top of a broader intrasellar base. The full extent of the suprasellar component is well appreciated, with compression of the inferior portion of the third ventricle *(arrows)*. A rim of enhancing tumor fills the prominently depressed sellar floor as it bulges into the sphenoid sinus.

Case 86

55-year-old man found by optometrist to have bilaterally reduced visual acuity.

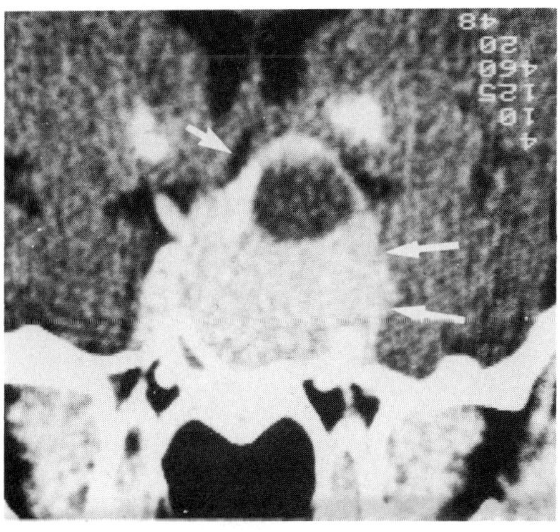

Again, the coronal plane gives an integrated image of suprasellar, infrasellar, and parasellar extension. The bulk of this large adenoma enhances uniformly, although it contains a prominent nonenhancing area.

The superior margin of the tumor displaces the anterior third ventricle *(short arrow)*. The sellar floor is markedly depressed, obliterating the sphenoid sinus. Parasellar extension into the medial portion of the middle cranial fossa is seen on the left *(long arrows)*. Such parasellar extension may pass under, through, or over the cavernous sinus.

The high density regions superior to the adenoma represent idiopathic calcification in the basal ganglia.

PITUITARY MICROADENOMAS

Case 87A

32-year-old woman presenting with amenorrhea and galactorrhea. Prolactinoma (coronal scan).

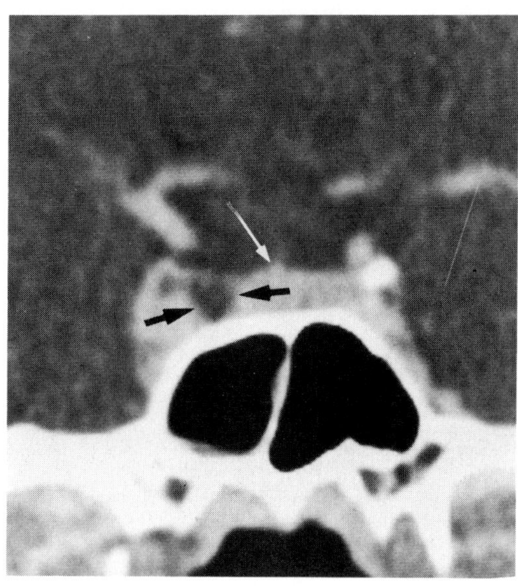

Secreting adenomas of the pituitary may cause significant endocrine symptoms despite small tumor size. (Contrast this case with the nonsecreting adenoma in Case 90.) Tumors less than 10 mm in diameter have been termed "microadenomas." Prolactinomas are the most frequent microadenomas to produce clinical symptoms, usually amenorrhea and/or galactorrhea in young women.

Axial scans are often normal in the presence of a microadenoma. Coronal scans performed immediately after a bolus injection of contrast material offer the best CT definition of these tumors.

A microadenoma may be directly imaged as a relatively low-attenuation lesion within the otherwise enhancing pituitary tissue *(arrows)*. This appearance must be correlated with secondary findings and the clinical presentation, since other low-density regions (e.g., small cysts) are common within the gland.

The lateral location of the tumor in this case is common for prolactinomas. Extension into the cavernous sinus may be associated with very high serum prolactin levels.

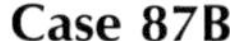

Case 87B

Same patient. Scan slightly more posterior (coronal scan).

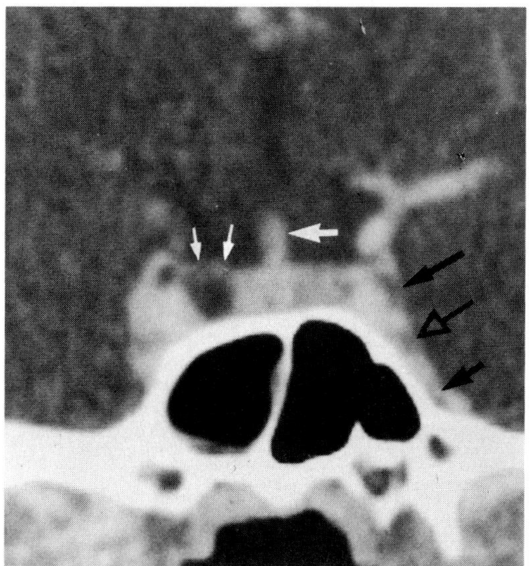

Secondary findings of a pituitary microadenoma on coronal scans include increased height of the gland, prominent superior convexity, deviation of the pituitary infundibulum, and focal erosion of the sellar floor. Each of these features can be an isolated normal finding, but their association suggests a responsible mass. Here the small adenoma causes a localized superior bulge *(small white arrows)* but does not displace the enhancing infundibulum *(large white arrow)*.

The superior surface of the pituitary gland may normally be "tented" in the midline at the junction with the infundibulum (*white arrow,* Case 87A). Occasionally, the entire superior surface of a normal gland is prominently convex (see Case 88), but the contour is smoothly symmetric, as opposed to the focal, eccentric deformity in this case. Conversely, microadenomas may be present within glands demonstrating no superior convexity, as is almost true on this scan.

Several cranial nerves are seen in cross-section as filling defects within the enhancing cavernous sinus (third nerve, *long black arrow;* fourth and/or sixth nerves, *open black arrow;* fifth nerve, *short black arrow*).

DIFFERENTIAL DIAGNOSIS: LOW-ATTENUATION AND SUPERIOR CONVEXITY OF PITUITARY TISSUE

Case 88

18-year-old woman.

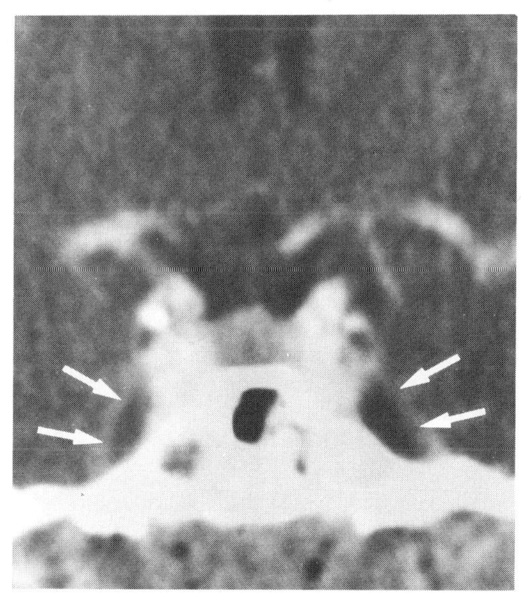

Normal Pituitary (Coronal Scan).

Case 89

24-year-old woman.

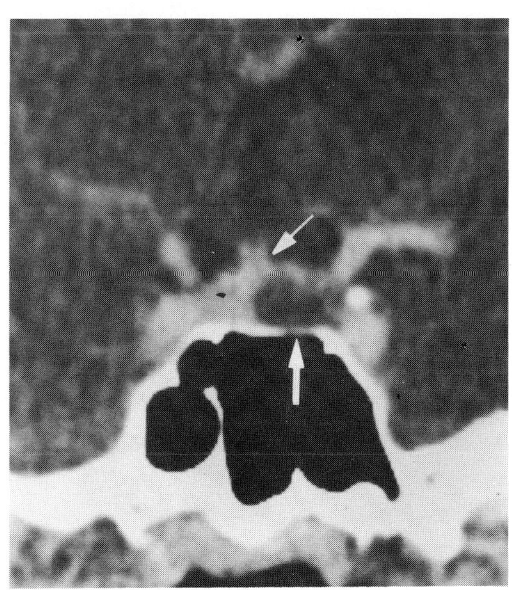

Microadenoma (Coronal Scan).

Pituitary enhancement may be less intense than the contrast density of the cavernous sinuses. The gland then appears as a relatively low-attenuation region, as seen in Case 88.

Superior convexity may be a normal feature of pituitary morphology, particularly in young women. In Case 88 the sella is narrow, probably accounting for the relatively tall gland with a prominent superior margin. This normal convexity is smoothly uniform and centered in the midline.

By contrast, the low-density adenoma in Case 89 asymmetrically distorts the superior margin of the gland. In addition, the infundibulum is displaced slightly toward the opposite side *(small white arrow),* and the sellar floor is thinned beneath the tumor *(large white arrow).*

Meckel's caves containing the fifth nerve ganglia are well seen within the posterior cavernous sinuses *(arrows)* in Case 88.

Case 90

32-year-old man with a long history of "nasal" voice and a two-week history of impaired vision.

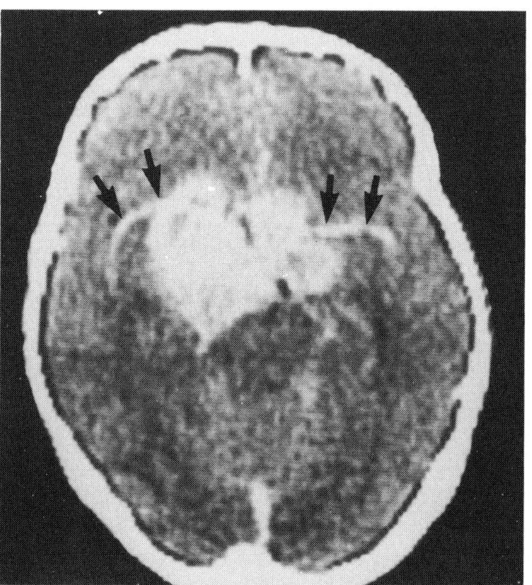

Nonsecreting pituitary adenomas may become very large before compression of the optic chiasm causes symptoms. This huge, lobulated suprasellar mass was accompanied by an equally large extracranial component filling the nasopharynx (and accounting for the history of nasal speech).

At the geographic center of the mass was the faintly seen "ghost" of an expanded sella turcica, a hallmark of intrasellar origin. The diagnosis of giant pituitary adenoma was made and confirmed by biopsy in the pharynx.

The horizontal segments of the middle cerebral arteries are elevated by the suprasellar mass *(arrows),* which is somewhat restrained by the vessels and grows in lobulations around the vascular grooves. Encasement of basal arteries is characteristic of parasellar meningiomas but can also be seen in large pituitary adenomas.

Case 91

55-year-old woman.

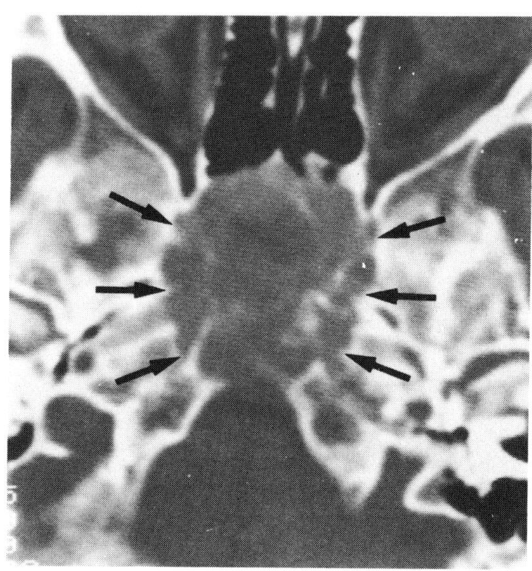

Inferior extension of a pituitary adenoma may fill the sphenoid sinus and continue eroding through the skull base to reach the nasopharynx. This case demonstrates a large defect in the middle of the sphenoid bone and clivus *(arrows)* due to inferior growth of a pituitary tumor. Such bone destruction may mimic the skull invasion of a nasopharyngeal neoplasm.

The relative amounts of suprasellar and infrasellar extension may depend on the comparative resistance to tumor expansion in the superior (diaphragma sellae) vs. inferior (sphenoid sinus and skull base) directions.

THE "EMPTY SELLA SYNDROME"

Case 92

59-year-old woman with headache, found to have a large sella on skull roentgenograms (coronal scan).

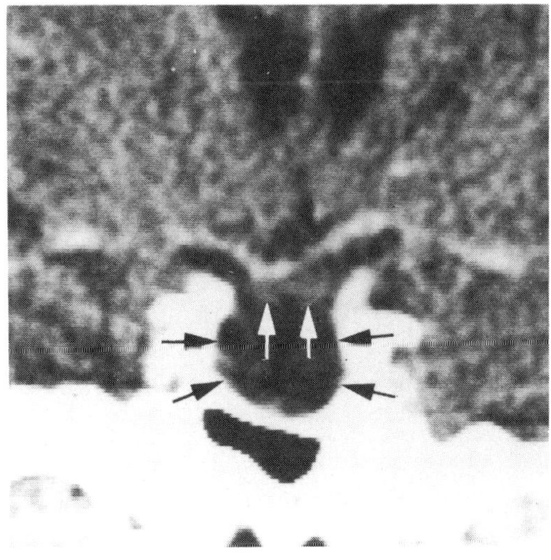

An unusually large aperture in the diaphragma sellae may allow spinal fluid from the suprasellar cistern to extend into the sella. The intrasellar cistern participates in normal CSF pulsations and can cause gradual expansion of the sella, closely resembling the enlargement seen with pituitary adenomas.

This "empty sella syndrome" is often discovered in otherwise healthy, middle-aged, overweight patients (especially women) with vague complaints (especially headache). Associated pituitary dysfunction is rare. Occasional visual symptoms may be caused by prolapse of the optic chiasm, more commonly seen with "secondary" empty sellas following necrosis or removal of pituitary tumors.

In this case the sella is clearly enlarged, with depression of the floor and lateral bowing of the cavernous sinuses *(black arrows)*. The sella is filled with CSF density, and no pituitary tissue is defined. The position of the optic chiasm *(white arrows)* is somewhat low.

Case 93

44-year-old woman. Metrizamide study of "empty sella" (coronal scan).

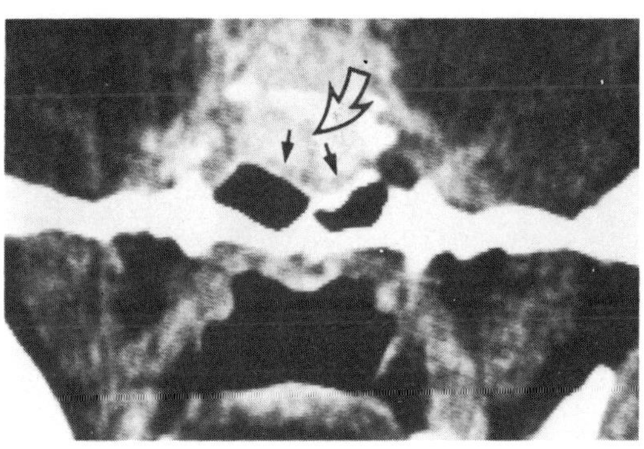

A number of low-attenuation lesions can occur within the sella turcica, including some pituitary adenomas, abscesses, cysts, craniopharyngiomas, and dermoid cysts. An "empty sella" must be distinguished from these low-density intrasellar masses.

The diagnosis of a true "empty sella" can be made on a routine coronal scan if the thin pituitary infundibulum can be seen to traverse the low-density area to reach the pituitary gland at the floor of the sella. The infundibulum is best seen on postcontrast scans due to enhancement of the hypophyseal portal venous system.

If this finding cannot be demonstrated, opacification of the subarachnoid spaces with contrast material will determine whether the sellar content is spinal fluid or a low-density lesion. Here, metrizamide fills the enlarged "empty sella," outlining the pituitary infundibulum *(curved, open arrow)* as it extends to the inferiorly flattened pituitary gland *(small arrows)*.

Occasionally a small pituitary adenoma may be found within an otherwise "empty" sella. This possibility reinforces the need for careful examination of such cases.

CRANIOPHARYNGIOMAS

Case 94

6-year-old girl (noncontrast scan).

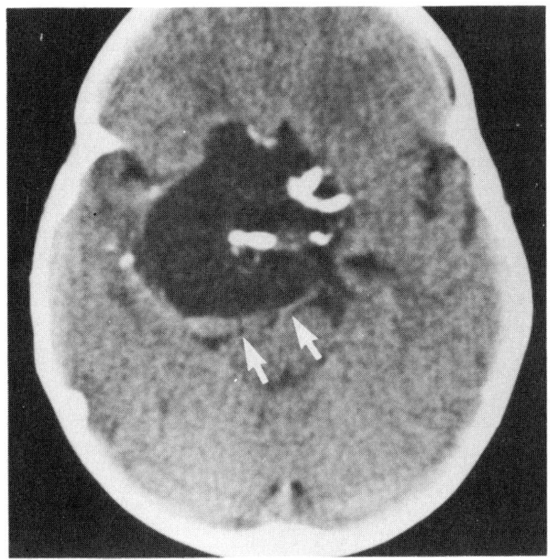

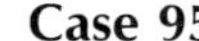

Case 95

12-year-old boy (postcontrast scan).

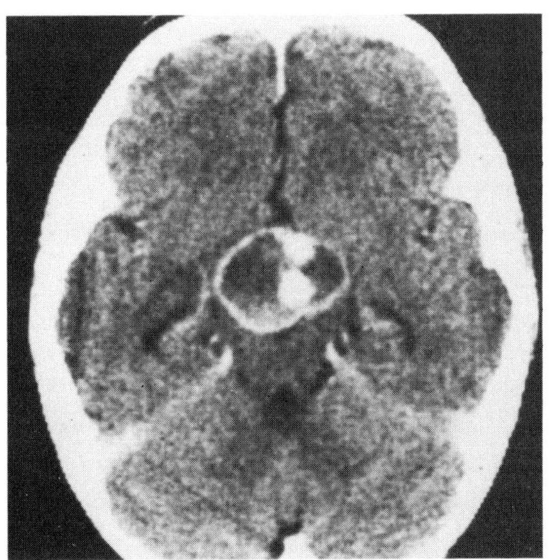

Craniopharyngiomas are typically seen as mixed-attenuation lesions in a suprasellar location. Low-attenuation regions may be due to cyst formation or low-density tissue. Calcification is characteristic and may take the form of arcs in the periphery of cystic lesions or dense nodules within areas of solid tumor (see Case 109).

Parasellar and retrosellar extension are common. In this case, the tumor occupies the medial portion of the right middle cranial fossa, with a retrosellar component displacing the brain stem posteriorly *(arrows)*.

Contrast enhancement in craniopharyngiomas may be minimal or intense. Patterns include homogeneous enhancement of solid tumors and rim enhancement surrounding cystic components. The target appearance in this case resembles a partially thrombosed giant aneurysm (see Case 318).

Although midline suprasellar location is characteristic of craniopharyngiomas, eccentric tumors are common (see Case 97), and occasional lesions are found within the sella or third ventricle.

ATYPICAL CRANIOPHARYNGIOMAS

Case 96

55-year-old man presenting with diabetes insipidus and bitemporal hemianopia. Solid craniopharyngioma.

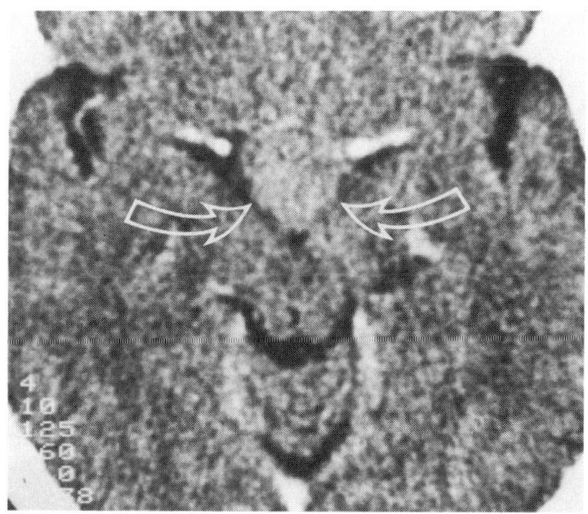

This mass occupies a suprasellar location but lacks other features of craniopharyngiomas. No cyst, calcification, or contrast enhancement is present. The nondescript appearance resembles a low-grade glioma of the hypothalamus or optic chiasm (see Case 107), although such tumors are rare in adults.

About 30% of craniopharyngiomas are found in adults and about 25% are solid masses.

Case 97

15-year-old boy presenting with growth arrest and temporal headaches. Cystic craniopharyngioma.

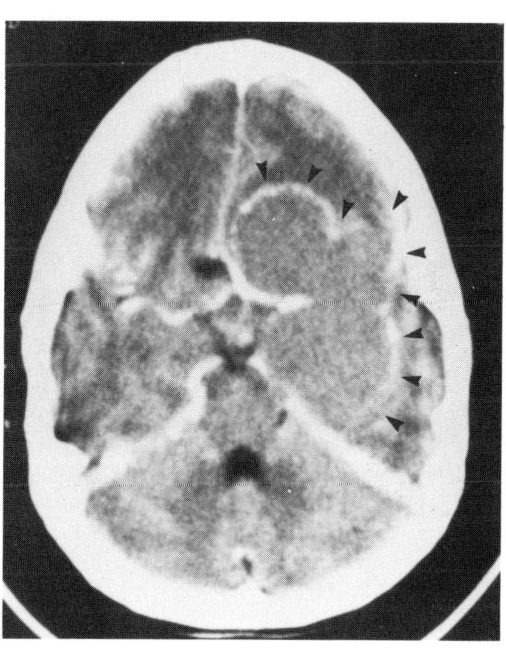

Cystic craniopharyngiomas do not always present as low-attenuation lesions. Hemorrhage or high protein levels may cause tumor cysts to appear isodense or even hyperdense.

Here a trilobed mass in the frontotemporal region demonstrates calcification and enhancement within rims of tissue surrounding homogeneous, isodense, nonenhancing central material. Despite the high attentuation values, the homogeneity of the lesion suggests a cyst. Scans at lower levels connected the eccentric mass with a small suprasellar component. The combination of rim calcification, central cyst, and relationship to the suprasellar area favors the diagnosis of craniopharyngioma.

Occasional craniopharyngiomas are filled with high-attenuation material mimicking an aneurysm or meningioma on precontrast scans. The lack of central contrast enhancement within cystic craniopharyngiomas aids the differential diagnosis in such cases.

DIFFERENTIAL DIAGNOSIS: LOW-ATTENUATION SUPRASELLAR MASS

Case 98

47-year-old woman.

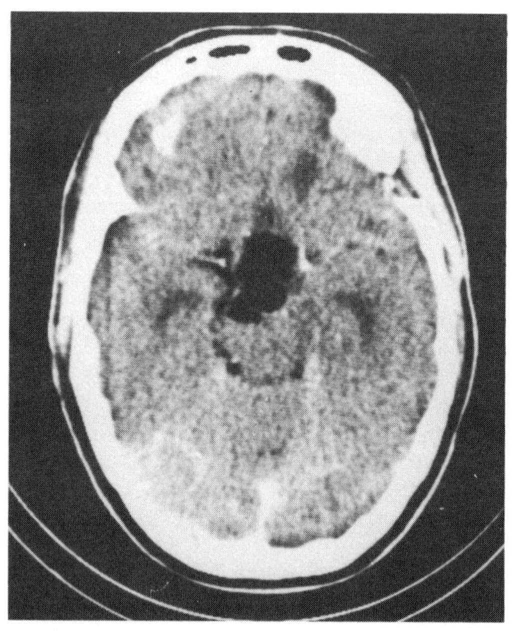

Dermoid Cyst.

Case 99

42-year-old woman.

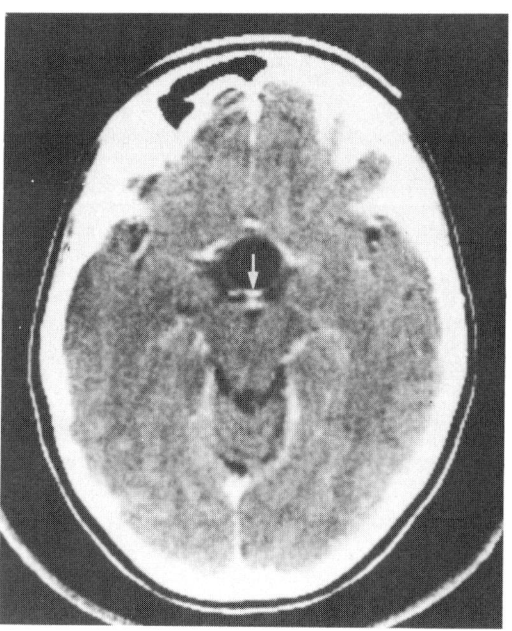

Pituitary Cyst With Suprasellar Extension.

Craniopharyngiomas are one of several low-attenuation lesions that may be found in the suprasellar region. Dermoid and epidermoid cysts and arachnoid cysts are frequently located at this site.

Dermoid cysts often contain very low attenuation values due to their fat content, as in Case 98 (see also Cases 125 and 127). These low values contrast with the less extreme low density of craniopharyngiomas or epidermoid cysts (see Case 369).

Calcification is common in dermoid cysts as well as in craniopharyngiomas (see Cases 127 and 128). The combination of fat content and marginal calcification may also be seen with simple lipomas (see Case 377), but these are less frequent in the suprasellar area.

Case 99 is an unusual example of a simple pituitary cyst extending into the suprasellar region, mimicking a cystic tumor or arachnoid cyst (see Case 348). The focal enhancement along the midposterior rim of the cyst *(arrow)* is the flattened pituitary infundibulum.

Gliomas of the hypothalamus may also present as low-attenuation suprasellar masses (see Case 349).

DIFFERENTIAL DIAGNOSIS: MIXED-ATTENUATION SUPRASELLAR MASS

Case 100

18-year-old man.

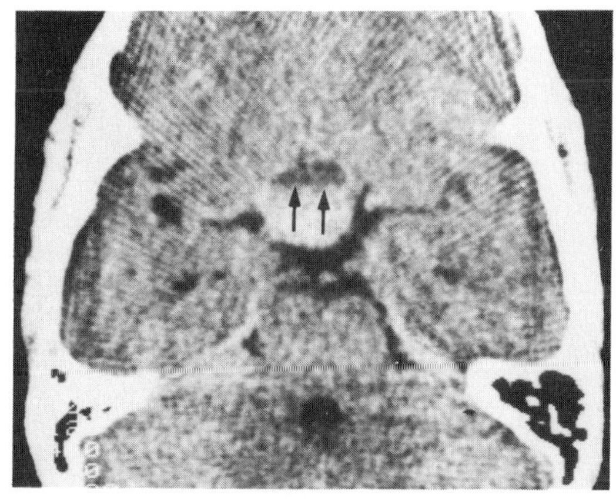

Cystic Pituitary Adenoma.

Case 101

55-year-old man (same patient as Case 96).

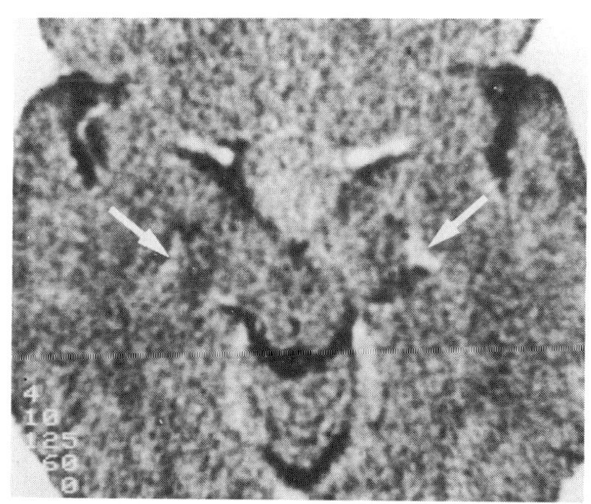

Craniopharyngioma.

As in Cases 83 and 84, the interpretation of lesions with this appearance depends on the age of the patient. In children, the leading possibilities would be hypothalamic-chiasmatic glioma and craniopharyngioma. The rare hamartomas of the tuber cinereum present slightly more posteriorly in the interpeduncular region. Histiocytosis is an infrequent cause of a suprasellar mass in childhood.

In an adult, the differential diagnosis includes suprasellar extension of pituitary adenoma, craniopharyngioma, epidermoid cyst, thrombosed aneurysm (see Case 313), or a rare, low-grade hypothalamic/optic glioma. Inflammatory lesions (e.g., sarcoidosis, tuberculosis, sphenoid mucocele) may cause a suprasellar mass, but other clinical clues are usually present.

The sedimentation level in Case 100 *(arrows)* indicates a cystic tumor, and the appearance is actually more suggestive of craniopharyngioma than the mass in Case 101. In Case 100, associated enlargement of the sella turcica was present and favored the diagnosis of pituitary adenoma.

The densities within the temporal horns in Case 101 *(arrows)* represent normal enhancement of choroid plexus. A composite "ring" of enhancement formed by the temporal horn choroid plexus and the adjacent tentorial margin may be misinterpreted as a rim-enhancing lesion.

Case 102A

23-year-old man presenting with reduced visual acuity.

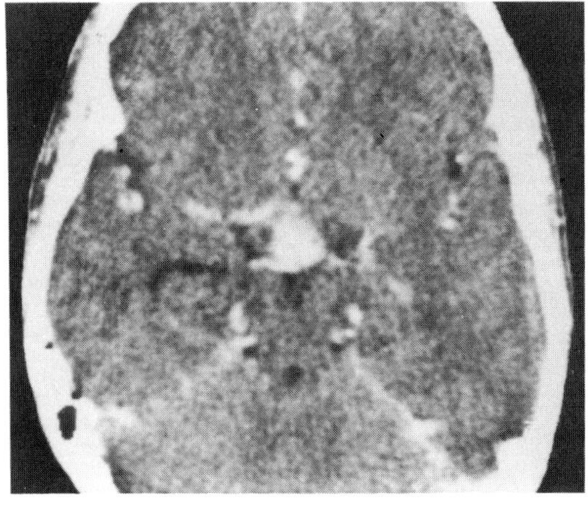

Germinomas are the most common tumors of the pineal region (see Case 117). They may also occur in a suprasellar location, where they have been called "ectopic pinealomas." (The term "atypical teratoma" is also used to refer to germinomas.) Most patients with suprasellar germinomas are teenagers or young adults presenting with diabetes insipidus or visual impairment.

Germinomas usually enhance uniformly and intensely, mimicking suprasellar pituitary adenoma, meningioma, or aneurysm. (Compare this scan with Cases 82 to 84.)

Case 102B

Same patient (coronal scan).

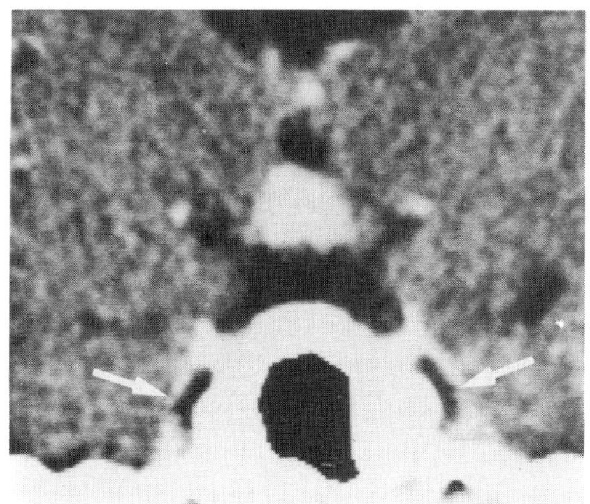

The coronal view clearly identifies the mass as a midline, suprasellar lesion, separated from the sella by uninvolved cistern. The inferior portion of the third ventricle is compressed by the tumor, while the region of the foramen of Monro is normal. (Compare with Case 114.)

Meckel's caves containing the trigeminal ganglia are seen as filling defects within the cavernous sinuses *(arrows)*.

DIFFERENTIAL DIAGNOSIS:
ENHANCING MASS WITH SUPRASELLAR AND INTRASELLAR COMPONENTS

Case 103

14-year-old girl with poor school performance due to hypothyroidism and markedly reduced visual acuity.

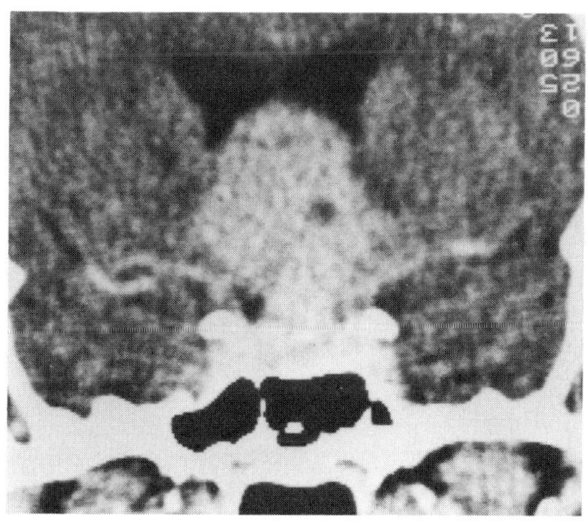

Germinoma.

Case 104

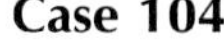

55-year-old man.

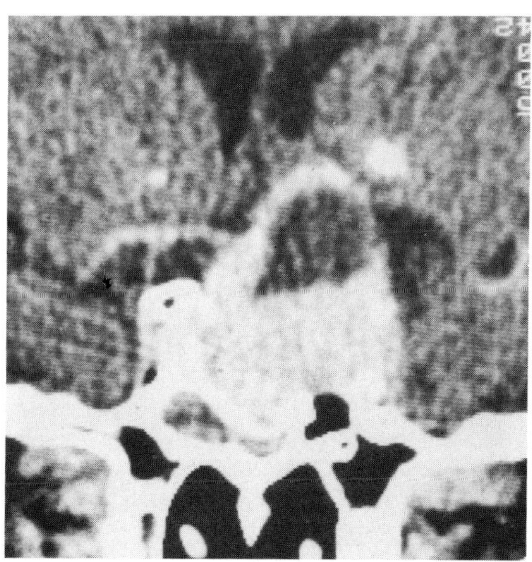

Pituitary Adenoma.

The distinction between a pituitary tumor with suprasellar extension and a suprasellar mass reaching into the sella may be difficult. In Case 104, the marked enlargement of the sella and the broad continuity between the intrasellar and suprasellar components favor a pituitary adenoma.

Although the enhancing suprasellar mass in Case 103 seems to merge with pituitary enhancement, there is a "waist" at the apparent junction. Furthermore, the center of the tumor bulk is suprasellar and the sella itself is not grossly expanded. (And the patient's age favors germinoma or hypothalamic glioma.) The same CT features usually allow the distinction between suprasellar meningiomas and pituitary adenomas.

The adenoma in Case 104 demonstrates eccentric parasellar and suprasellar growth and contains a large low-density region superiorly. An axial scan through the suprasellar component would appear as a parasagittal, rim-enhancing lesion resembling a thrombus-filled aneurysm.

The germinoma in Case 103 extends superiorly through the region of the third ventricle to deform the inferior portions of the lateral ventricular bodies. The internal cerebral veins were grossly elevated at angiography.

OPTIC CHIASM GLIOMAS

Case 105

3-year-old girl being evaluated for suspected "battered child syndrome." The child's mother was subsequently noted to have multiple cafe-au-lait spots.

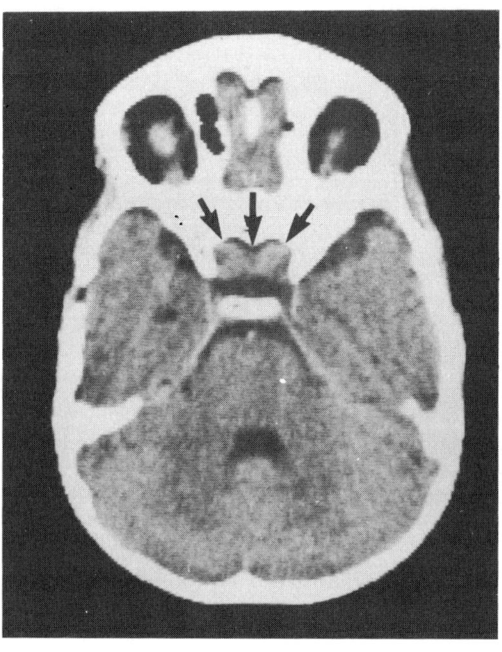

Optic gliomas are a common manifestation of neurofibromatosis, along with acoustic schwannomas (see Case 70), meningiomas (see Case 295), and increased incidence of glial tumors (see Case 349). The optic gliomas of neurofibromatosis are typically low-grade lesions that act more like hyperplasia than neoplasms. Contrast enhancement in this type of glioma may be minimal.

Erosion and enlargement of the chiasmatic sulcus at the entrance to the optic canals *(arrows)* is a hallmark of masses involving the chiasm and extending toward the optic nerves. This finding may be useful in distinguishing optic gliomas from other suprasellar lesions. Similarly, posterior extension of tumor into the optic tracts favors the diagnosis of chiasmatic glioma (see Case 110).

Case 106

5-year-old boy.

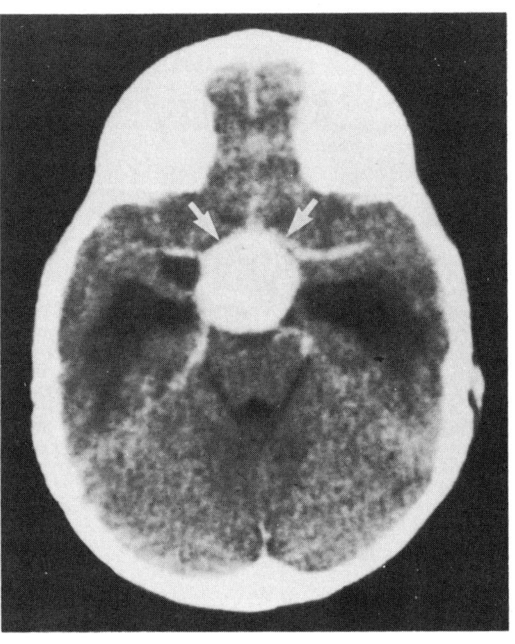

Gliomas of the optic chiasm in children without neurofibromatosis are more aggressive lesions. The tumors frequently demonstrate intense, uniform contrast enhancement, as in this case.

Here a midline mass fills the suprasellar cistern, the normal home of the optic chiasm. The A-1 segments of the anterior cerebral arteries are stretched across the anterosuperior surface of the tumor *(arrows)*. Greatly enlarged temporal horns indicate hydrocephalus due to compression of the third ventricle.

HYPOTHALAMIC GLIOMAS

Case 107

5-year-old boy with "gelastic" seizures (laughing spells). Coronal scan.

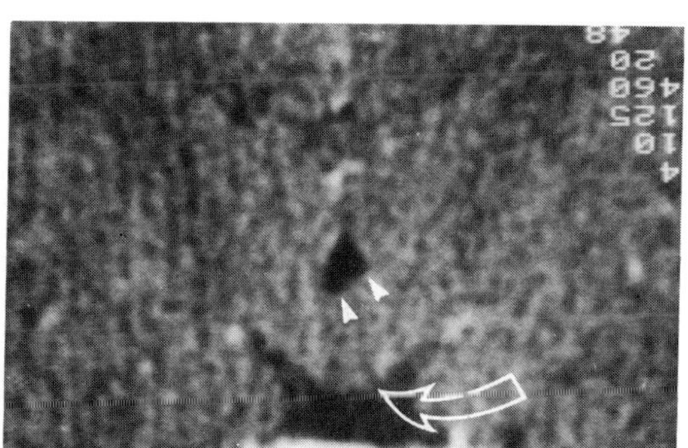

Hypothalamic gliomas rank with optic gliomas and craniopharyngiomas as the most common suprasellar masses in children. Some of these tumors are low-grade lesions demonstrating isodensity and minimal contrast enhancement. Their diagnosis depends on distortions of anatomy caused by displacements of the suprasellar cistern or the anterior third ventricle.

When axial scans are ambiguous in the suprasellar region, coronal scans may define a mass by simultaneously demonstrating its interfaces with cistern *(large arrow)* and ventricle *(small arrows),* as in this case.

A solid, noncalcified, nonenhancing craniopharyngioma is unusual in a child (see Case 96 for an example in an adult).

Case 108

5-year-old boy (different patient).

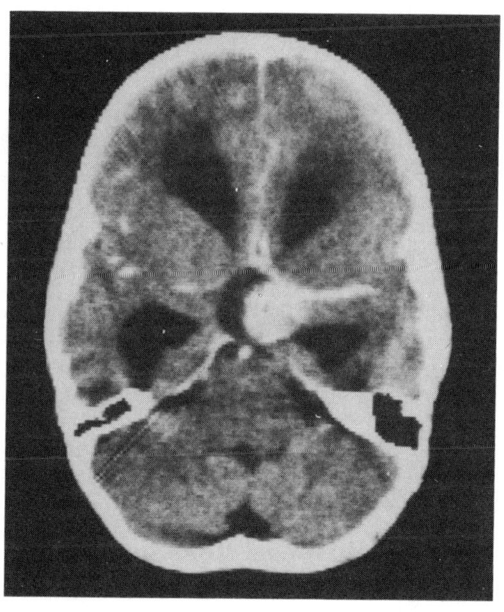

Hypothalamic gliomas may present as densely enhancing suprasellar masses. This appearance resembles that of optic chiasm gliomas, as seen in Case 106.

It may be difficult or impossible to distinguish between hypothalamic and chiasmatic gliomas on CT scans. Eccentric location (as in this case) suggests that the tumor arose along the wall of the third ventricle (i.e., hypothalamus), while erosion of the chiasmatic sulcus discussed in Case 105 would favor a mass originating in the chiasm.

Obstructive hydrocephalus is severe in this case, with transependymal CSF passage causing the appearance of edema around the frontal horns (see Cases 355 and 356).

DIFFERENTIAL DIAGNOSIS: CALCIFIED SUPRASELLAR MASS

Case 109

58-year-old woman.

Case 110

7-year-old girl.

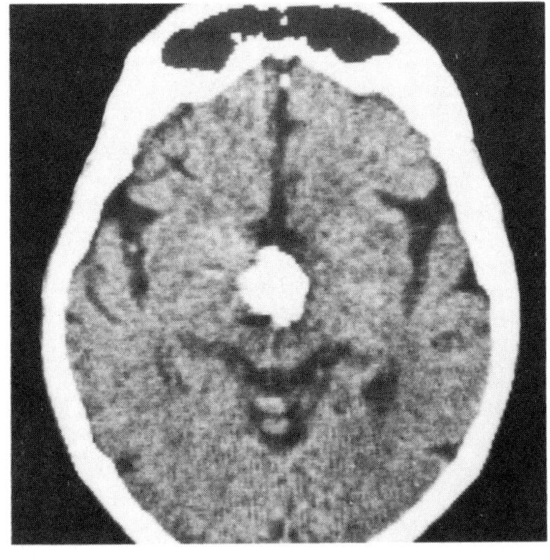

Craniopharyngioma (Noncontrast Scan).

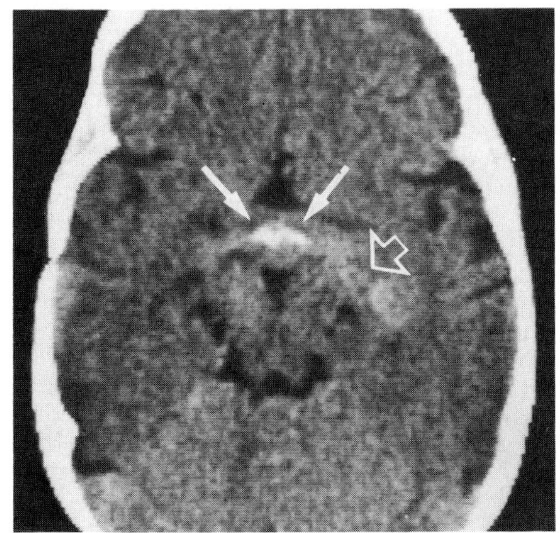

Optic Glioma (Noncontrast Scan).

Craniopharyngiomas are characterized by suprasellar calcification, which is occasionally dense and solid as in Case 109.

Many other suprasellar lesions may also contain calcium. The calcification of the optic glioma in Case 110 is most dense in the chiasm *(long arrows),* with faint calcification extending along the optic tracts *(open arrow).* Other suprasellar masses containing calcium include aneurysms, dermoid cysts (see Case 127), and occasional meningiomas.

PARASELLAR METASTASES

Case 111

56-year-old man. Metastatic prostate carcinoma arising from the anterior clinoid process.

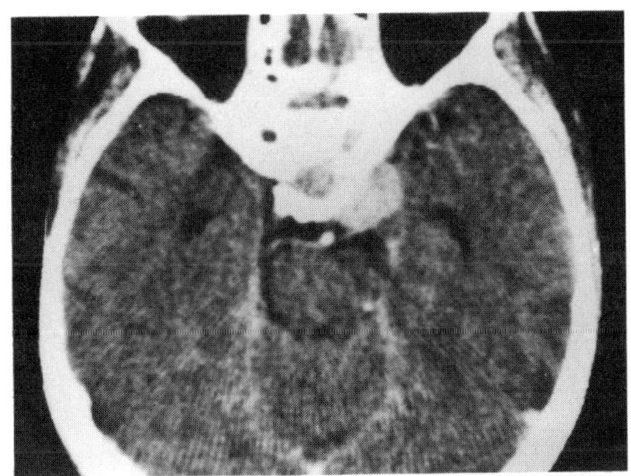

Several sellar and parasellar structures may be involved by metastatic disease. Metastases to the pituitary gland and infundibulum (e.g., breast carcinoma) may mimic the appearance of pituitary adenomas or other suprasellar masses. Metastatic involvement of the sphenoid bone may produce parasellar masses resembling benign lesions such as aneurysms or meningiomas.

In this case, mixed sclerosis and destruction of the anterior clinoid process was seen at wide window widths. Rapid tumor growth confirmed the diagnosis of metastatic disease (Case 31 presents a later scan of this lesion).

Case 112

67-year-old man. Systemic lymphoma involving the cavernous sinus.

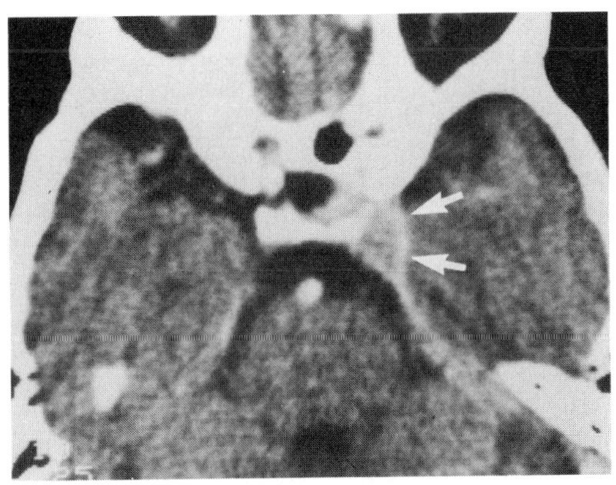

Metastatic involvement of the cavernous sinus may resemble other parasellar masses. An appearance similar to that in this case could be caused by a trigeminal schwannoma (see Case 133A), a carotid artery-cavernous sinus fistula, an aneurysm of the internal carotid artery, or parasellar inflammatory disease. Metastatic lymphoma frequently involves the meninges or ventricular surfaces (see Case 55).

REFERENCES

1. Banna M., Baker H.L., Houser O.W.: Pituitary and parapituitary tumours on computed tomography. *Br. J. Radiol.* 53:1123–1143, 1980.
2. Bonneville J.F., Cattin F., Moussa-Balha K., et al.: Dynamic computed tomography of the pituitary gland: The "tuft sign." *Radiology* 149:145–148, 1983.
3. Braun I.F., Pinto R.S., Epstein F.: Dense cystic craniopharyngiomas. *A.J.N.R.* 3:139–141, 1982.
4. Cabezudo J.M., Vaquero J., Garcia-de-Sola R., et al.: Computed tomography with craniopharyngiomas: A review. *Surg. Neurol.* 15:422–427, 1981.
5. Chambers E.F., Turski P.A., LaMasters D., et al.: Regions of low density in the contrast-enhanced pituitary gland: normal and pathological processes. *Radiology* 144:109–113, 1982.
6. Daniels D.L., Williams A.L., Thornton R.S., et al.: Differential diagnosis of intrasellar tumors by computed tomography. *Radiology* 141:697–701, 1981.
7. Diebler C., Ponsot G.: Hamartoma of the tuber cinereum. *Neuroradiology* 25:93–101, 1983.
8. Dietemann J.L., Bonneville J.F., Buchheit F., et al.: CT findings in symptomatic Rathke's cleft cysts of the pituitary gland. *Neuroradiology* 24:263–267, 1983.
9. Dominque J.N., Wing D.S., Wilson C.B.: Coexisting pituitary adenomas and partially empty sellas. *J. Neurosurg.* 48:23–28, 1978.
10. Fitz C.T., Wortzman G., Harwood-Nash D.C., et al.: Computed tomography in craniopharyngioma. *Radiology* 127:687–691, 1978.
    contrast enhancement. *Neuroradiology* 20:241–247, 1981.
11. Floyd J.L., Dorwart R.H., Nelson M.J., et al. Pituitary hyperplasia secondary to thyroid failure: CT appearance. *A.J.N.R.* 5:469–471, 1984.
12. Gardeur D., Naidich T.P., Metzer J.: CT analysis of intrasellar pituitary adenomas with emphasis on patterns of contrast enhancement. *Neuroradiology* 20:241–247, 1981.
13. Ghoshhajra K.: High resolution metrizamide CT cisternography in sellar and suprasellar abnormalities. *J. Neurosurg.* 54:232–239, 1981.
14. Hall K., McAllister V.L.: Metrizamide cisternography in pituitary and juxtapituitary lesions. *Radiology* 134:101–108, 1980.
15. Hatam A., Bergstom M., Greitz T.: Diagnosis of sellar and parasellar lesions by computed tomography. *Neuroradiology* 18:249–258, 1979.
16. Haughton V.M., Rosenbaum A.E., Williams A.L., Drayer B.P.: Recognizing the empty sella by CT: The infundibulum sign. *A.J.N.R.* 1:527–529, 1980.
17. Hemminghytt S., Kalkoff R.K., Daniels D.L., et al.: Computed tomographic study of hormone-secreting microadenomas. *Radiology* 146:65–69, 1983.
18. Kapila A., Chakeres D.W., Blanco E.: The Meckel cave: Computed tomographic study. *Radiology* 152:425–433, 1984.
19. Kline L.B., Acker J.D., Post J.D., et al.: The cavernous sinus: A computed tomographic study. *A.J.N.R.* 2:299–305, 1981.
20. Leeds N.E., Naidich T.P.: Computerized tomography in the diagnosis of sellar and parasellar lesions. *Semin. Roentgenol.* 12:121–135, 1977.
21. Lin S.R., Bryson M.M., Gobien R., et al.: Radiologic findings of hamartoma of the tuber cinereum and hypothalamus. *Radiology* 127:697–703, 1978.
22. Macpherson P., Anderson D.E.: Radiological differentiation of intrasellar aneurysms from pituitary tumors. *Neuroradiology* 21:177–183, 1981.
23. Numaguchi Y., Kishikawa T., Ikeda J., et al.: Neuroradiological manifestations of suprasellar pituitary adenomas, meningiomas, and craniopharyngiomas, *Neuroradiology* 21:67–72, 1981.
24. Peyster R.G., Hoover E.D.: CT of the abnormal pituitary stalk. *A.J.N.R.* 5:49–52, 1984.
25. Post M.J.D., David J.N., Glaser J.S., et al.: Pituitary apoplexy: Diagnosis by computed tomography. *Radiology* 134:665–670, 1980.
26. Roppolo H.M., Latchaw R.E., Meyer J.D., et al.: Normal pituitary gland: I. Macroscopic anatomy-CT correlation. *A.J.N.R.* 4:927–935, 1983.
27. Roppolo H.M., Latchaw R.E.: Normal pituitary gland: II. Microscopic anatomy-CT correlation. *A.J.N.R.* 4:937–944, 1983.
28. Sage M.R., Chan E.S., Reilly P.L.: The clinical and radiographic features of the empty sella syndrome. *Clin. Radiol.* 31:513–519, 1980.
29. Savoiardo M., Harwood-Nash D.C., Tadmor R., et al.: Gliomas of the intracranial anterior optic pathways in children. *Radiology* 138:601–610, 1981.
30. Steinberg G.K., Koenig G.H., Golden J.B.: Symptomatic Rathke's cleft cysts. *J. Neurosurg.* 56:290–295, 1982.
31. Swartz J.D., Russell K.B., Basile B.A., et al.: High resolution computed tomographic appearance of the intrasellar contents in women of childbearing age. *Radiology* 147:115–117, 1983.
32. Swenson S.A., Forbes G.S., Younge B.R., et al.: Radiologic evaluation of tumors of the optic nerve. *A.J.N.R.* 3:319–326, 1982.
33. Syvertsen A., Haughton V.M., Williams A.L., et al.: The computed tomographic appearance of the normal pituitary gland and pituitary microadenomas. *Radiology* 133:385–391, 1979.
34. Takeuchi J., Handa H., Otsuka S., et al.: Neuroradiological aspects of suprasellar germinoma. *Neuroradiology* 17:153–158, 1979.
35. Taylor S.: High resolution computed tomography of the sella. *Radiol. Clin. North. Am.* 20:207–236, 1982.
36. Tibbs P.A., Challa V., Mortara R.: Isolated histiocytosis X of the hypothalamus. *J. Neurosurg.* 49:929–934, 1978.
37. Wakai S., Fukushima T., Teramoto A., et al.: Pituitary apoplexy: Its incidence and clinical significance. *J. Neurosurg.* 55:187–193, 1981.
38. Wolpert S.M., Molitch M.E., Goldman J.A., et al.: Size, shape and appearance of the normal female pituitary gland. *A.J.N.R.* 5:263–267, 1984.

CHAPTER 6

OTHER MASSES

COLLOID CYSTS OF THE THIRD VENTRICLE

Case 113

55-year-old man with a history of unexplained falls while jogging (noncontrast scan).

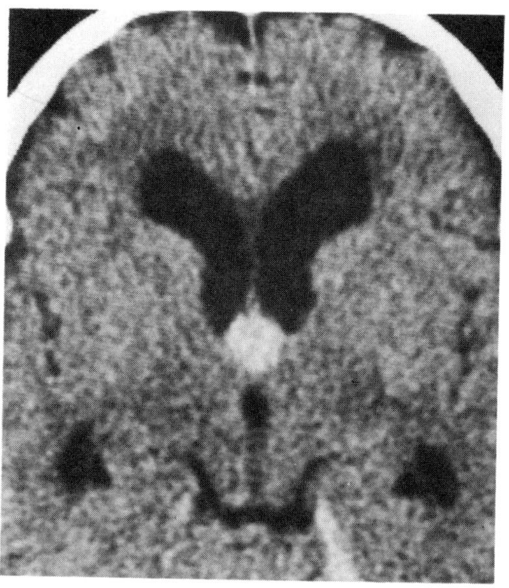

A well-defined, high-attenuation midline mass at the foramina of Monro is highly characteristic of a colloid cyst. This lesion typically arises from the anterior roof of the third ventricle. The mass usually demonstrates precontrast high attenuation due to dense protein content, which may be pathologically gelatinous or caseous.

Colloid cysts are occasionally isodense or even low-density lesions. Contrast enhancement is rare but can be seen both peripherally and centrally.

The paired columns of the fornix form a normal bulge along the anteromedial margin of the foramina of Monro and should not be confused with an isodense mass (see Cases 35, 121, 164, and 181).

Case 114

57-year-old man with episodic acute headache, nausea, and vomiting (coronal noncontrast scan).

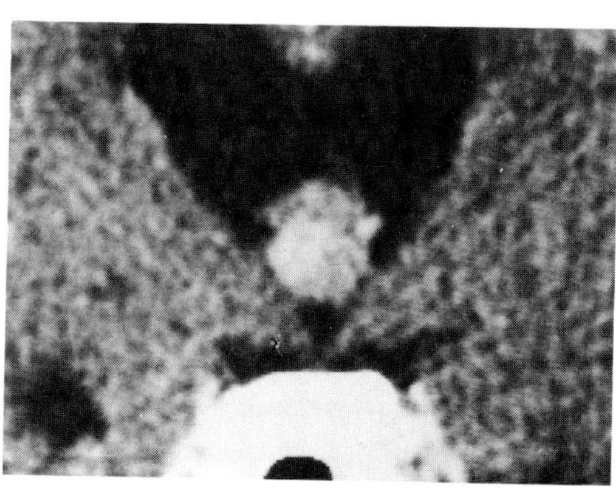

The strategic position of colloid cysts leads to hydrocephalus as the masses enlarge. Some patients experience episodic positional headaches, thought to be due to intermittent ventricular obstruction caused by shifts in position of mobile cysts. (However, similar histories are obtained from patients with large, apparently immobile lesions.)

Compare the superior third ventricular location of this colloid cyst with the more inferior location of germinomas and hypothalamic gliomas, as in Cases 102B and 107.

DIFFERENTIAL DIAGNOSIS: DENSE LESION NEAR THE FORAMEN OF MONRO

Case 115

58-year-old man.

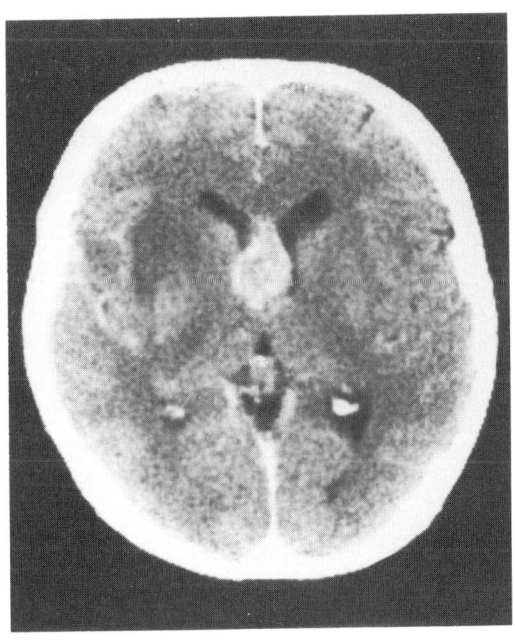

Glioblastoma Of The Septum Pellucidum (Postcontrast Scan).

Case 116

39-year-old woman.

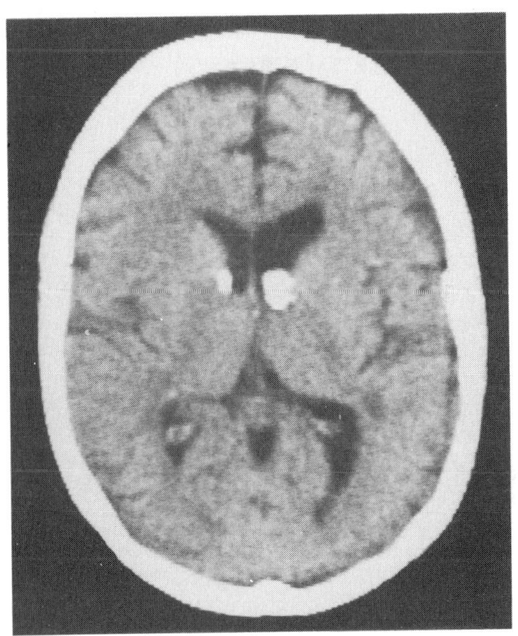

Tuberous Sclerosis (Noncontrast Scan).

Colloid cysts are among many dense or enhancing lesions that may occur near the foramen of Monro. Some masses project superiorly from the skull base to reach this level, e.g., suprasellar extension of pituitary adenomas, craniopharyngiomas, aneurysms, or dolichoectatic basilar arteries. Other lesions may arise within the third ventricle or frontal horns, e.g., intraventricular meningiomas, choroid plexus tumors or granulomas, or arteriovenous malformations involving the septal, thalamostriate, or internal cerebral veins.

Gliomas are commonly seen near the frontal horns and frequently invade the septum pellucidum, as in Case 115. Thickening of the septum suggests intra-axial origin of a deep frontal lesion. The finding is most common in gliomas but can also be seen with other pathologies (e.g., primary CNS lymphoma; see Case 136).

Tuberous sclerosis is discussed in Case 154. Calcified, subependymal tubers often occur lateral to the foramen of Monro, as in Case 116 (although their occurrence is frequently unilateral). Subependymal tubers may develop into giant cell astrocytomas, characterized on CT scans by an enlarging and enhancing mass (see Cases 156 and 157). The tumors may obstruct the foramen of Monro to cause unilateral or bilateral hydrocephalus, but they behave otherwise as low-grade neoplasms.

Case 117

22-year-old man presenting with headache, nausea, and vomiting (postcontrast scan).

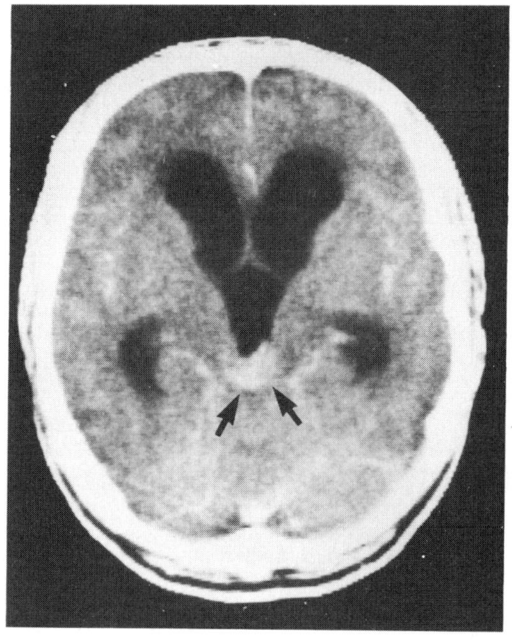

Germ cell tumors form the most common group of pineal masses. Within this category, germinomas are the most frequent pathology. (Other pineal germ cell tumors include teratoma, choriocarcinoma, embryonal cell carcinoma, and endodermal sinus tumor.) Pineal germinomas are common in boys but relatively rare in girls, who more often have suprasellar versions of this tumor (see Case 103).

Germinomas (sometimes called "atypical teratomas") usually demonstrate homogeneous high attenuation on precontrast scans and uniform, intense enhancement following contrast injection.

Case 118

14-year-old girl with headache and poor school performance (postcontrast scan).

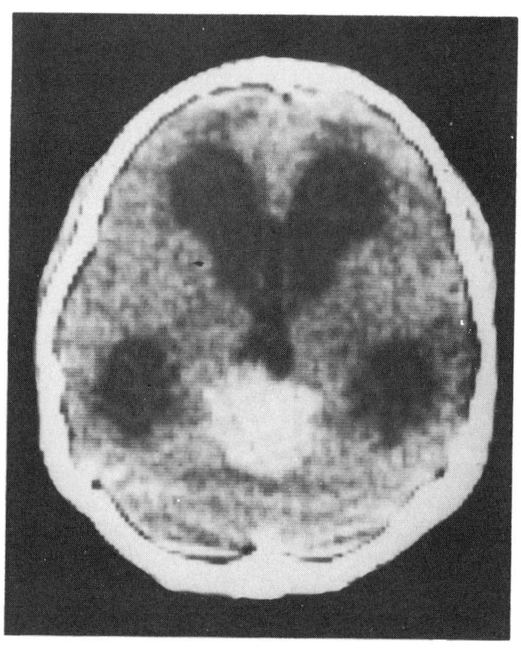

The characteristic homogeneous enhancement of pineal germinomas may be mimicked by meningiomas of the quadrigeminal plate (see Case 295) or "aneurysms" of the vein of Galen (see Case 296). Hydrocephalus is often present due to obstruction of the posterior third ventricle and proximal aqueduct.

Germinomas are usually radiosensitive. The mass in this case disappeared with radiation therapy and has not reappeared in six years of follow-up.

OTHER PINEAL REGION TUMORS

Case 119

38-year-old man with nystagmus and Parinaud's syndrome. Dermoid cyst.

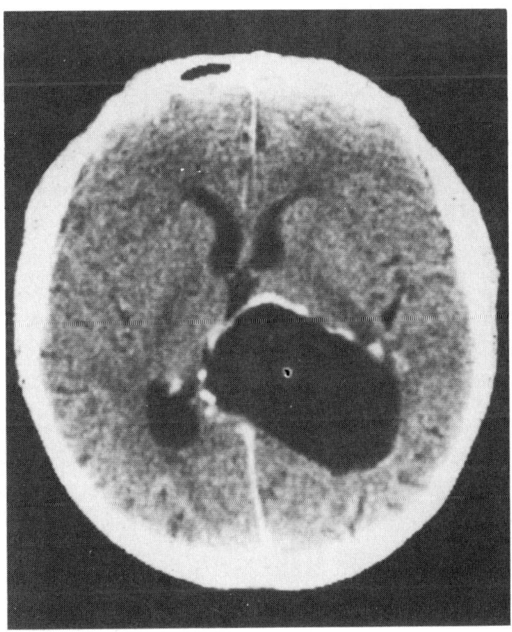

Dermoid cysts and teratomas may contain a mixture of fat and protein with an average attenuation value resembling spinal fluid (see Case 125). Rim calcification may surround a low-density center in both of these lesions (see Cases 98, 125, and 127). Teratomas often contain additional densely calcified or ossified elements within the substance of the tumor.

Epidermoid cysts present a similar low-attenuation appearance but are less frequently calcified (see Case 367). Small lipomas commonly occur in the quadrigeminal cistern, but have very low-density values indicating homogeneous fat content (see Case 377).

Case 120

23-year-old woman. Astrocytoma of the thalamus and brain stem.

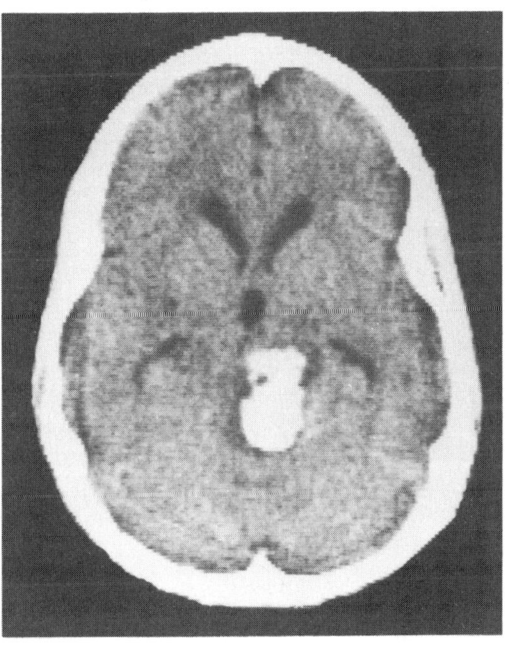

In addition to germ cell lesions, pineal region masses may be glial tumors or tumors of true pineal cell origin (pineoblastoma and pineocytoma; see Case 121).

In this case, a densely calcified astrocytoma obliterates the posterior third ventricle like a pineal neoplasm. However, the mass is eccentric and appears to involve the midbrain and thalamus. These features suggest an intra-axial glioma, which was confirmed at biopsy.

DIFFERENTIAL DIAGNOSIS: INTENSELY ENHANCING MASS IN THE PINEAL REGION

Case 121

17-year-old boy with behavioral change.

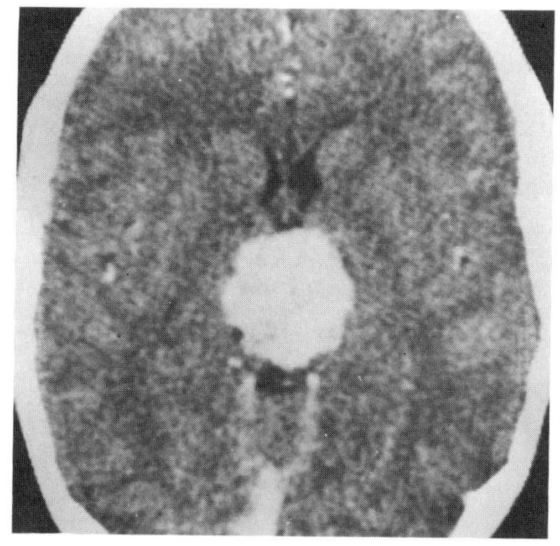

Pineocytoma.

Case 122

17-year-old girl with headache and paresis of upward gaze.

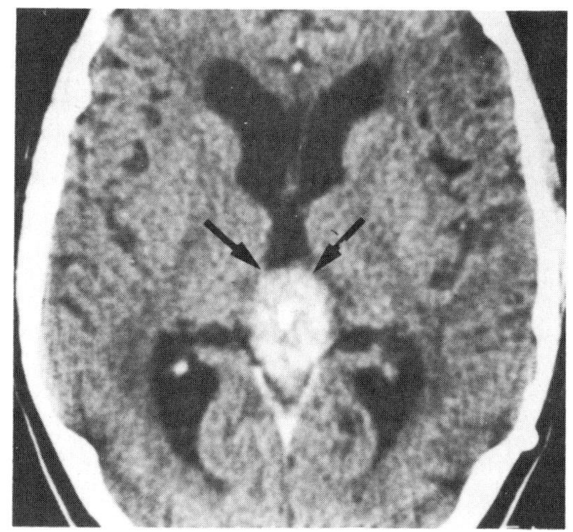

Brain Stem Astrocytoma.

The most common pineal tumors with this appearance are germinomas (see Cases 117 and 118). The rare pineocytoma in Case 121 has grown anteriorly to occupy the third ventricle, in contrast to the usual enlargement of pineal masses within the quadrigeminal cistern. Hydrocephalus is, remarkably, absent.

Gliomas of the brain stem or thalamus may extend into the pineal region to mimic a primary pineal tumor (see Case 120). In Case 122, the midline mass has displaced the pineal superiorly while obstructing the posterior third ventricle *(arrows)*. More caudal sections demonstrated the mass arising within the midbrain and extending exophytically into the quadrigeminal cistern.

Other lesions in this diagnostic group include subsplenial meningiomas and the so-called vein of Galen aneurysm (see Cases 295 and 296).

CHOROID PLEXUS PAPILLOMAS

Case 123

11-month-old boy with an enlarging head (postcontrast scan).

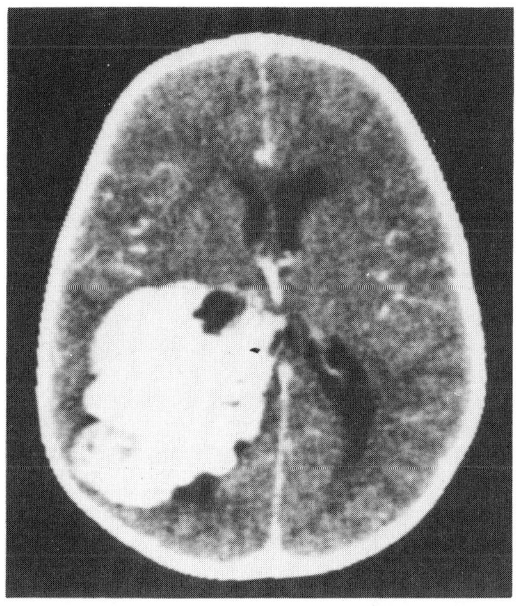

Choroid plexus papillomas are among the intracranial tumors that may be present at birth. (Others include medulloblastoma, craniopharyngioma, ependymoma, astrocytoma, and teratoma.) They are often associated with hydrocephalus, sometimes due to excessive production of spinal fluid. More commonly, a secondary communicating hydrocephalus develops from repeated tumor hemorrhages with high cerebrospinal fluid loads of protein and cells.

Choroid plexus papillomas in children are most common in the lateral ventricles, particularly on the left. They usually arise from the trigone and are often massive when discovered.

Most choroid plexus papillomas demonstrate uniform, mildly increased density on noncontrast scans. Intense, homogeneous contrast enhancement is common. These features may mimic primitive neuroectodermal tumors or intraventricular meningiomas (see Case 52), but the latter are rare in infancy and childhood.

Case 124

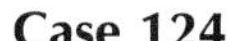

68-year-old woman.

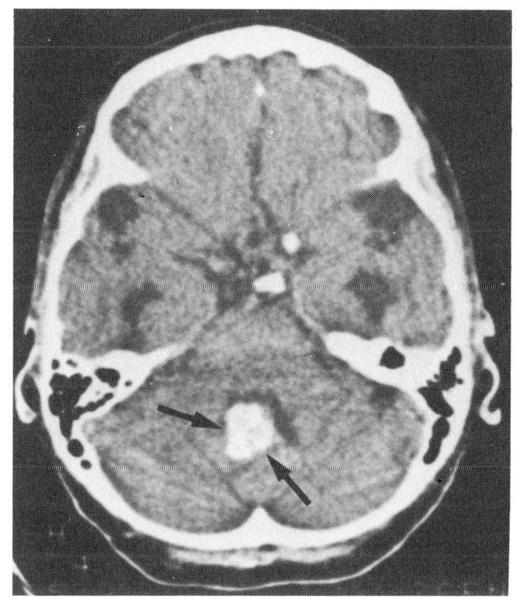

In adults, choroid plexus papillomas occur most commonly in the fourth ventricle. This location can suggest the diagnosis, with the differential diagnosis including hemangioblastoma, ependymoma, vermian metastasis, unusual glioma, and arteriovenous malformation (see also Case 62).

A lateral ventricular tumor in an adult is unlikely to be a choroid plexus papilloma and should suggest meningioma, metastasis, ependymoma, AVM, or an inflammatory lesion (e.g., granuloma, parasitic or fungal mass).

Choroid plexus tumors occasionally contain or degenerate into carcinomas.

DERMOID CYSTS

Case 125

61-year-old woman with a history of seizures since age 19 years.

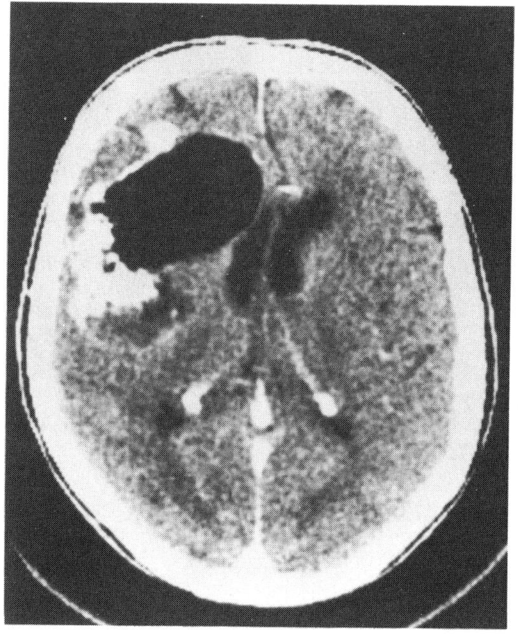

Case 126

68-year-old man with subtotal resection of a parasellar dermoid cyst 15 years before admission.

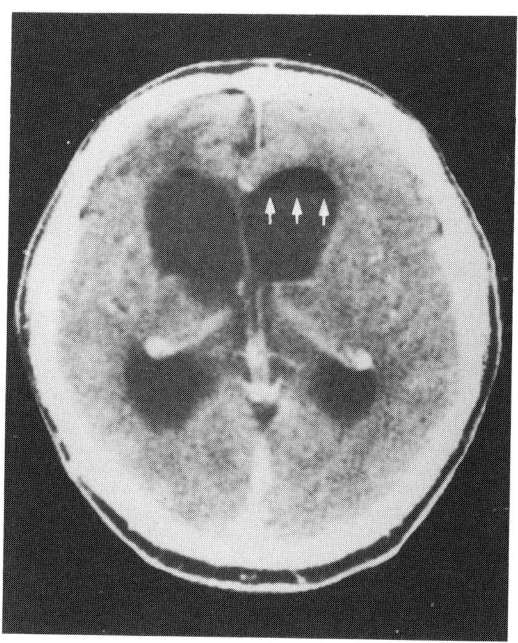

Dermoid tumors or "cysts" are benign masses arising from epithelial cells enclosed intracranially during embryogenesis. In addition to squamous epithelium, dermoid cysts contain mesodermal cells, which may form skin appendages such as hair follicles, sweat glands, and sebaceous glands. Slow proliferation of these tissues leads to gradual accumulation of a pilosebaceous mass, causing the congenital lesions to appear in adulthood.

The CT appearance of dermoid cysts is usually a characteristic combination of central fat and dense peripheral calcification. Some regions of the mass may have intermediate attenuation values (as seen posteriorly in this case) due to the presence of hair or other proteinaceous material. Contrast enhancement is rare.

The mass in this case arose from the parasellar region, with large lobulations occupying the anterior and middle cranial fossae.

Dermoid cysts may rupture into the ventricular system, causing a characteristic appearance of floating fat. The free fat may be seen as tiny black droplets or as fat-fluid levels crossing ventricular chambers *(arrows)*. Fat-fluid levels may also be seen with leaking epidermoid cysts and teratomas. In this case, the recurrent right parasellar dermoid cyst has ruptured into the adjacent frontal horn. Associated hydrocephalus is present with obstruction at the aqueductal level.

Intraventricular rupture or leakage of fatty material is often clinically silent. However, some patients experience a severe chemical meningitis, particularly when the contents of a ruptured cyst extend beyond the ventricles to involve the subarachnoid spaces.

DIFFERENTIAL DIAGNOSIS: SUPRASELLAR MASS WITH CALCIFICATION AND LOW ATTENUATION

Case 127

60-year-old man.

Case 128

6-year-old girl.

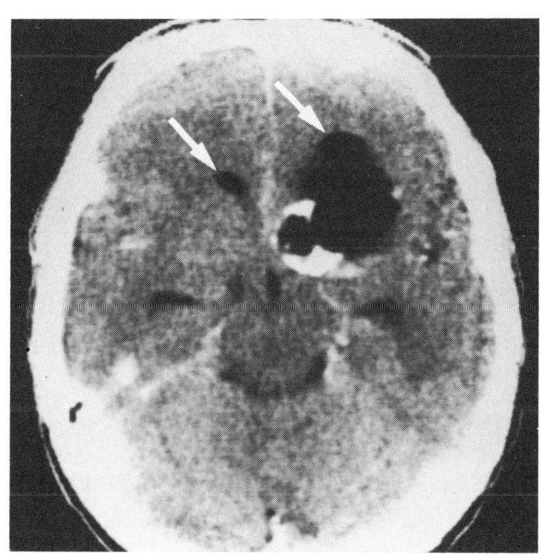

Dermoid Cyst.

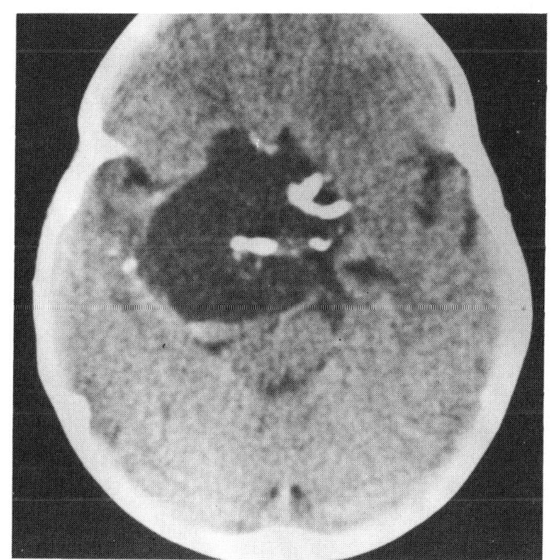

Craniopharyngioma.

Many dermoid cysts are found in the parasellar or suprasellar regions (see also Case 98). Another common location is in the midline of the posterior fossa, either within the fourth ventricle or between the cerebellar hemispheres.

The heavy calcification and low density of a parasellar dermoid cyst may resemble a craniopharyngioma, as in Case 128. However, the extreme low attenuation of fat within dermoid cysts usually distinguishes these lesions from the fluid and debris within craniopharyngiomas. Craniopharyngiomas often contain cholesterol, but the cyst content rarely matches the homogeneous fatty nature of a dermoid cyst.

The tumor in Case 127 has ruptured into the ventricular system, with fat droplets floating in the frontal horns *(arrows)*.

Hypothalamic gliomas may also present with low attenuation (cystic or solid; see Case 349) and calcification, resembling these other suprasellar lesions.

EPIDERMOID CYSTS

Case 129

50-year-old woman with tic douloureux
and facial nerve paresis.

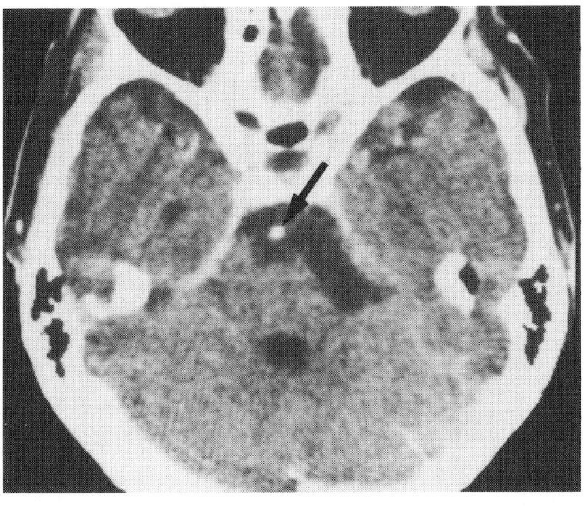

Epidermoid cysts are usually low-attenuation, nonenhancing, extra-axial lesions. The density of the masses represents the average of mixed cholesterol and keratin components. Occasional high-attenuation epidermoids are seen, probably reflecting a preponderance of dense keratin over low-attenuation cholesterol.

The low density of most epidermoids may resemble subarachnoid cysts or cisterns (see Cases 367 through 370). In this case, the expansion of peripontine cisterns could be mistaken for widened CSF spaces due to brain stem displacement by an extra-axial mass. (Compare with Cases 69 and 74). Narrow window width displays and histogram analysis will usually show an epidermoid cyst to be less homogeneous than a true cyst.

Epidermoid cysts are often soft, extensively infiltrating lesions that surround vessels and cranial nerves. Here, a portion of the tumor has insinuated itself between the basilar artery *(arrow)* and the pons.

Case 130

52-year-old man with a three-year history of memory
loss culminating in arrest for shoplifting
(scan after metrizamide administration).

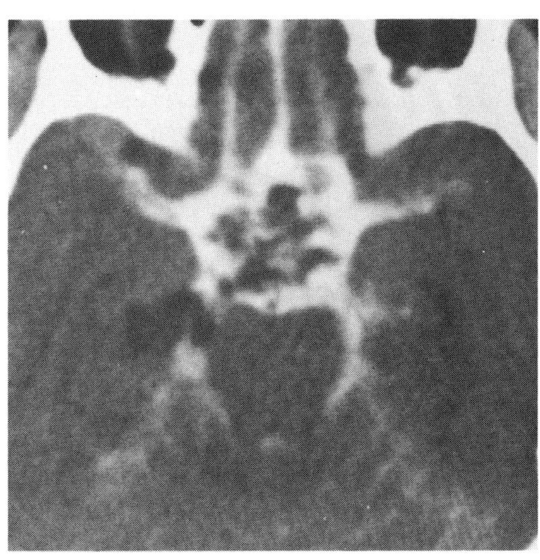

The surface of epidermoid cysts is typically papillary or frondlike, resembling a cauliflower. This characteristic irregularity cannot be appreciated when the tumor is surrounded by CSF of similar density.

The addition of subarachnoid contrast material outlines the tumor interstices and provides the diagnosis. This technique is useful for distinguishing epidermoid cysts from arachnoid cysts when a low-density extra-axial lesion is encountered.

In this case, a routine scan had demonstrated a low-attenuation suprasellar mass splaying the cerebral penduncles and compressing the medial temporal lobes (see Case 369). The metrizamide study outlines the typical irregular surface of an epidermoid cyst.

Normal gyral anatomy is also well demonstrated on such scans. Here the gyrus rectus of the inferior frontal lobe is outlined anterior to the suprasellar cistern. Distortions of the adjacent sulci may be a secondary finding associated with CSF rhinorrhea from the cribriform region (see Case 224).

DIFFERENTIAL DIAGNOSIS: LOW-ATTENUATION, EXTRA-AXIAL LESION IN THE CEREBELLOPONTINE ANGLE

Case 131

74-year-old man.

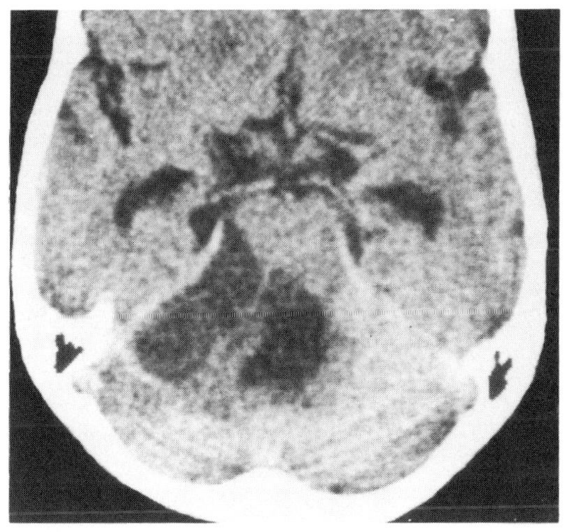

Acoustic Schwannoma (Noncontrast Scan).

Case 132

40-year-old man.

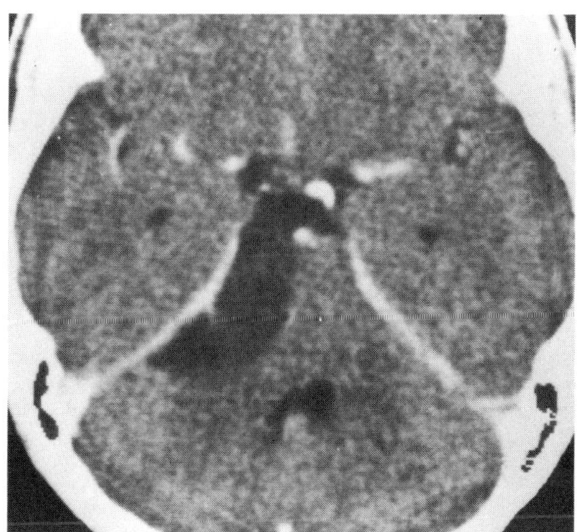

Epidermoid Cyst (Postcontrast Scan).

Several low-attenuation lesions may occupy the cerebellopontine angle. Some acoustic schwannomas contain low-density components, either solid or cystic. Only minimal contrast enhancement occurred in Case 131. (Case 71 presents a postcontrast scan of this patient.)

The cerebellopontine angle is a common location for epidermoid cysts, such as in Case 132.

Arachnoid cysts may also be found at this site and should be included in the differential diagnosis (see Case 363).

Case 133A

48-year-old man presenting with diminished facial sensation and ipsilateral masseter atrophy.

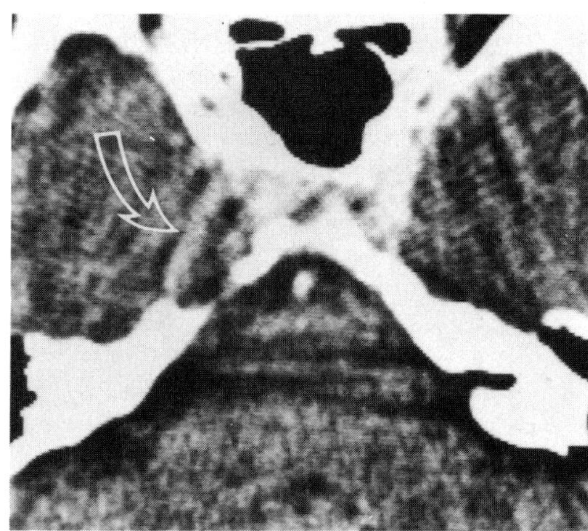

Case 133B

Same patient (coronal view).

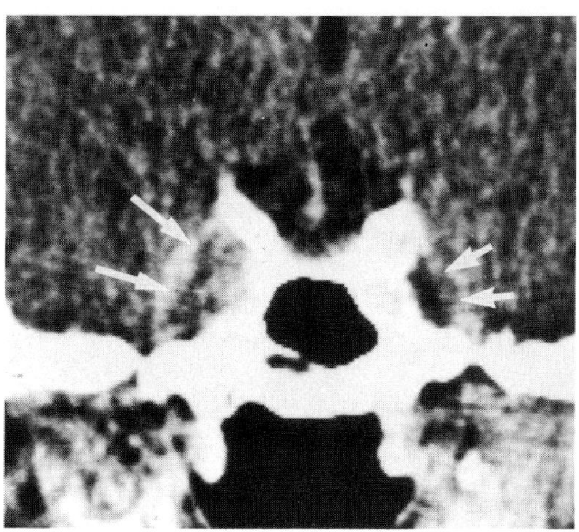

Trigeminal schwannomas commonly arise near the gasserian ganglion. The ganglion is located within the posterior portion of the cavernous sinus, occupying a shallow depression on the anterosuperior surface of the petrous apex (see Cases 88 and 102B).

Small trigeminal schwannomas appear as filling defects expanding the cavernous sinus, as in this case. Larger tumors may demonstrate contrast enhancement and acquire a "dumbbell" shape with parasellar and posterior fossa components (see Case 134).

Trigeminal schwannomas are among the lesions to be sought in patients with tic douloureux. A more classic finding in such cases is looping of a vessel (e.g., vertebral or basilar artery) near the "entry zone" of the fifth cranial nerve as it joins the pons (see Case 279). In most cases of trigeminal neuralgia the CT scan is unremarkable.

Coronal scans are useful for demonstrating the asymmetry between normal *(short arrows)* and enlarged *(long arrows)* trigeminal ganglia. The coronal plane also defines extracranial extension of large trigeminal neuromas through the floor of the middle cranial fossa near the foramen ovale.

Other processes that can expand the cavernous sinus include pituitary adenomas, internal carotid artery aneurysms, carotid-cavernous fistulas, parasellar metastases, and parasellar meningiomas (see Cases 111, 112, 315 and 316).

DIFFERENTIAL DIAGNOSIS: ENHANCING MASS SPANNING THE PETROUS APEX

Case 134

15-year-old girl.

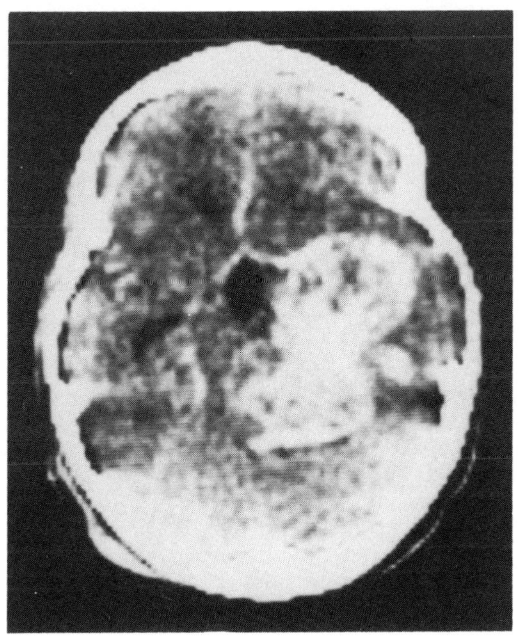

Trigeminal Schwannoma.

Case 135

50-year-old man.

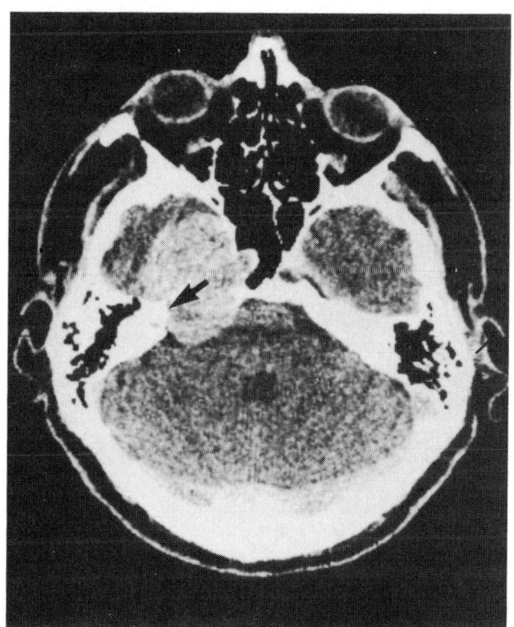

Meningioma.

Large trigeminal schwannomas may expand from the petrous apex to involve both the middle and posterior cranial fossae. A tumor extending from the trigeminal ganglion into the middle fossa is extradural, while a tumor extending along the trigeminal nerve into the posterior fossa is intradural. The combined "dumbbell" configuration demonstrates a "waist" where the tumor passes through the tentorial hiatus. Contrast enhancement of large neuromas is often inhomogeneous or patchy, resembling the typical stain at angiography.

Meningiomas may extend through the tentorial hiatus from origins in either the parasellar region or the cerebellopontine angle. Case 135 illustrates the former mechanism, with homogeneously enhancing tumor eroding the petrous bone *(arrow)* to enter the posterior fossa. Transtentorial meningiomas originating from the posterior fossa often demonstrate a "comma" shape (see Case 19).

Epidermoid cysts may also span the petrous apex with a bilobed configuration, but they are usually low-attenuation lesions with little contrast enhancement.

Case 136

59-year-old woman presenting with dementia and facial weakness.

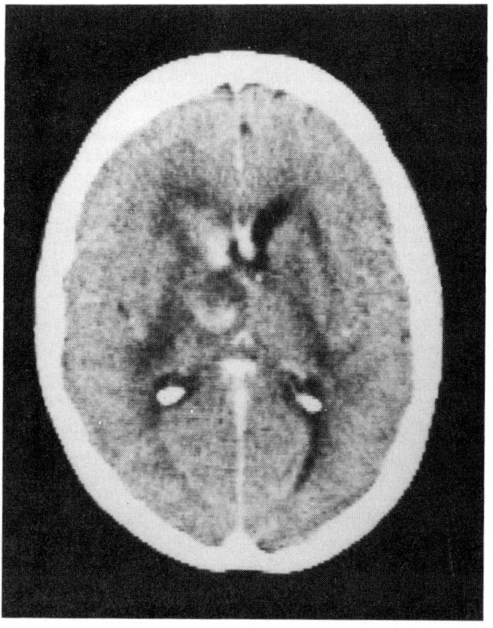

Primary CNS lymphomas ("reticulum cell sarcoma," "microglioma," "immunoblastic lymphoma") usually present as one or more deep hemisphere masses. Frequent areas of involvement include the basal ganglia, corpus callosum, cerebellar vermis, and paraventricular white matter. The tumor in this case infiltrates the septum pellucidum (compare to Cases 41 and 115).

On precontrast scans the lesions are often isodense but may show decreased or increased attenuation. Contrast enhancement may be solid or peripheral. CT findings often regress in response to steroid therapy and may wax and wane spontaneously.

Clues to the diagnosis include multicentric involvement of deep hemisphere structures, steroid response, and a clinical association with immunosuppression (see Case 138).

Case 137

58-year-old man presenting with hemiparesis.

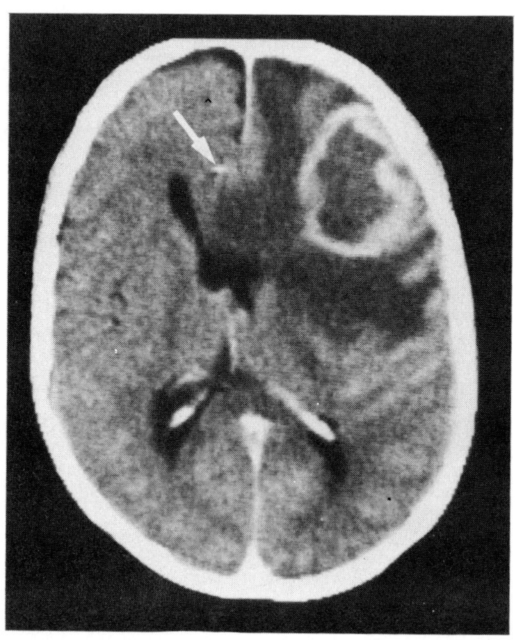

Primary CNS lymphomas can assume a variety of appearances and may mimic other pathologies. This large, rim-enhancing, solitary lesion closely resembles a glioblastoma. Lobar location of primary CNS lymphoma is probably not as unusual as originally believed.

Primary lymphoma of the CNS is more common than parenchymal involvement by systemic lymphoma, which more typically infiltrates the meninges.

This case is a good example of subfalcial herniation. The edematous frontal lobe passes beneath the falx and deforms the frontal horns. The pericallosal arteries are markedly displaced *(arrows).*

DIFFERENTIAL DIAGNOSIS: MULTIPLE ENHANCING CEREBRAL AND CEREBELLAR NODULES

Case 138

32-year-old woman with a renal transplant.

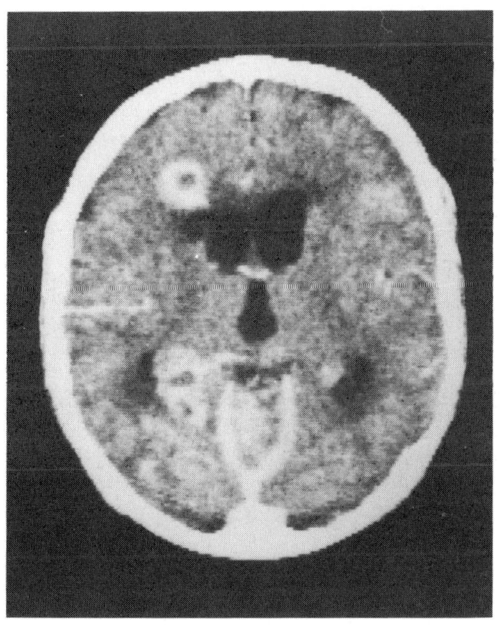

Primary CNS Lymphoma.

Case 139

53-year-old woman from Southeast Asia with fever and pulmonary infiltrates.

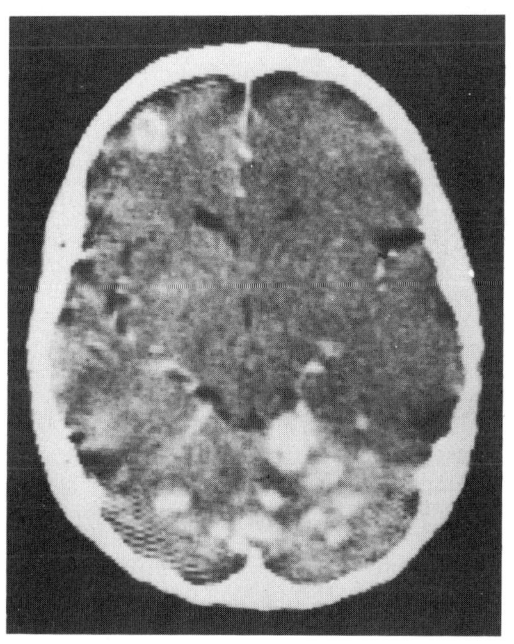

Metastatic Adenocarcinoma.

Multiple, focal-enhancing lesions may be inflammatory (e.g., multiple sclerosis, disseminated infection, neurosarcoidosis), vascular (e.g., multifocal infarctions, hemangiomas), or neoplastic (see Cases 4, 172, 173, and 236). In the latter category, metastases and primary CNS lymphomas are the leading possibilities.

Primary CNS lymphomas are rare in otherwise healthy individuals. They are much more common in patients who are immunosuppressed due to disease (e.g., lymphoma) or medication (e.g., transplant regimens).

Infection was a primary consideration in Case 139, but the pulmonary and cerebral lesions proved to represent adenocarcinoma. The CT scan had been performed because of an acute cerebrovascular accident, and the left hemisphere shows slightly decreased attenuation with a conspicuous lack of enhancing metastases.

Case 140

24-year-old man. Clivus chordoma (wide window width).

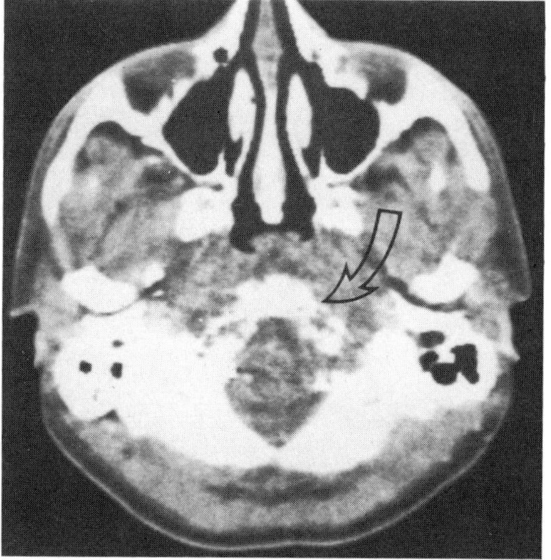

Case 141

24-year-old woman. Parasellar chordoma (wide window width).

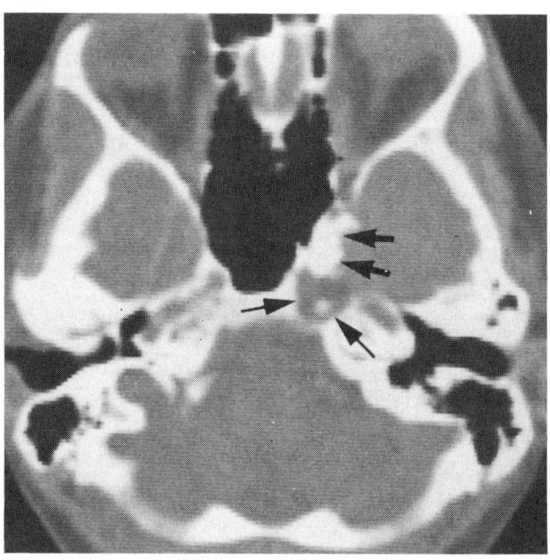

Chordomas arise from remnants of the primitive notochord and most frequently involve the clivus or sacrum. Clivus chordomas may appear as calcified masses projecting intracranially from an intact skull base. Such tumors may mimic a clivus meningioma (see Case 320).

Other chordomas have a more destructive appearance, as illustrated by the permeation in this case. Large soft-tissue components may expand intracranially or into the nasopharynx.

Chordomas may also originate in the parasellar region, appearing as a calcified mass that mimics parasellar meningioma or aneurysm (see Cases 315 and 316). In this case, an area of bone destruction at the petrous apex *(thin arrows)* is associated with dense calcification more anteriorly *(thick arrows)*.

Chondromas are rare tumors of the skull base. Their appearance on CT scans (and skull roentgenograms) may closely resemble that of chordoma, with a mixture of lytic and calcified components.

Case 142

14-year-old girl. Uremic encephalopathy.

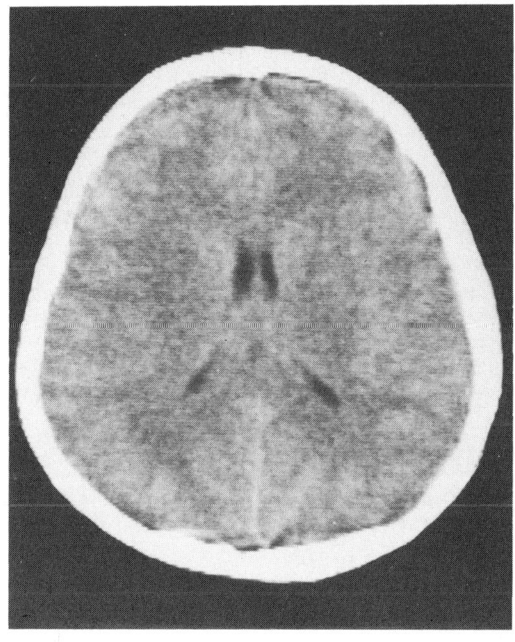

Several categories of diffuse encephalopathy may present with increased intracranial pressure mimicking a mass lesion. In these cases, scans may show cerebral swelling with compression of ventricles and sulci.

The differential diagnosis for diffusely swollen hemispheres includes metabolic encephalopathy (e.g., uremia, Reye's syndrome), hypertensive encephalopathy, pseudotumor cerebri, and superior sagittal sinus thrombosis. Head trauma, anoxia, and encephalitis may present a similar appearance but are usually evident clinically (see Cases 219, 271, 273, and 274).

The ventricles may normally be quite small in young patients (especially women), and compression may be difficult to judge. In this case, the ventricles are small enough to suggest cerebral swelling. They returned to a normal size following resolution of the patient's uremia.

Case 143

35-year-old woman with headaches and papilledema. Pseudotumor cerebri.

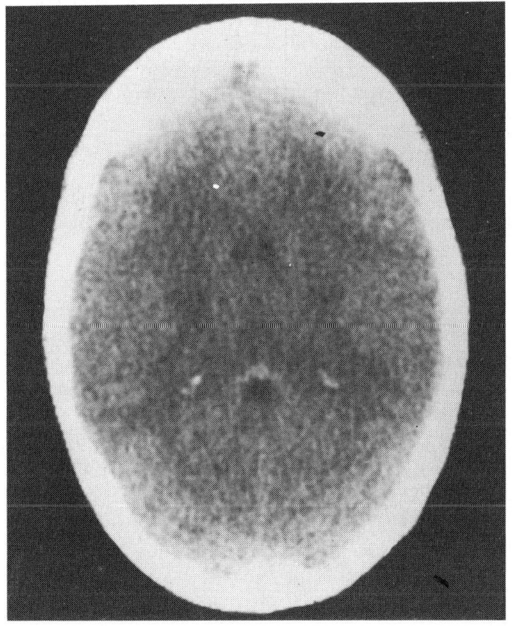

The syndrome of "benign intracranial hypertension" or "pseudotumor cerebri" may be considered in young patients (especially overweight women) with papilledema and symptoms of elevated intracranial pressure. Apart from a few specific associations, (e.g., hypervitaminosis A, tetracycline toxic reaction), the cause of the syndrome is undefined and controversial. It is characterized by the typical clinical picture in the absence of specific intracranial pathology.

In such patients, CT serves the primary purpose of excluding a mass lesion or hydrocephalus. The secondary finding of small ventricles suggesting cerebral swelling is seen in a minority of patients.

REFERENCES

1. Cecchini A., Pezzotta S., Paoletti P., et al.: Dense dermoids in craniovertebral region. *J. Comput. Assist. Tomogr.* 7:479–483, 1983.
2. Chakeres D.W., LaMasters D.L.: Paragangliomas of the temporal bone: High-resolution CT studies. *Radiology* 150:749–753, 1984.
3. Chambers E.F., Turski P.A., Sobel D., et al.: Radiologic characteristics of primary cerebral neuroblastoma. *Radiology* 139:101–104, 1981.
4. Futrell N.N., Osborn A.G., Cheson B.D.: Pineal region tumors: Computed tomographic-pathologic spectrum. *A.J.N.R.* 2:415–420, 1981.
5. Ganti S.R., Antures J.L., Louis K.M., et al.: Computed tomography in the diagnosis of colloid cysts of the third ventricle. *Radiology* 138:385–391, 1981.
6. Gardeur D., Palmieri A., Mashaly R.: Cranial computed tomography in the phakomatoses. *Neuroradiology* 25:293–304, 1983.
7. Giannotta S.L., Hopkins J., Kindt G.W.: CT in Reye syndrome. *Neurosurgery* 2:201–204, 1978.
8. Goldberg R., Byrd S., Winter J., et al.: Varied appearance of trigeminal neuroma on CT. *A.J.R.* 134:57–60, 1980.
9. Hildenbrand P.G., Gabrielsen T.O., Dorouini-Zis K., et al.: Radiology of primary intracranial yolk-sac (endodermal sinus) tumors. *A.J.N.R.* 4:991–993, 1983.
10. Hinshaw D.B., Ashwal S., Thompson J.R., et al.: Neuroradiology of primitive neuroectodermal tumors. *Neuroradiology* 25:87–92, 1983.
11. Holtas S., Nyman V., Cronqvist S.: Computed tomography of malignant lymphoma of the brain. *Neuroradiology* 26:33–38, 1984.
12. Jooma R., Kendall B.E.: Diagnosis and management of pineal tumors. *J. Neurosurg.* 58:654–665, 1983.
13. Kaye A.H., Hahn J.F., Kinney S.E., et al.: Jugular foramen schwannomas. *J. Neurosurg.* 60:1045–1053, 1984.
14. Kazner E., Stochdorph O., Wende S., et al.: Intracranial lipoma: Diagnostic and therapeutic considerations. *J. Neurosurg.* 52:234–245, 1980.
15. Kendall B., Reider-Grosswasser I., Valentine A.: Diagnosis of masses presenting within the ventricles on computed tomography. *Neuroradiology* 25:11–22, 1983.
16. Krol G., Sundaresan H., Deck M.: Computed tomography of axial chordomas. *J. Comput. Assist. Tomogr.* 7:286–289, 1983.
17. Laster D.W., Moody D.M., Ball M.R.: Epidermoid tumors with intraventricular and subarachnoid fat. *A.J.R.* 128:504–507, 1977.
18. Latchaw R.E., L'heureux P.R., Young G., et al.: Neuroblastoma presenting as central nervous system disease. *A.J.N.R.* 3:623–630, 1982.
19. Lo W.M., Solti-Bohman L.G., Lambert P.R.: High resolution CT in the evaluation of glomus tumors of the temporal bone. *Radiology* 150:737–742, 1984.
20. Lukin R., Tomsick T.A., Chambers A.A.: Lymphoma and leukemia of the central nervous system. *Semin. Roentgenol.* 15:246, 1980.
21. Mendenhall N.P., Thar T.L., Agee O.F., et al.: Primary lymphoma of the central nervous system: Computerized tomography scan characteristics and treatment results for 12 cases. *Cancer* 52:1993–2000, 1983.
22. Neuwelt E.A., Glasberg M., Frenkel E., et al.: Malignant pineal region tumors: A clinico-pathological study. *J. Neurosurg.* 51:597–607, 1979.
23. Palacios E., Gorelick P.B., Gonzalez C.F., et al.: Malignant lymphoma of the nervous system. *J. Comput. Assist. Tomogr.* 6:689–701, 1982.
24. Silver A.J., Ganti S.R., Hilal S.K.: Computed tomography of tumors involving the atria of the lateral ventricles. *Radiology* 145:71–78, 1982.
25. Sklar F.H., Beyer C.W., Ramanathan M., et al.: Cerebrospinal fluid dynamics in patients with pseudotumor cerebri. *Neurosurgery* 5:208–216, 1979.
26. Tubman D.E., Frick M.P., Hanto D.W.: Lymphoma after organ transplantation; Radiologic manifestation in the central nervous system, thorax, and abdomen. *Radiology* 149:625–631, 1983.
27. Weingarten K.L., Zimmerman R.D., Leeds N.E.: Spontaneous regression of intracerebral lymphoma. *Radiology* 149:721–724, 1983.
28. Zimmerman R.A., Bilaniuk L.T.: CT of primary and secondary craniocerebral neuroblastoma. *A.J.N.R.* 1:431–434, 1980.
29. Zimmerman R.A., Bilaniuk L.T., Wood J.H., et al.: Computed tomography of pineal, parapineal, and histologically related tumors. *Radiology* 137:669–677, 1980.

CHAPTER 7

INFLAMMATORY AND DEGENERATIVE DISEASES

HERPES ENCEPHALITIS

Case 144

37-year-old man with fever and reduced level of consciousness.

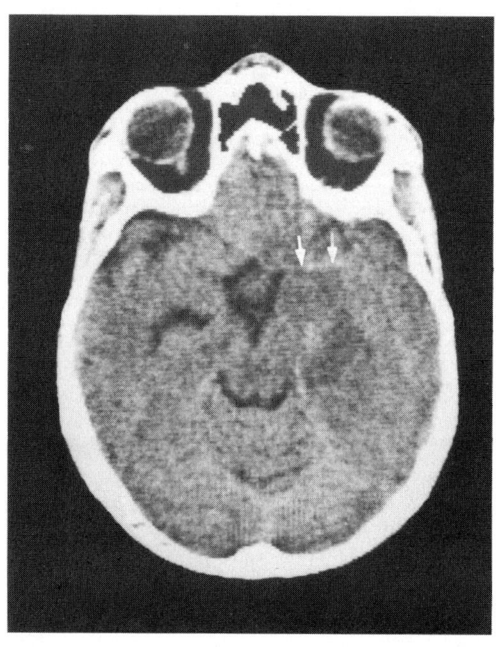

Encephalitis due to herpes simplex (type 1) typically begins in the medial anterior temporal and posteroinferior frontal lobes. Initial CT findings are limited to subtle, low attenuation and mass effect. As the disease progresses, patchy hemorrhage and abnormal contrast enhancement are common.

The characteristic CT pattern may not develop until the patient has become comatose. Close attention to the frontotemporal regions on early scans often demonstrates mild edema, which can support the clinical diagnosis and guide biopsy.

Involvement is unilateral in this case, with vague, low density and mass effect in the medial left frontotemporal region. (Compare this scan with that of the low-grade glioma in Case 33.) The ipsilateral temporal horn is compressed, and the uncus is swollen and displaced medially. The proximal middle cerebral artery *(arrows)* appears relatively dense due to surrounding low attenuation (and possible stasis; compare with Case 270).

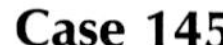

Case 145

36-year-old man scanned ten days after the onset of symptoms.

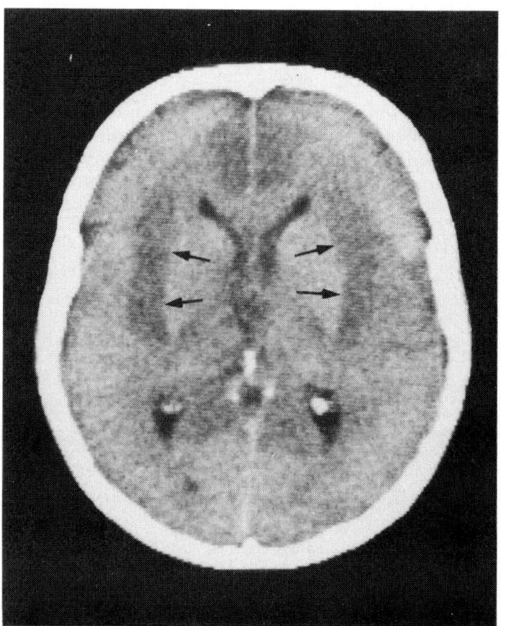

In this case, involvement is bilateral. Lower sections demonstrated mass effect and poorly defined low attenuation in the medial frontotemporal lobes.

At this level there is symmetrical involvement of the parasagittal frontal lobes and the deep sylvian regions. The striking margination of the lenticular nucleus *(arrows)* is characteristic of herpes encephalitis.

Pyogenic or fungal cerebritis may initially appear as a nonspecific region of low attenuation and swelling similar to that seen in viral encephalitis. Patchy contrast enhancement may occur. Peripheral enhancement may be seen prior to the formation of a true abscess capsule (see discussion of Case 146).

CEREBRAL ABSCESSES

Case 146

4-year-old girl with hypoplastic right heart syndrome treated in infancy by creation of a right-to-left atrial shunt. Pyogenic abscess.

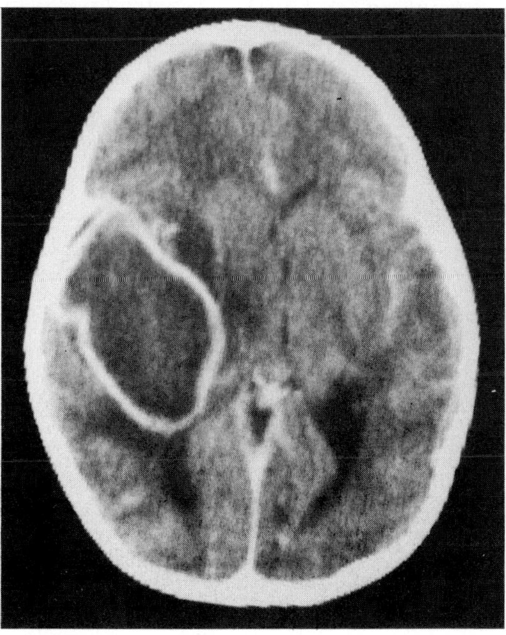

Pyogenic cerebral abscesses typically demonstrate a thin, uniform rim of contrast enhancement surrounding a low-attenuation center. The usually smooth contour of the enhancing periphery contrasts with the thicker, more irregular margin of most cerebral neoplasms (but see Cases 44, 47, and 150).

The formation of a true abscess capsule is preceded by a stage of cerebritis that may demonstrate peripheral enhancement. Clues to the lack of an organized capsule include nonvisualization of the capsule on precontrast scans and diffusion of contrast material into the center of the lesion on postcontrast images.

Attenuation values within an abscess are usually higher than CSF density due to the content of cells and protein. Associated edema is often prominent, and additional "daughter" abscesses may be seen near the primary lesion.

Many abscesses can be aspirated with CT guidance and followed to resolution by serial CT scans during antibiotic therapy. Enhancement of the abscess capsule may persist for weeks or months during successful treatment. In this case, aspiration yielded 40 ml of pus containing streptococci and gram-negative anaerobic rods. The abscess disappeared over a two-month treatment period.

Case 147

47-year-old diabetic man. Mucormycosis.

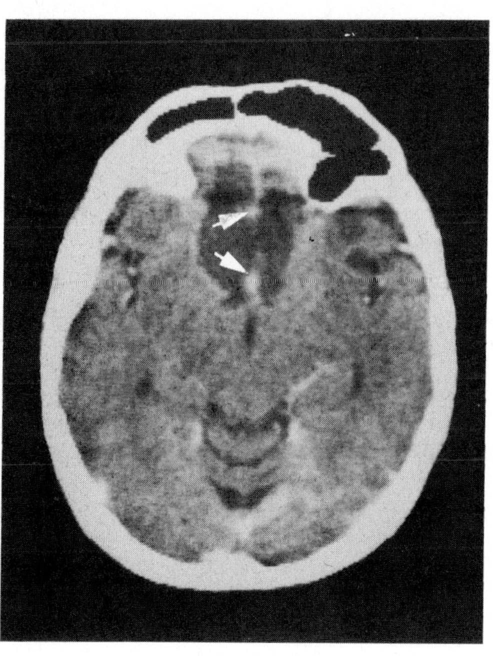

Fungal abscesses are rare in otherwise healthy individuals. They more commonly occur in immunosuppressed hosts and are a feared cerebral complication of diabetes mellitus.

In this case, the infection has crossed the cribriform plate from the ethmoid sinus to the inferior frontal regions. The abscess cavity bridges the interhemispheric fissue to involve both medial frontal lobes. The proximal segments of the anterior cerebral arteries are stretched above the bridging portion of the abscess, serving to restrain its lobulations (*arrows;* compare with Case 90).

Several fungi (including *Aspergillus* and *Mucor*) have a tendency for vascular invasion. This patient later suffered infarction in the anterior cerebral artery distributions. At postmortem examination the arterial lumens were occluded by hyphae.

DIFFERENTIAL DIAGNOSIS: SUPERFICIAL, RIM-ENHANCING MASS WITH EDEMA

Case 148

80-year-old woman.

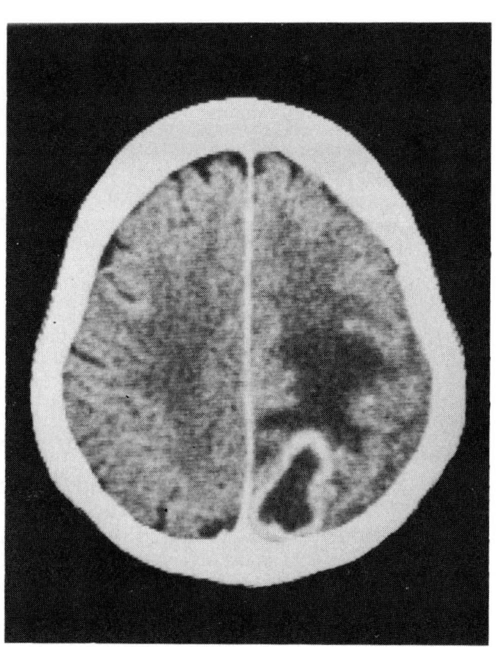

Glioblastoma.

Case 149

28-year-old Asian male immigrant.

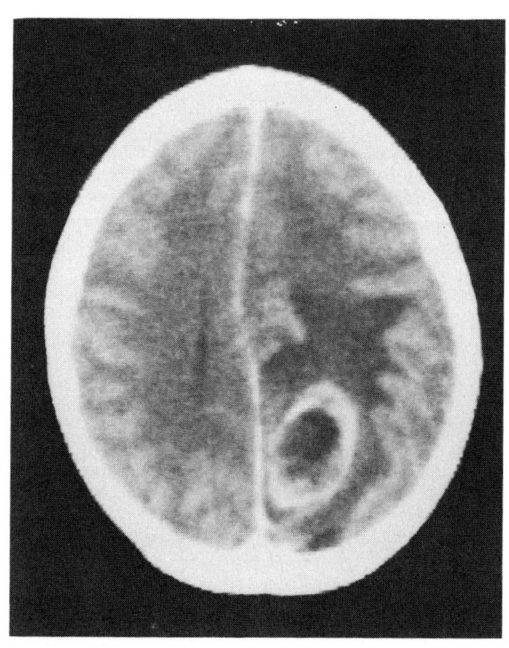

Pyogenic Abscess.

The enhancing rim of some malignant gliomas is fairly uniform and may mimic the capsule of an abscess (see Cases 150 and 151).

Conversely, some pyogenic abscesses (such as in Case 149) develop a relatively thick capsule, which resembles the periphery of a high-grade glioma or metastasis. Fungal abscesses may also demonstrate a thick-walled, loculated, or semisolid morphology.

The relatively poor inflammatory response of deep hemispheric white matter may cause the capsule of an abscess to be less developed along the medial wall than along the lateral margin. When present, this feature may aid in distinguishing an abscess from a neoplasm.

DIFFERENTIAL DIAGNOSIS: CYSTIC MASS WITH UNIFORM, THIN WALLS

Case 150

32-year-old man.

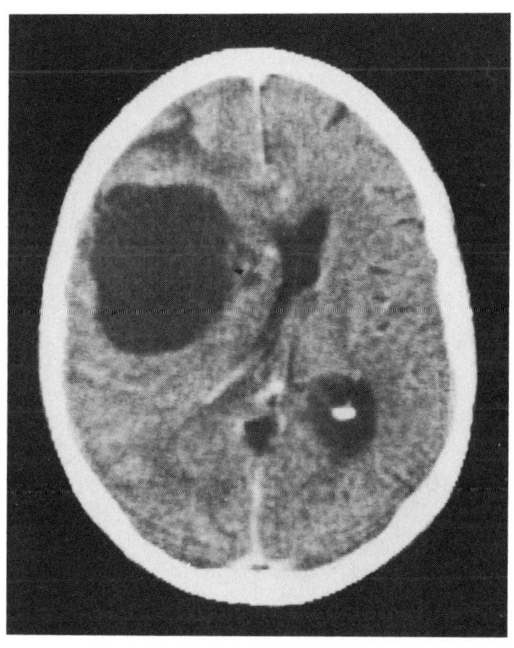

Glioblastoma.

Case 151

56-year-old alcoholic man presenting with headache.

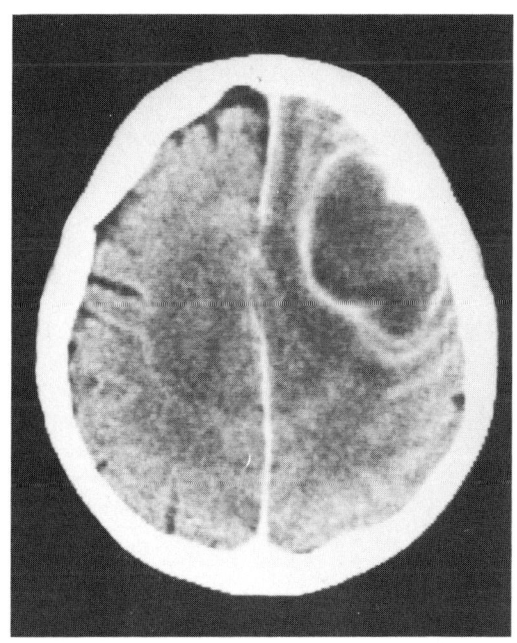

Pyogenic Abscess.

A cystic glioma with an unusually smooth, thin rim may closely resemble a large abscess (Case 150; see Cases 44 and 47 for other examples). However, an abscess should remain the first diagnostic consideration when such a thin-walled cystic lesion is encountered.

Porencephalic cysts can reach similar proportions but lack peripheral enhancement and contain lower-density fluid (see Cases 371 and 372). Arachnoid cysts are usually more angular in morphology and are clearly extra-axial (see Cases 361 and 362).

PERINATAL VIRAL MENINGOENCEPHALITIS: SEQUELAE

Case 152

5-month-old girl with a history of neonatal meningitis, now presenting with seizures and developmental delay.

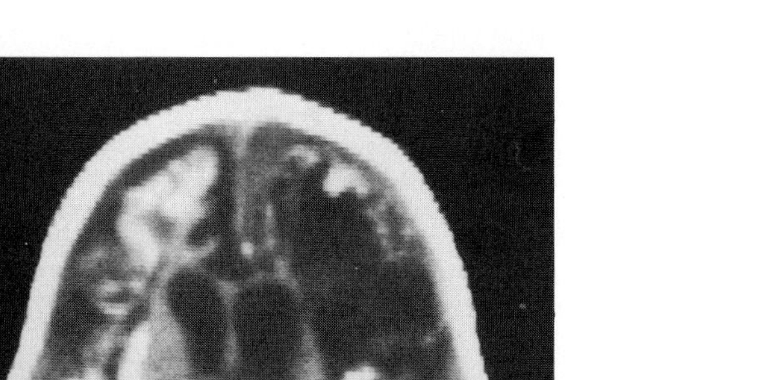

Scans performed after perinatal meningoencephalitis may demonstrate a combination of patchy encephalomalacia and extensive intracerebral calcification. The pattern is nonspecific and can be seen with many viruses.

Calcification may develop rapidly (weeks to months) and may include a gyriform cortical pattern resembling Sturge-Weber syndrome (see Case 189). Widespread encephalomalacia may be caused by perinatal anoxia without infection, but extensive calcification, as in this case, suggests an infectious insult.

Case 153

4-month-old boy with a history of neonatal herpes encephalitis.

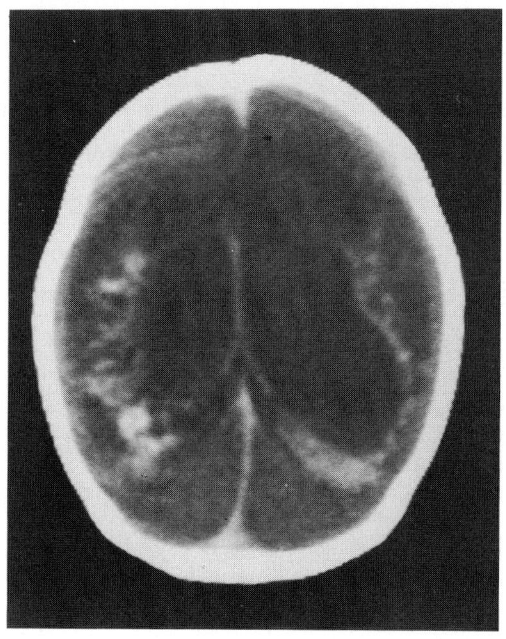

Neonatal herpes encephalitis is a panencephalitis caused by type 2 virus acquired from the birth canal. (Case 273 presents the acute phase of this disease.) The sequelae of the infection include parenchymal loss and calcification. It may be difficult to distinguish the acute and chronic effects of cerebritis from the ischemic consequences of associated meningitis and arteritis.

Widespread cortical encephalomalacia has developed in this case. Only periventricular fringes of calcified "normal" parenchymal density remain, in contrast to Case 152. The "ghost" of cerebral tissue along the margins of enlarged ventricles distinguishes the appearance from hydranencephaly (see Case 338).

DIFFERENTIAL DIAGNOSIS: PERIVENTRICULAR CALCIFICATION IN A CHILD

Case 154

6-year-old boy with seizures.

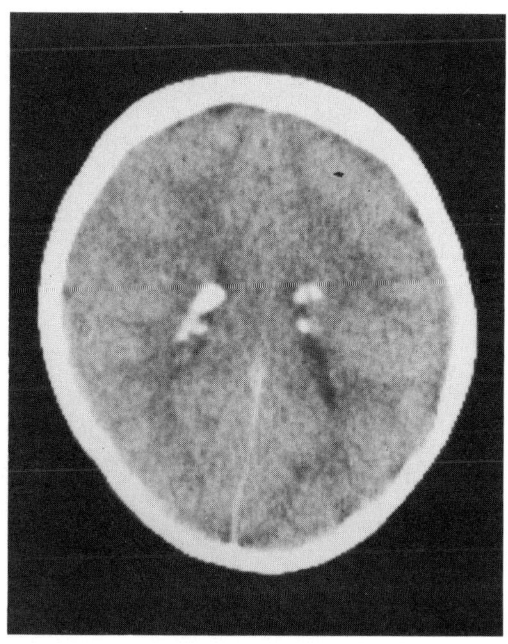

Tuberous Sclerosis.

Case 155

13-month-old girl with microcephaly and developmental delay.

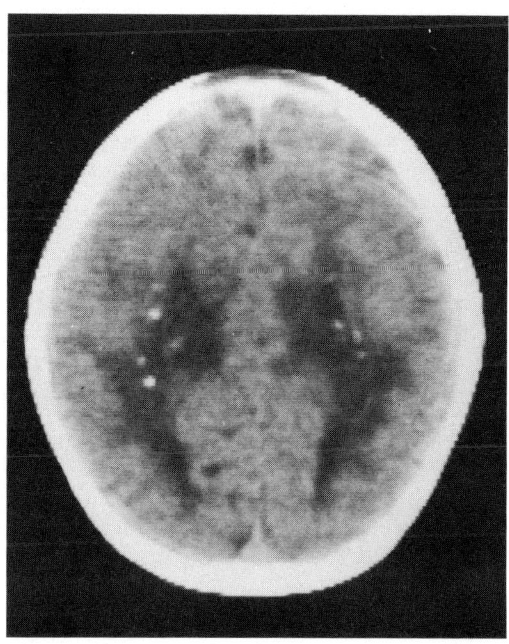

Congenital Infection With Cytomegalovirus.

Subependymal calcifications are a hallmark of tuberous sclerosis. This disease is one of the neurocutaneous syndromes or "neurophacomatoses" and is inherited as an autosomal dominant trait with frequent sporadic cases. (The father of the child in this case also had seizures.)

Calcifications occur in hyperplastic nodules of malformed neuroglial tissue called "tubers." Tubers may develop into giant cell astrocytomas, often occuring near the foramen of Monro. These low-grade gliomas exhibit benign growth characteristics, but may cause obstructive hydrocephalus because of strategic location.

Other potential CT findings in tuberous sclerosis include calcifications in cerebral cortex, localized low-attenuation regions of abnormal myelination within white matter, and patchy regions of calvarial sclerosis.

Congenital infections with cytomegalovirus (CMV) typically cause periventricular calcification and microcephaly. The ventricles are often enlarged due to cerebral damage.

Congenital toxoplasmosis may also produce cerebral calcifications and ventricular enlargement. The calcifications of toxoplasmosis tend to be scattered and the ventricular enlargement often represents true hydrocephalus. However, subependymal calcification and microcephaly may occur and be indistinguishable from CMV.

DIFFERENTIAL DIAGNOSIS: PERIVENTRICULAR MASS IN AN ADULT

Case 156

38-year-old woman.

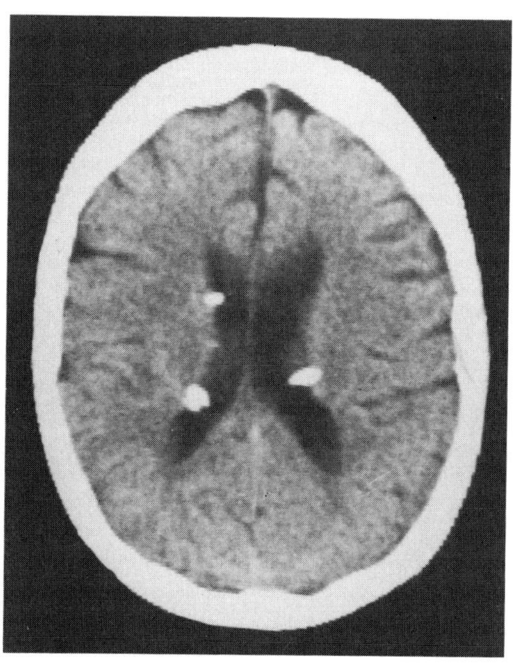

Tuberous Sclerosis (Noncontrast Scan).

Case 157

67-year-old man.

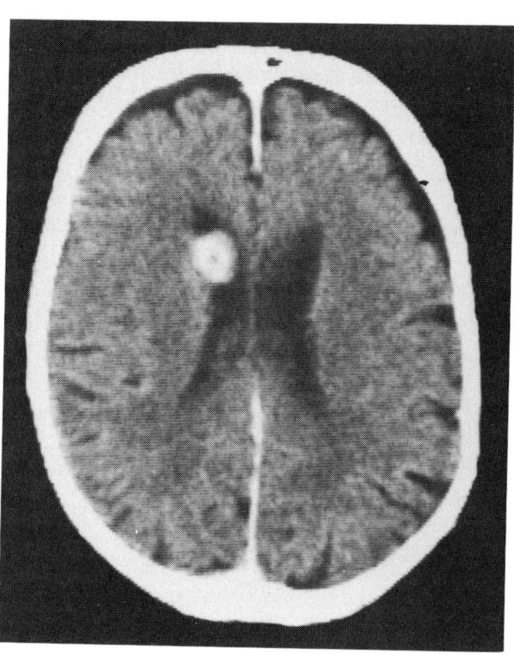

Metastatic Squamous Cell Carcinoma Of The Lung (Postcontrast Scan).

The pattern of multiple periventricular calcifications without contrast enhancement in Case 156 is characteristic of uncomplicated tuberous sclerosis in adults as well as in children. Subependymal tubers may develop into enhancing astrocytomas, and a solitary lesion could have an appearance indistinguishable from that of Case 157.

Intraventricular metastases may arise from choroid plexus or from subependymal tumor deposits (see Case 12). The differential diagnosis in Case 157 would include ependymoma, AVM, and rare inflammatory granuloma. The location would be atypical for intraventricular meningioma (see Case 52) or choroid plexus papilloma (see Cases 123 and 124).

Heterotopic gray matter may occur along the lateral ventricular margins in children or adults. These "masses" appear as slightly dense subependymal nodules without calcification or prominent contrast enhancement. Associated developmental anomalies (e.g., absence of the septum pellucidum) may be present.

Case 158

24-year-old Mexican woman with seizures. Parenchymal cysticercosis.

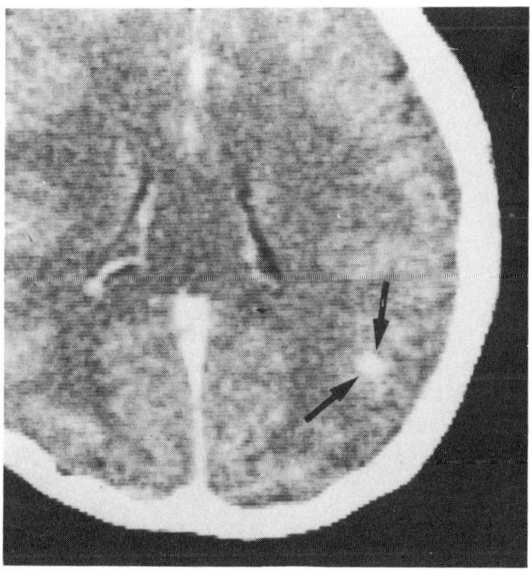

Case 159

17-year-old girl with hydrocephalus. Intraventricular cysticercosis (scan with Intraventricular metrizamide).

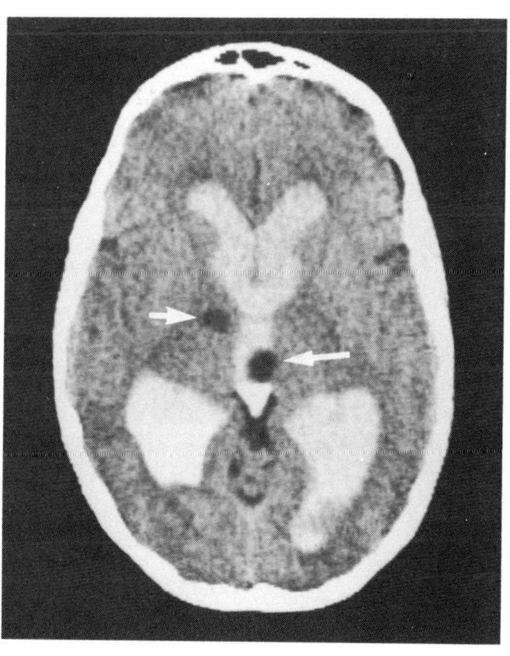

Cysticercosis ranks as the most important parasitic infection of the CNS in this hemisphere. The disease occurs when man serves as an intermediate host for the larval form of the pork tapeworm, *Taenia solium*.

The encysting larvae of cysticercosis can cause a wide spectrum of cerebral lesions. Cisternal, ventricular, and parenchymal involvement may be seen separately or in combination. Lesions may be cystic or solid, calcified or enhancing, solitary or multiple.

In this case, a small, calcified parenchymal lesion demonstrated minimal contrast enhancement.

Cysts of cysticercosis may be found within the cerebral ventricles, cranial subarachnoid spaces (especially basal cisterns), and spinal canal, as well as within brain parenchyma. They may be seen as solitary lesions or clustered aggregates.

Cysticercosis cysts often blend with surrounding spinal fluid, requiring subarachnoid contrast material for demonstration. In this case, the ganglionic cyst *(small arrow)* was apparent on a routine scan, but the third ventricular lesion *(large arrow)* was not identified until the metrizamide study.

Case 160

64-year-old man with a history of lung resection for histoplasmosis. Histoplasmoma.

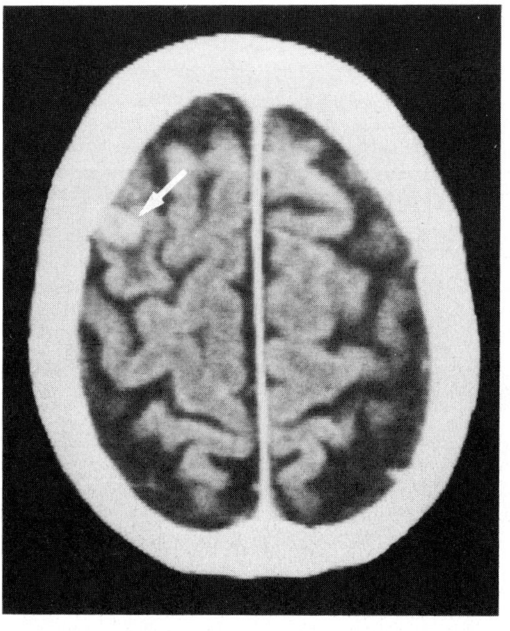

Fungal infections may cause a wide variety of CT abnormalities. The simplest lesions are solitary parenchymal granulomas, as seen in this case *(arrow)*. The superficial location, edema, and frequent multiplicity often mimic metastases.

In other cases, a region of fungal cerebritis may evolve to a frank abscess, similar to the development of a pyogenic infection (see Case 147). Fungal meningitis (e.g., coccidiomycosis, histoplasmosis) may present as a densely enhancing process filling the basal cisterns. Ependymal (or subependymal) infection may also be seen (see Case 163).

Case 161

26-year-old woman with immunodeficiency and disseminated pulmonary histoplasmosis. *Nocardia* brain abscess.

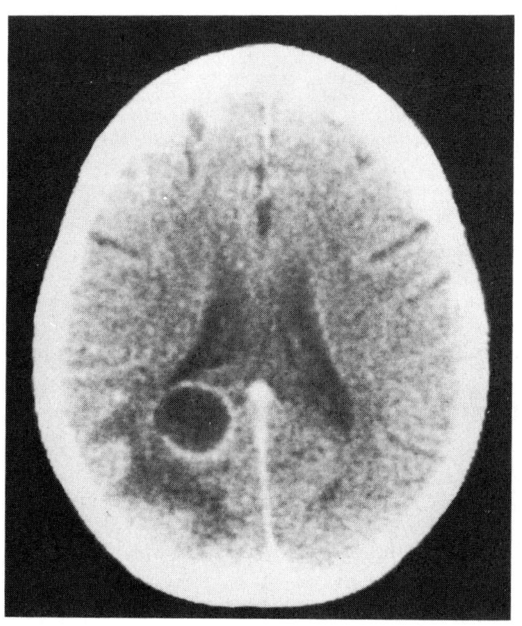

A variety of opportunistic infections may develop in immunosuppressed hosts. Fungal pathogens (e.g., aspergillosis) are common in such cases. Cerebral lesions may also be caused by unusual bacteria (e.g., *Nocardia,* as seen here) or mycobacteria. Protozoal infection in the form of toxoplasmosis has been frequently observed in the acquired immune deficiency syndrome (AIDS).

Nocardial cerebral abscesses are often multiloculated or numerous, unlike the single cavity in this case. The possibility of primary CNS lymphoma (see Cases 136 through 138) or progressive multifocal leukoencephalopathy (see Case 179) should also be considered when numerous lesions are encountered in an immunodeficient host.

INFECTIONS INVOLVING CSF SURFACES

Case 162

42-year-old man with a history of pulmonary tuberculosis, now presenting with multiple left-sided cranial nerve palsies. Tuberculous meningitis (coronal scan).

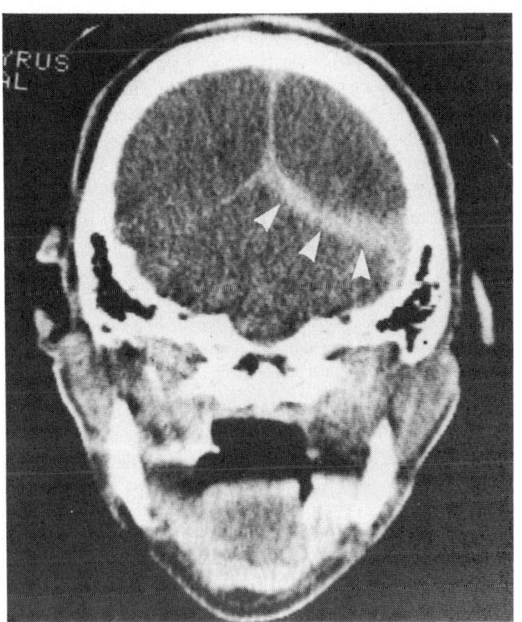

Case 163

49-year-old man admitted to the hospital in a coma. Ventriculitis due to aspergillosis (with obstruction of the foramina of Monro).

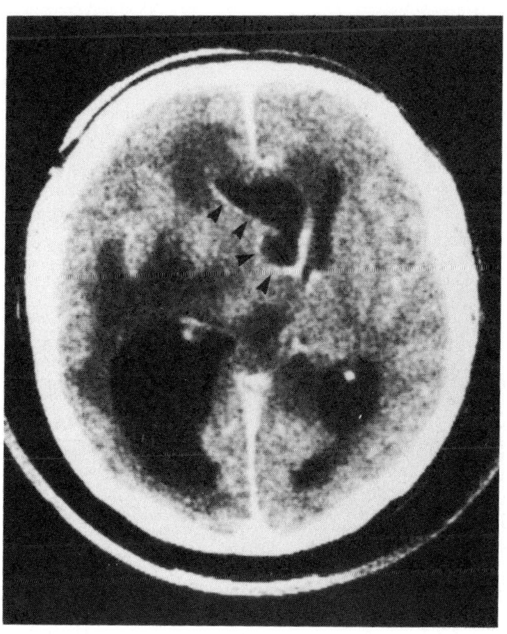

A wide range of organisms may cause clinical meningitis. Viral infections are often associated with encephalitis (see Cases 152 and 153); they rarely present meningeal findings on CT scans. Bacterial infections may elicit a thick exudate that fills the basal cisterns or sulci, causing them to appear isodense.

Prominent meningeal enhancement may be seen in pyogenic, fungal, and tuberculous meningitis. Here, a coronal scan demonstrates enhancement of the grossly thickened tentorium *(arrows),* proved surgically to represent tuberculous pachymeningitis. (The CT appearance alone could also be compatible with an "en plaque" meningioma of the tentorium or a tentorial subdural hematoma; see Case 191.)

When thick meningeal enhancement is found in the basal cisterns, the differential diagnosis includes tuberculosis, fungal disease (e.g., coccidiomycosis), pyogenic meningitis, cysticercosis, sarcoidosis, and meningeal tumor (e.g., carcinomatosis, seeding from a primary CNS malignancy, lymphoma, and leukemia).

Bacterial, fungal, or parasitic infections may involve the ventricular lining. Findings on CT scan in ventriculitis include enhancement of the ependymal or subependymal tissues, as seen surrounding the right frontal horn in this case. Secondary hydrocephalus may be present due to obstructing tissue or septations.

Here, the right foramen of Monro has been compromised to a greater extent than that on the left. The resulting asymmetrical hydrocephalus is associated with unilateral transependymal CSF edema (see Cases 355 and 356) and a marked midline shift (subfalcial herniation).

The ventricle on the side of the mass effect is enlarged rather than compressed. This finding indentifies unilateral hydrocephalus as a major component of the lesion and places the inciting process at the foramen of Monro.

Enhancing ventricular margins may also be seen with primary or metastatic tumor (see Cases 12, 54, and 55) and in noninfectious inflammatory disease, such as sarcoidosis.

Case 164

5-month-old boy with meningitis due to *Hemophilus influenzae*. Subdural effusion.

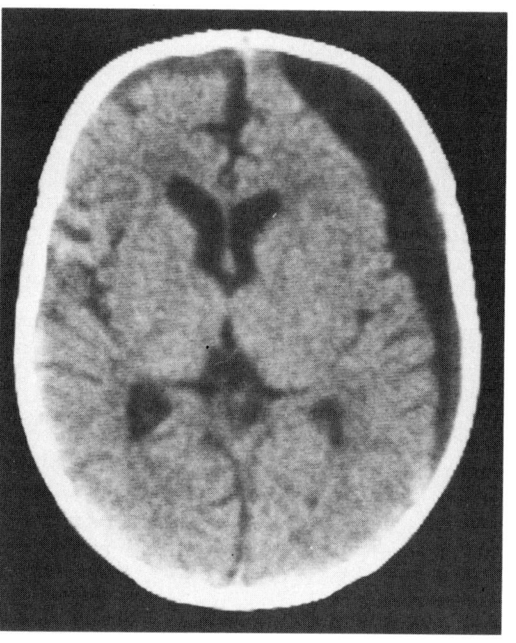

Subdural effusions are commonly associated with infection by *H influenzae*, the leading cause of meningitis in this country. The effusions typically contain large amounts of protein but few cells. Their appearance is nonspecific and resembles other subdural fluid collections.

Subdural effusions may persist beyond successful treatment of the meningitis. They may increase in size like chronic subdural hematomas. Infection of the effusion produces a subdural empyema in occasional cases.

Case 165

20-year-old man. Subdural empyema associated with mastoiditis.

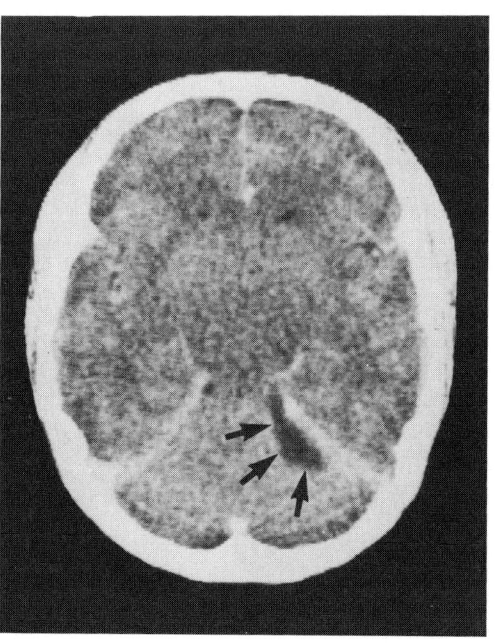

Intracranial infection may arise from sinusitis or mastoiditis of the skull base (see also Case 147). This spread of infection often involves retrograde thrombophlebitis, which can lead to subdural empyema and/or cerebritis.

In this case, infection has extended from the petrous bone to form a pocket of subdural empyema along the inferior surface of the tentorium *(arrows)*. (Compare the location of this process with that of the subdural hematoma seen along the superior surface of the tentorium in Case 191.)

Case 166

27-year-old woman with headache and fever.
Acute sinusitis (wide window width).

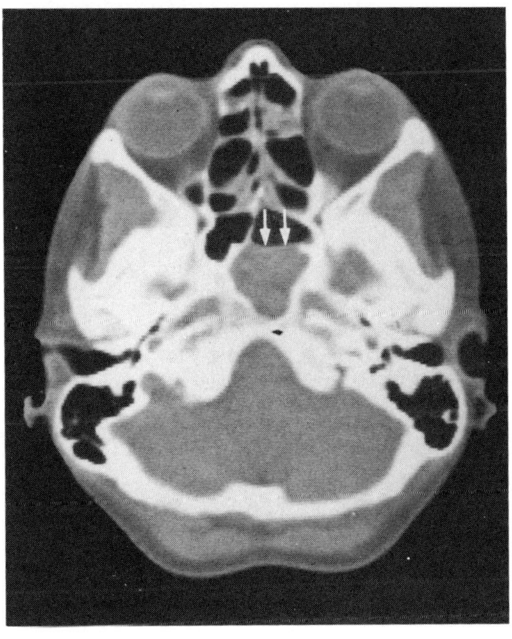

The skull base and sinuses should be evaluated with wide window widths on all scans. Many patients referred for possible cerebral abscesses are instead suffering from sinusitis. Findings on CT scan include mucosal thickening (seen here in the ethmoid sinuses) and air-fluid levels (seen here in the sphenoid sinus; *arrows*).

An air-fluid level is the standard radiographic criterion for diagnosis of acute sinusitis in the appropriate clinical context. In the setting of trauma, the same finding suggests a basal skull fracture (see Case 222).

Infections spreading from the sphenoid sinus may mimic other parasellar lesions. For example, aspergillosis may cause sclerosis of bone and encasement of vessels resembling a meningioma. An expanding mucocele of the sphenoid sinus is also in the differential diagnosis of a parasellar mass.

Case 167

20-year-old man (same patient as Case 165).
Chronic mastoiditis (wide window width).

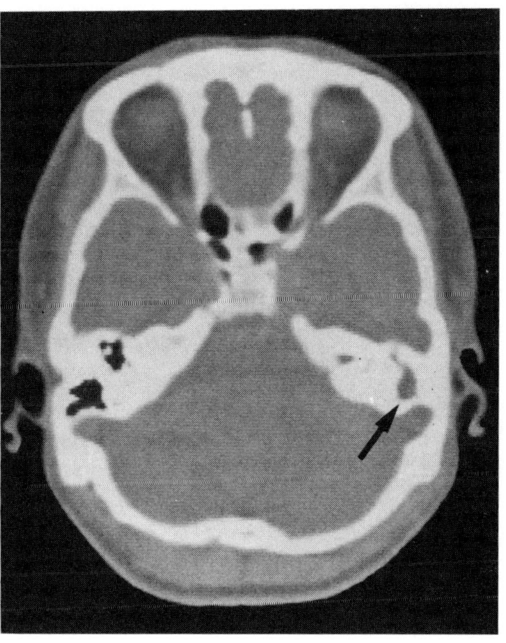

Mastoiditis causes opacification of petrous air cells, often with associated involvement of the middle ear. Chronic infection leads to generalized sclerosis surrounding focal areas of bone erosion. Cholesteatomas often accompany chronic mastoiditis, with eventual destruction of middle ear structures.

Here the normally pneumatized right petrous bone contrasts with the opacification seen on the left. No ossicles were visible in the left tympanic cavity.

Case 165 illustrates the infratentorial subdural empyema that arose from the left petrous bone in this case. Mastoiditis infrequently leads to thrombosis of the adjacent sigmoid sinus, which may in turn cause increased intracranial pressure or hydrocephalus ("otitic hydrocephalus").

MULTIPLE SCLEROSIS

Case 168

29-year-old woman presenting with optic neuritis.

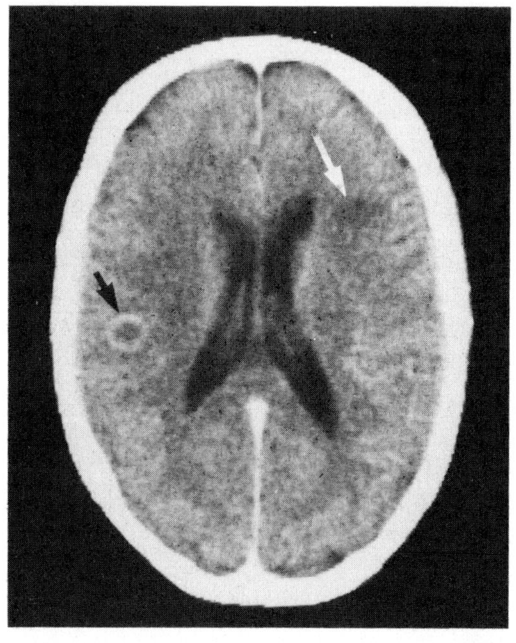

Multiple sclerosis may present a variety of lesions on CT scans. Nonenhancing plaques are often seen as small areas of decreased attenuation within white matter *(white arrow)*. These are particularly common in periventricular regions and can be confused with small infarctions in the corona radiata (see Cases 175 and 248).

Active demyelinating plaques may present as focal areas of nodular or ring-like contrast enhancement *(black arrow)*. Although most of these lesions are small, occasional solid or rim-enhancing plaques are large enough to resemble neoplasms (see Case 171). Serial scans may demonstrate the evolution of a plaque from an active enhancing phase to a quiescent, low-attenuation lesion.

Magnetic resonance imaging is superior to CT imaging in detecting and quantitating demyelinating disease. The CT scan may be normal in some patients with clinically obvious multiple sclerosis. Alternatively, CT scans may be dramatically abnormal in patients with minimal symptoms.

Case 169

30-year-old woman.

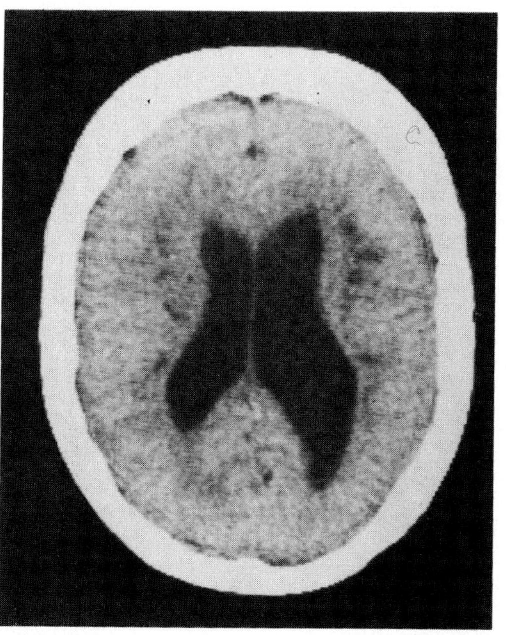

Long-standing multiple sclerosis is often associated with ventricular and sulcal enlargement. These findings in a young patient may suggest the diagnosis even if individual plaques are not defined. (See Cases 186 and 187 for discussion of other causes of prominent CSF spaces in young patients.)

In this case, rows of low-attenuation plaques parallel the enlarged ventricles. The appearance resembles that of "lacunar" infarction in the corona radiata (compare with Case 248), but the clinical settings are widely dissimilar.

CONTRAST ENHANCEMENT IN MULTIPLE SCLEROSIS

Case 170

38-year-old woman.

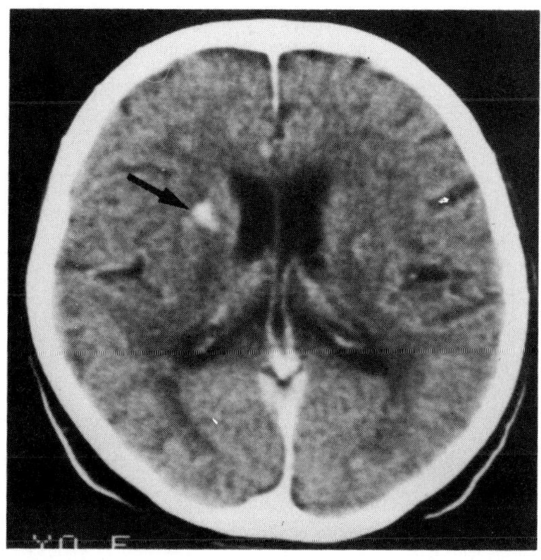

Acute or subacute demyelinating plaques often demonstrate contrast enhancement. The most common pattern is solid enhancement of a small lesion in the periventricular white matter, as illustrated in this case *(arrow)*.

Plaques occasionally show ring enhancement (see Case 168). Multiplicity is common (see Case 172). The intensity and multiplicity of enhancing lesions may be increased on delayed scans after large amounts of contrast material have been administered.

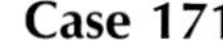

Case 171

29-year-old woman.

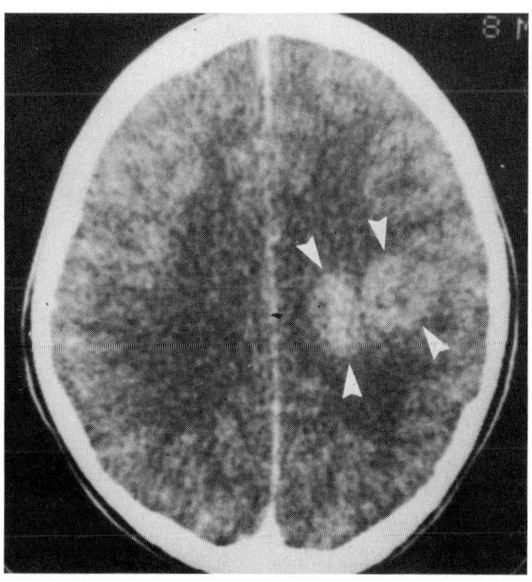

Large regions of active demyelination may cause atypical patterns of contrast enhancement. The enhancement may be solid (as in this case) or peripheral, and may measure several centimeters in diameter. The resulting appearance resembles a malignant neoplasm. Such lesions are usually located in the centrum semiovale, but may also occur in the corpus callosum.

DIFFERENTIAL DIAGNOSIS: MULTIPLE ENHANCING CEREBRAL NODULES

Case 172

45-year-old woman.

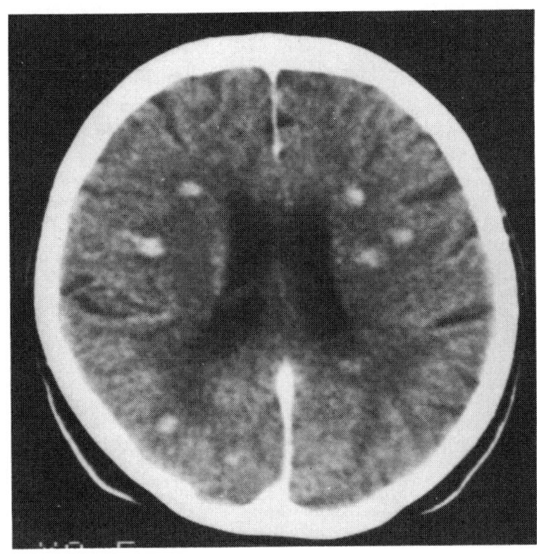

Multiple Sclerosis.

Case 173

50-year-old woman.

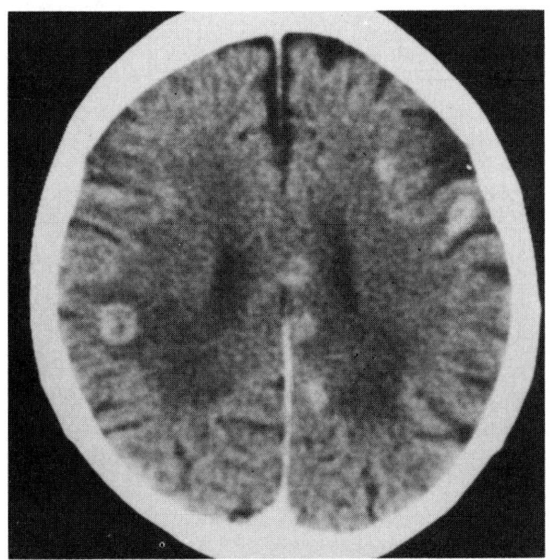

Metastases (Unknown Primary Neoplasm).

The enhancing plaques of multiple sclerosis may be numerous and uniform in size, as in Case 172. The pattern of the lesions then resembles the appearance of multiple metastases, as in Case 173.

Plaques usually occupy a midhemisphere location. This distribution is more central than the peripheral position of metastases near the gray-white matter junction. The clinical setting also distinguishes these two processes in most cases.

Additional pathologies in the differential diagnosis of multiple, enhancing nodules include disseminated infection (e.g., cysticercosis, tuberculosis, histoplasmosis, toxoplasmosis), primary CNS lymphoma (see Case 138), and subacute, multifocal infarction (arterial or venous; see Cases 236 and 276).

Case 174

79-year-old woman presenting with transient ischemic attack. "Old white matter" (possible "Binswanger's disease").

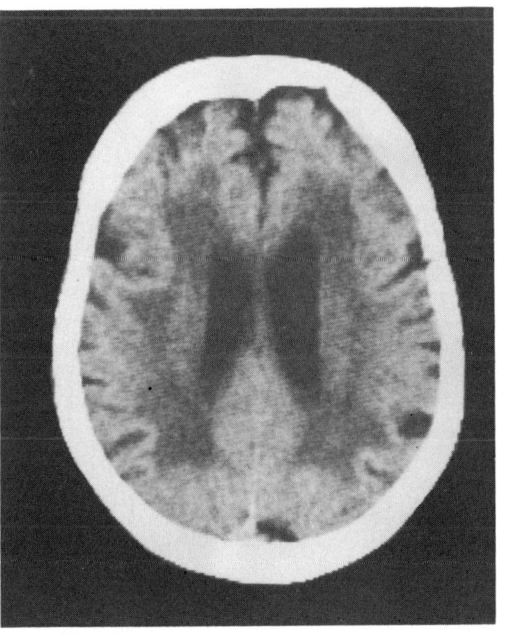

Striking low attenuation is commonly seen in the deep white matter of elderly patients. The symmetry of this low-density change distinguishes it from focal edema or infarction. Involvement may be limited to periventricular regions near the frontal horns and trigones, or may extend diffusely throughout the centrum semiovale.

This white matter pattern has been considered to represent Binswanger's disease (subcortical arteriosclerotic encephalopathy). However, most cases lack a characteristic history, and the involvement is predominantly periventricular rather than subcortical. Together with the very common occurrence of this finding in elderly patients, these factors suggest that the pattern may alternatively represent a more generalized leukoencephalopathy associated with aging.

Case 175

69-year-old man with a history of hypertension and diabetes mellitus. Deep hemisphere infarctions.

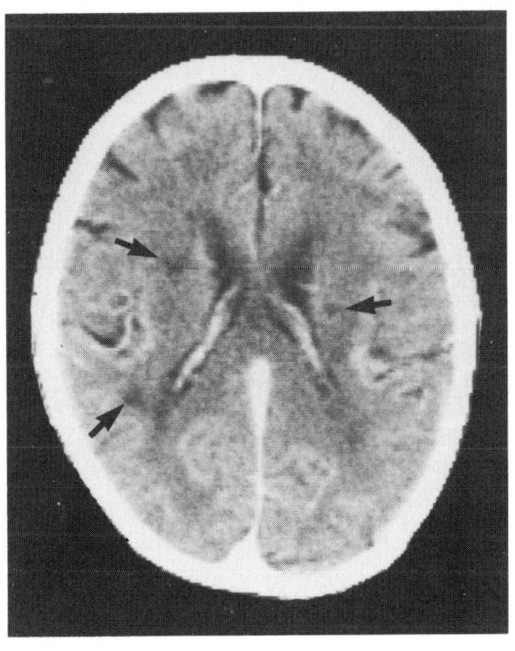

Focal infarctions in periventricular white matter are a common manifestation of small-artery disease. These lesions are analogous to "lacunar" infarctions of the basal ganglia (see Cases 248 and 250) and are most frequently seen in diabetic and/or hypertensive patients.

Like hydrocephalus (see Case 356), deep hemisphere infarction is a common pathology which could be considered a form of white matter disease. The small lesions in this case might be viewed as one end of a spectrum leading toward Binswanger's disease at the opposite extreme.

Here, the scattered infarcts in and near the corona radiata mimic the appearance of demyelinating plaques in multiple sclerosis (see Case 169).

Case 253 discusses central pontine myelinolysis, another white matter disease seen in adults.

Case 176

Newborn boy delivered at 26 weeks' gestation. Normal immature white matter.

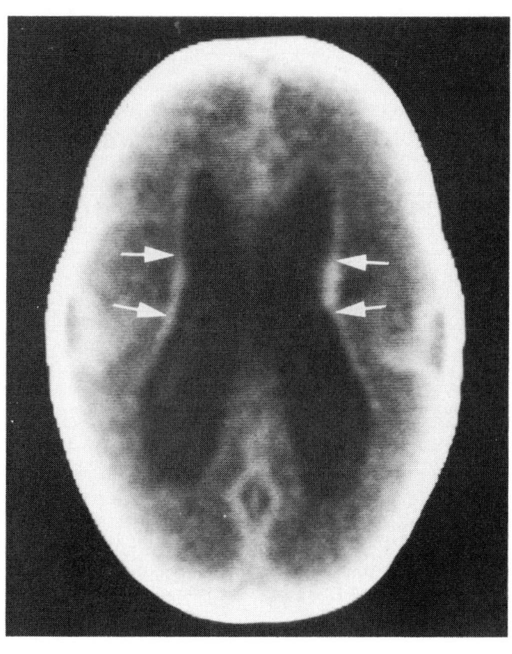

CT scans of premature infants demonstrate diffuse, low attenuation throughout the white matter. This normal low density is associated with immature myelination and high water content. It does not imply (or exclude) anoxic or ischemic damage. Even full-term neonates may demonstrate prominent low density in white matter for several months.

In this case, the smooth cortical ribbon is best seen in the medial occipital and sylvian regions. The dense subependymal layer of germinal matrix *(arrows)* is often prominent in premature infants and should not be mistaken for periventricular hemorrhage.

The dural sinuses often appear unusually dense in neonates, probably due to hemoconcentration seen against a background of parenchymal low density. This diffuse vascular prominence should not be confused with the focal density of superior sagittal sinus thrombosis (see Case 275).

Case 177

13-year-old boy with poor school performance and hyperkinesia. Adrenoleukodystrophy (postcontrast scan).

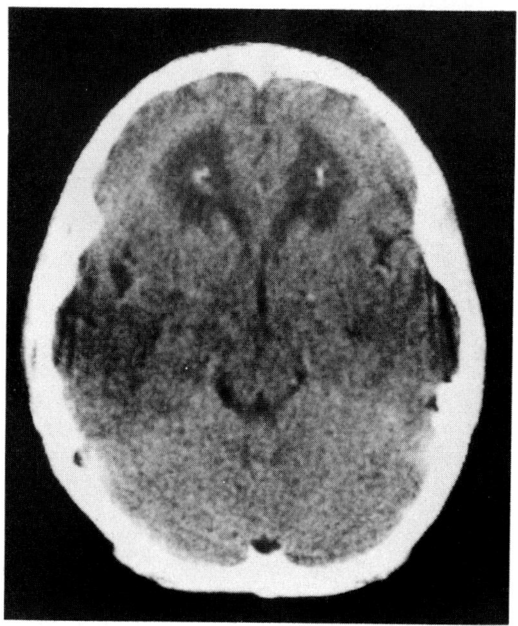

Adrenoleukodystrophy is a rare demyelinating process affecting young males. It seems to be a sex-linked recessive disorder of lipid metabolism, usually associated with adrenal hypofunction.

The typical CT pattern consists of symmetrical areas of demyelination beginning in the parieto-occipital regions and spreading anteriorly. A zone of peripheral contrast enhancement is often present at the advancing margin of demyelination.

Many atypical appearances have been reported. In this case, the frontal lobe predominance and the central contrast enhancement are unusual.

TOXIC AND INFECTIOUS LEUKOENCEPHALOPATHIES

Case 178

7-year-old boy, four years after radiation and chemotherapy (with vincristine, Adriamycin, and prednisone) for medulloblastoma. Disseminated necrotizing leukoencephalopathy.

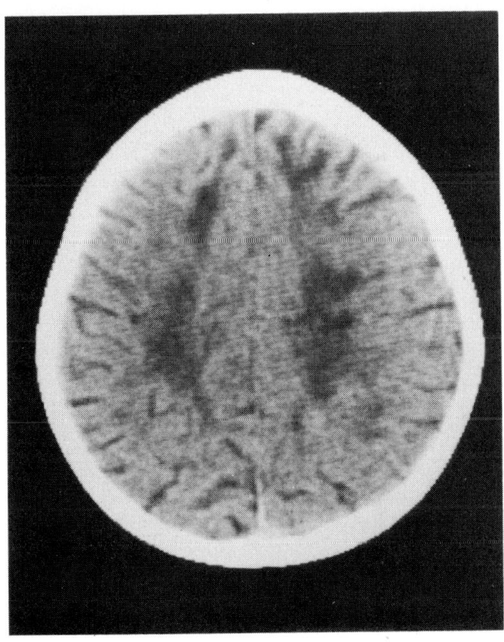

White matter damage has been noted pathologically and on CT scans following chemotherapy and/or cerebral radiation, particularly in children. The combination of radiation and chemotherapy may carry a higher risk of leukoencephalopathy than either treatment alone.

Methotrexate leukoencephalopathy has been identified in leukemia patients receiving radiotherapy, but the toxicity of other chemotherapeutic agents is less well established. The phrase "disseminated necrotizing leukoencephalopathy" is used for methotrexate-associated disease, but may apply to other combinations of chemotherapy and/or radiation. Evidence of radiation-induced demyelination may be seen on CT scans in the absence of associated chemotherapy.

Case 179

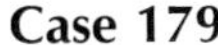

43-year-old man with a renal transplant. Progressive multifocal leukoencephalopathy.

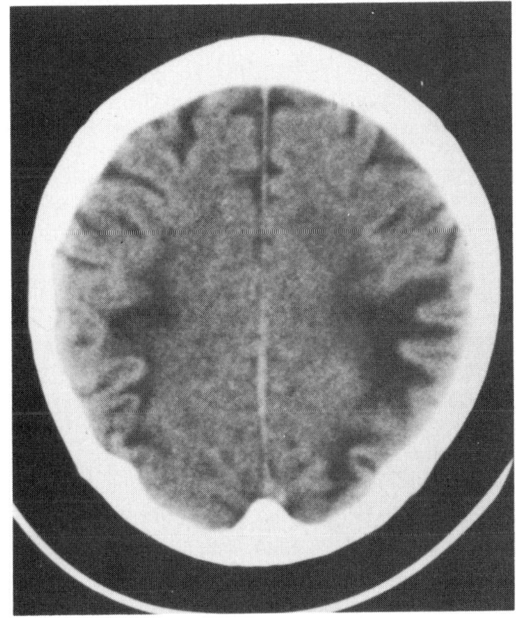

Progressive multifocal leukoencephalopathy (PML) is a demyelinating disease representing infection by a papovavirus. The disease is usually seen in immunosuppressed hosts. Lymphoma and leukemia are the most common predisposing conditions, but iatrogenic immunosuppression may also be implicated (compare with discussion of primary CNS lymphoma, Cases 136 and 138).

The multifocal demyelination is often most prominent in the parieto-occipital white matter, as seen here. Mass effect and contrast enhancement are rare.

The CT appearance of PML may resemble early cerebritis or tumor-related edema. Diagnosis is aided by the limitation of findings to white matter and the lack of contrast enhancement. A progressive clinical course and characteristic follow-up scans are confirmatory.

Case 180

10-year-old girl presenting with ataxia. Friedreich's ataxia.

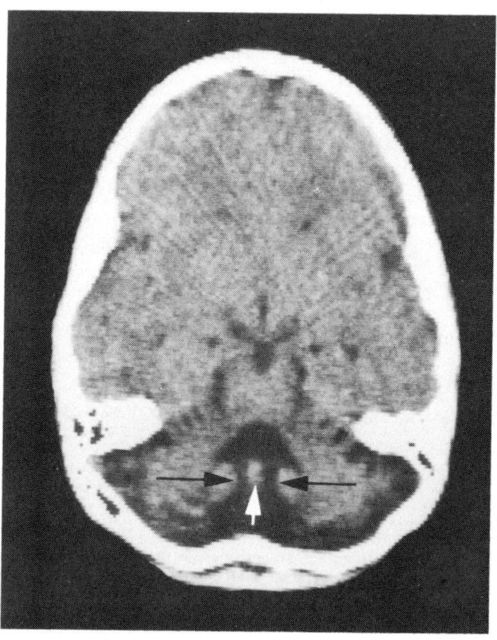

Atrophy is well defined on CT scans, with the loss of parenchymal volume clearly outlined by expanded subarachnoid spaces. In this case, the greatly enlarged posterior fossa cisterns, cerebellar sulci, and fourth ventricle contrast with the normally inconspicuous CSF spaces above the tentorium.

A number of familial syndromes (e.g., olivopontocerebellar degeneration, Marie's ataxia) may cause cerebellar degeneration with or without brain stem atrophy. Friedreich's ataxia usually presents with spinal cord involvement and less impressive cerebellar findings. Examples of acquired cerebellar atrophy include alcohol abuse, paraneoplastic syndromes, and the phenytoin/seizure combination.

Enlarged subarachnoid spaces highlight surface anatomy. Here the inferior vermis is clearly seen *(white arrow)* as a small nodule of tissue forming the posterior wall of the fourth ventricle and residing between the cerebellar tonsils *(black arrows).*

Case 181

60-year-old woman presenting with dementia and movement disorder. Huntington's chorea.

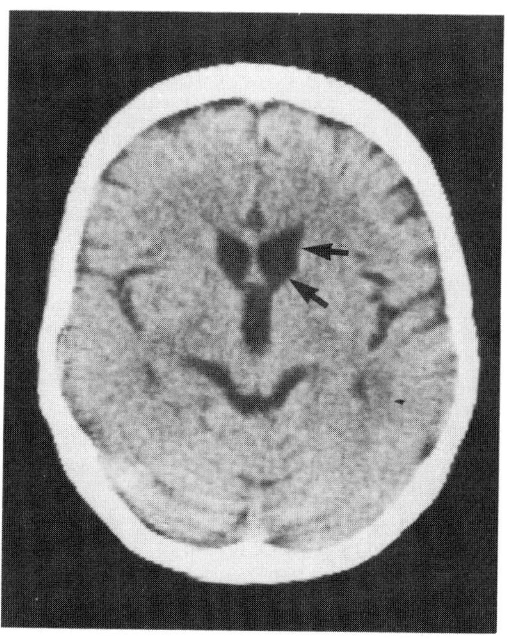

The normal caudate head bulges into the lateral aspect of the frontal horns to cause a medially convex margin. Atrophy of the caudate nucleus in advanced Huntington's disease causes this curvature to flatten and reverse, leaving a concave surface as seen here *(arrows)*. Associated ventricular and sulcal enlargement is often present.

This characteristic CT finding is a late development in the disease and is not seen in presymptomatic carriers. Positron emission tomography can identify abnormal caudate metabolism before atrophy appears on CT scans.

CEREBRAL ATROPHY

Case 182

82-year-old man.

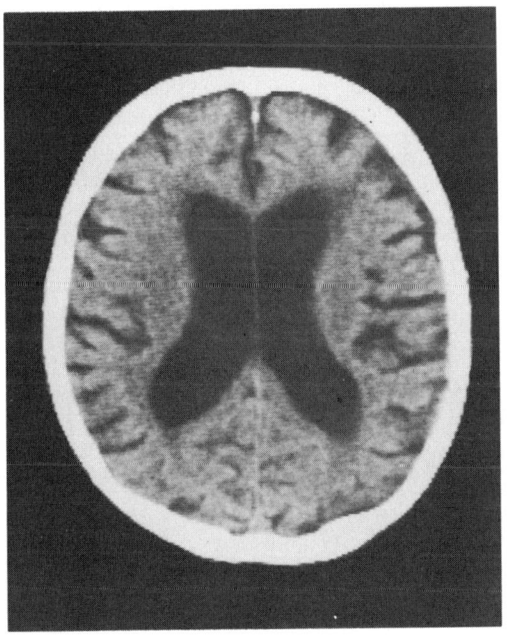

Cerebral atrophy is demonstrated on CT scans by diffuse enlargement of ventricles and subarachnoid spaces. The relative degree of ventricular and sulcal enlargement is usually similar. Prominence of the ventricular component raises the question of hydrocephalus (see Cases 351 and 354).

The correlation between enlarged CSF spaces and reduced intellectual capacity has been difficult to establish in group studies and cannot be applied to an individual case.

Case 183

74-year-old man. Possible Pick's disease.

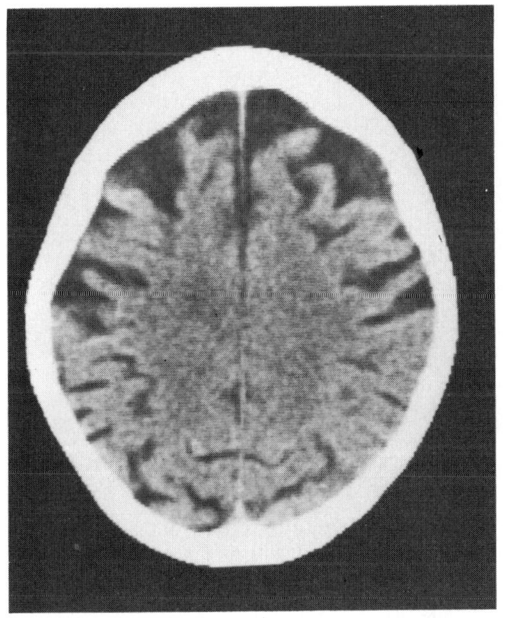

In some cases, the loss of cerebral volume predominantly involves the frontal lobes. The diagnosis of Pick's disease may be suggested when localized frontal atrophy is associated with prominent atrophy of the temporal lobes (inferior and middle temporal gyri).

Classic Pick's disease demonstrates strikingly thin gyri separated by gaping sulci in the frontal and temporal lobes. However, these knife-like gyri are not seen in all cases.

Alzheimer's disease may also give the appearance of focal frontal atrophy.

Case 184

80-year-old woman.

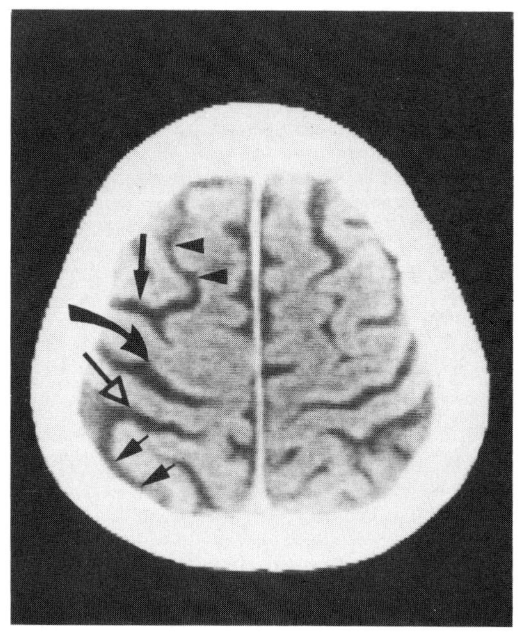

Atrophic enlargement of cerebral sulci demonstrates gyral landmarks on vertex scans.

The superior frontal sulcus *(black arrowheads)* follows a parasagittal course before intersecting posteriorly (at a right angle) with the precentral sulcus *(straight black arrow)*.

The intraparietal sulcus *(short black arrows)* angles obliquely across the posterior parietal vertex before merging anteriorly with the postcentral sulcus *(open black arrow)*.

The central sulcus *(curved black arrow)* lies between the precentral sulcus and postcentral sulcus as the middle member of the three major laterally directed sulci.

Case 185

74-year-old woman.

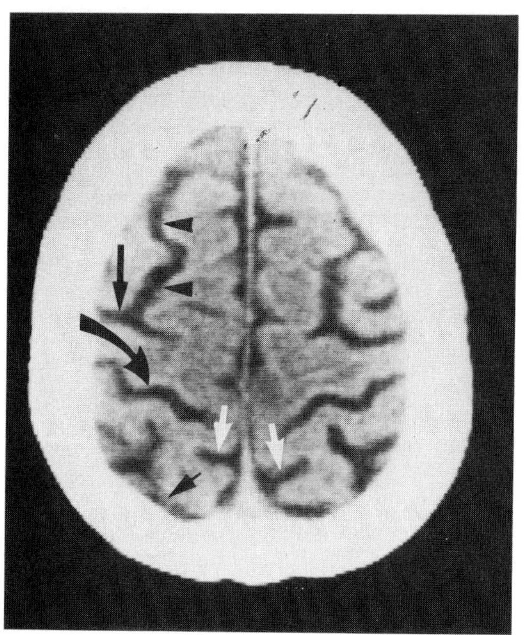

The landmarks discussed in Case 184 are labeled with the same key in this patient.

Another vertex landmark is the marginal ramus of the cingulate sulcus, seen as a short, paired sulcus on the medial surface of the hemisphere *(white arrows)*. The central sulcus is usually the next most anterior sulcus on the lateral surface of the convexity.

Usually one or more of these landmarks is apparent on vertex scans. Their recognition localizes lesions with respect to the motor and sensory gyri, regardless of head flexion or extension.

DIFFERENTIAL DIAGNOSIS: PSEUDOATROPHY

Case 186

32-year-old man weighing 87 lb.

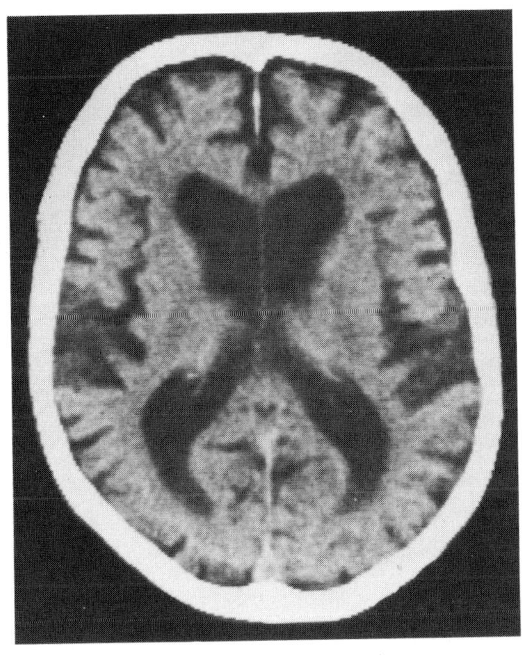

Malnutrition Due To Psychiatric Disorder.

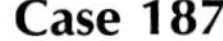

Case 187

30-year-old man.

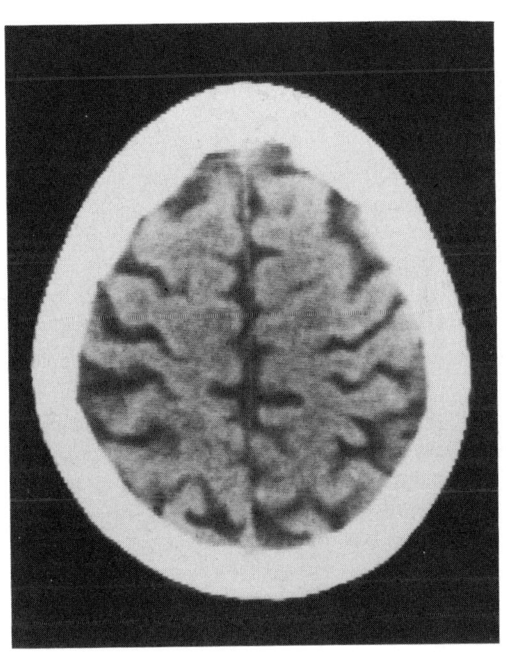

Alcoholism

A number of conditions may cause enlargement of cerebral sulci resembling atrophy. Alcoholic "atrophy" is common, possibly due to nutritional or hydration factors as well as to direct effects of ethanol. In some patients the enlarged sulci return to normal after successful treatment.

Other circumstances have also been associated with abnormal enlargement of cerebral sulci. These include malnutrition (anorexia nervosa or other psychiatric causes, as in Case 186), high doses of exogenous or endogenous steroids, multiple sclerosis, lupus cerebritis, acquired immune deficiency syndrome, and chronic renal disease (possibly related to dialysis and hydration or nutrition states).

When a young patient presents with enlarged sulci, these possibilities should be considered (along with presenile dementia disorders and toxic-anoxic insults).

CEREBRAL HEMIATROPHY WITH HEMICRANIAL HYPERTROPHY (DYKE-DAVIDOFF-MASSON SYNDROME)

Case 188A

69-year-old woman with a history of a "stroke" as an infant.

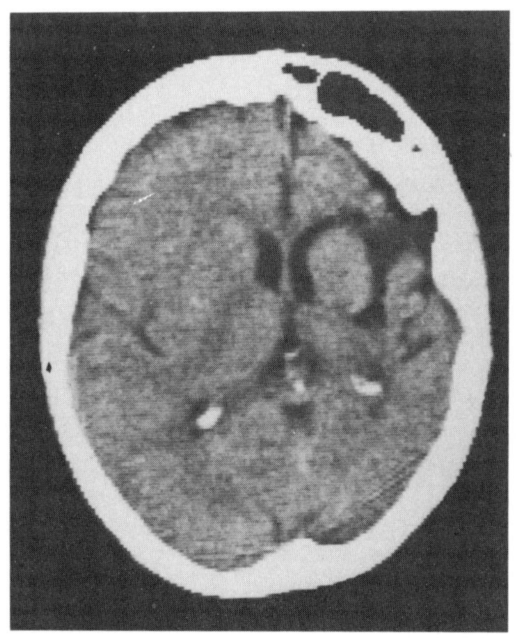

The interrelationship of brain growth and skull contour is demonstrated when a cerebrovascular accident in infancy or childhood damages one cerebral hemisphere, as in this case. The reduced cerebral volume leads to ipsilateral changes in calvarial morphology.

Here, the involved hemicranium is small, with eccentric falx position. The skull is thickened on the side of cerebral atrophy, and the ipsilateral sinuses and air cells are asymmetrically enlarged.

Case 188B

Same patient.

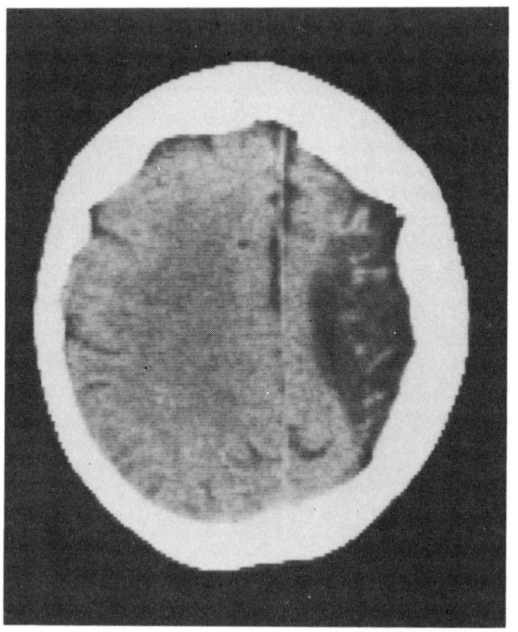

The small hemicranium, eccentric falx position, and thick calvarium on the side of cerebral atrophy are illustrated again.

STURGE-WEBER SYNDROME

Case 189A

24-year-old man with seizures.

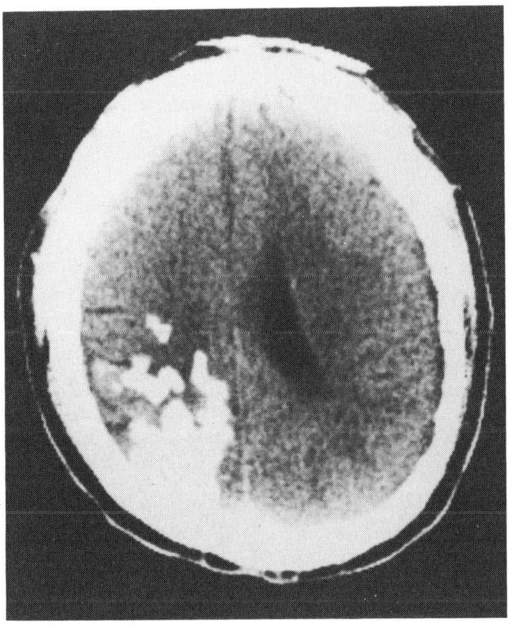

Case 189B

Same patient (wide window width).

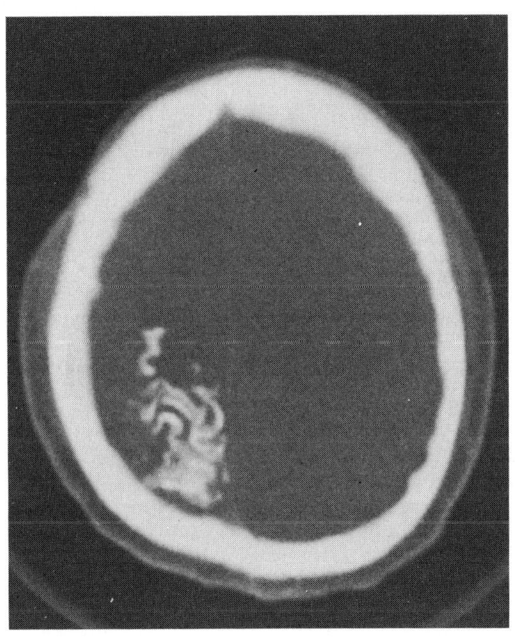

Sturge-Weber syndrome is one of the neurophacomatoses combining cutaneous and intracranial abnormalities. The external manifestation of the syndrome is a facial hemangioma or "port-wine stain" in the distribution of the first division of the trigeminal nerve.

This hallmark is associated with an ipsilateral venous angioma of the meninges, most common in the parieto-occipital region. (An alternative name for the syndrome is "encephalotrigeminal angiomatosis.") Cerebral cortex underlying the meningeal angioma exhibits a characteristic "tram-track" or "gyriform" pattern of dystrophic calcification. The calcification may be observed to develop in an infant or toddler over a period of weeks or months. Occasional patients with typical intracranial findings have no facial lesions.

Postcontrast scans may demonstrate vague, superficial enhancement in the region of calcification, possibly representing the meningeal angioma. Large superficial veins may be seen, reflecting an associated abnormality of cortical venous drainage with collateral flow away from the superior sagittal sinus.

Wide window settings demonstrate the typical gyriform pattern of calcification in this syndrome.

Associated cerebral atrophy is common and may be focal or hemispheric. In this case, atrophy of the hemisphere has resulted in a small hemicranium. The falx position is eccentric and the ipsilateral calvarium is thickened. The appearance is comparable with other examples of the Dyke-Davidoff-Masson syndrome, as seen in Case 188.

Gyriform calcification is probably a nonspecific response to cortical damage and can be seen in other circumstances (e.g., in children following encephalitis or meningitis [see Case 152], or after treatment for CNS leukemia).

REFERENCES

1. Allen J.H., Martin J.T., McLain L.W.: Computed tomography in cerebellar atrophic processes. *Radiology* 130:379–382, 1979.
2. Anders B.J., Lauer B.A., Foley L.C.: Computerized tomography to define CNS involvement in congenital cytomegalovirus infection. *Am. V. Dis. Child.* 134:795–797, 1980.
3. Artmann H., Gall M.V., Hacker H., et al.: Reversible enlargment of cerebral spinal fluid spaces in chronic alcoholics. *A.J.N.R.* 2:23–27, 1981.
4. Aubourg P., Diebler C.: Adrenoleukodystrophy—its diverse CT appearances and an evolutive or phenotypic variant; the leukodystrophy without adrenal insufficiency. *Neuroradiology* 24:33–42, 1982.
5. Bentson J., Reza M., Winter J., et al.: Steroids and apparent cerebral atrophy on computed tomography scans. *J. Comput. Assist. Tomogr.* 2:16–23, 1978.
6. Bhargava S., Tandon P.N.: Intracranial tuberculomas: A CT study. *Br. J. Radiol.* 53:935–945, 1980.
7. Bonstelle C.T.: Infectious processes of the brain, in Haaga J.R., Alfidi R.J. (eds.): *Computed Tomography of the Whole Body.* St. Louis, C.V. Mosby Co., 1983, pp. 110–135.
8. Byrd S.E., Locke G.E., Biggers S., et al.: The computed tomographic appearance of cerebral cysticercosis in adults and children. *Radiology* 144:819–823, 1982.
9. Carroll B.A., Lane B., Norman D., et al.: Diagnosis of progressive multifocal leukoencephalopathy by computed tomography. *Radiology* 122:137–141, 1977.
10. Centeno R.S., Bentson J.R., Mancuso A.A.: CT scanning in rhinocerebral mucormycosis and aspergillosis. *Radiology* 140:383–389, 1981.
11. Collins A.T., Cromwell L.D.: Computed tomography in the evaluation of congenital cerebral toxoplasmosis. *J. Comput. Assist. Tomogr.* 4:326–329, 1980.
12. Danziger A., Price H.I.: CT findings with cerebral hemiatrophy. *Neuroradiology* 19:269–271, 1980.
13. Danziger A., Price H., Schechter M.M.: An analysis of 113 intracranial infections. *Neuroradiology* 19:31–34, 1980.
14. De Leon M.J., George A.E., Ferris S.H., et al.: Positron emission tomography and computed tomography assessments of the aging human brain. *J. Comput. Assist. Tomogr.* 8:88–94, 1984.
15. Enzmann D.R., Britt R.H., Placone R.C. Jr.: Staging of human brain abscess by computed tomography. *Radiology* 146:703–708, 1983.
16. Enzmann D.R., Hayward R.W., Norman D., et al.: Cranial computed tomographic scan appearance of Sturge-Weber disease. *Radiology* 122:721–724, 1977.
17. Enzmann D.R., Norman D., Mani J., et al.: Computed tomography of granulomatous basal arachnoiditis. *Radiology* 120:341–344, 1976.
18. Gado M., Hughes C.P., Danziger W., et al.: Volumetric measurements of the cerebrospinal fluid spaces in demented subjects and controls. *Radiology* 144:535–538, 1982.
19. George A.E., de Leon M.J., Rosenbloom S., et al.: Ventricular volume and cognitive deficit; A computed tomographic study. *Radiology* 149:493–498, 1983.
20. Goto K., Ishii N., Fukasawa H.: Diffuse white matter disease in the geriatric population. *Radiology* 140:687–695, 1981.
21. Haughton V.M., Ho K.C., Williams A.L., et al.: CT detection of demyelinated plaques in multiple sclerosis. *A.J.R.* 132:213–215, 1979.
22. Heinz E.R., Drayer B.P., Haenggeli C.A., et al.: Computed tomography in white-matter disease. *Radiology* 130:371–378, 1979.
23. Heinz E.R., Martinez J., Haenggeli A.: Reversibility of cerebral atrophy in anorexia nervosa and Cushing's syndrome. *J. Comput. Assist. Tomogr.* 1:415–418, 1977.
24. Huckman M.S.: Computed tomography in the diagnosis of degenerative brain disease. *Radiol. Clin. North. Am.* 20:169–183, 1982.
25. Inoue Y., Fukuda T., Takashima S., et al.: Adrenoleukodystrophy: New CT findings. *A.J.N.R.* 4:951–954, 1983.
26. Kingsley D.P., Kendall B.E.: CT of the adverse effects of therapeutic radiation of the central nervous system. *A.J.N.R.* 2:453–460, 1981.
27. Kumpe D.A., Rao C.V., Garcia J., et al.: Intracranial neurosarcoidosis. *J. Comput. Assist. Tomogr.* 3:324–330, 1979.
28. LeMay M.: Radiologic changes of the aging brain and skull. *A.J.N.R.* 5:269–275, 1984.
29. Loizou L.A., Kendall B.E., Marshall J.: Subcortical arteriosclerotic encephalopathy: A clinical and radiological investigation. *J. Neurol. Neurosurg. Psych.* 44:294–304, 1981.
30. McCormick G.F., Zee C.S., Heiden J.: Cysticercosis cerebri: Review of 127 cases. *Arch. Neurol.* 39:534–539, 1982.
31. McGeachie R.E., Fleming J.O., Sharer L.R., et al.: Diagnosis of Pick's disease by computed tomography. *J. Comput. Assist. Tomogr.* 3:113–115, 1979.
32. Ostrov S.G., Quencer R.M., Gaylis N.B., et al.: Cerebral atrophy in systemic lupus erythematosis: Steroid or disease-induced phenomenon? *A.J.N.R.* 3:21–23, 1982.
33. Packer R.J., Bilaniuk L.T., Zimmerman R.A.: CT parenchymal abnormalities in bacterial meningitis: Clinical significance. *J. Comput. Assist. Tomogr.* 6:1064–1068, 1982.
34. Palacios E., Rodriquez-Carbajal J., Taveras J.M. (eds.): *Cysticercosis of the Central Nervous System.* Springfield, Ill., Charles C. Thomas, 1983.
35. Quencer R.M.: Maturation of normal primate white matter: Computed tomographic correlation. *A.J.N.R.* 3:365–372, 1982.
36. Reith K.G., DiChiro G., Cromwell L.D., et al.: Primary demyelinating disease simulating glioma of the corpus callosum. *J. Neurosurg.* 55:620–624, 1981.
37. Rosenbloom S., Buchholz D., Kumar A.J., et al.: Evolution of central pontine myelinolysis on CT. *A.J.N.R.* 5:110–112, 1984.
38. Rovira M., Romero F., Torrent D.: Study of tuberculous meningitis by CT. *Neuroradiology* 19:137–141, 1980.
39. Sadhu V.K., Handel S.F., Pinto R.S., et al.: Neuroradiologic diagnosis of subdural empyema and CT limitations. *A.J.N.R.* 1:39–44, 1980.
40. Stober T., Wussow W., Schimrigk K.: Bicaudate diameter: The most specific and simple CT parameter in the diagnosis of Huntington's disease. *Neuroradiology* 26:25–28, 1984.
41. Vinuela F.V., Fox A.J., Debrun G.M., et al.: New perspectives in computed tomography of multiple sclerosis. *A.J.N.R.* 3:277–281, 1982.
42. Wang A.M., Morris J.H., Hickey W.F., et al.: Unusual CT patterns of multiple sclerosis. *A.J.N.R.* 4:47–50, 1983.
43. Wang A.M., Skias D.D., Rumbaugh C.L., et al.: Central nervous system changes after radiation therapy and/or chemotherapy: correlation of CT and autopsy findings. *A.J.N.R.* 4:466–471, 1983.
44. Whelan M.A., Hilal S.K.: Computed tomography as a guide in the diagnosis and follow-up of brain abscesses. *Radiology* 135:663–671, 1980.
45. Whelan M.A., Kricheff I.I., Handler M., et al.: Acquired immunodeficiency syndrome: Cerebral computed tomographic manifestations. *Radiology* 149:477–484, 1983.
46. Whelan M.A., Stern J., deNapoli R.A.: The computed tomographic spectrum of intracranial mycosis: Correlation with histopathology. *Radiology* 141:703–707, 1981.
47. Zee C.S., Segall H.D., Miller C., et al.: Unusual neuroradiological features of intracranial cysticercosis. *Radiology* 137:397–407, 1980.
48. Zeumer H., Schonsky B., Sturm K.W.: Predominant white matter involvement in subcortical arteriosclerotic encephalopathy. *J. Comput. Assist. Tomogr.* 4:14–19, 1980.
49. Zimmerman R.D., Leeds N.E., Danziger A.: Subdural empyema: CT findings. *Radiology* 150:417–422, 1984.
50. Zimmerman R.D., Russell E.J., Leeds N.E.: CT in the early diagnosis of herpes encephalitis. *A.J.R.* 134:61–66, 1980.

CHAPTER 8

TRAUMATIC LESIONS

Case 190

2-year-old child injured in an auto accident.

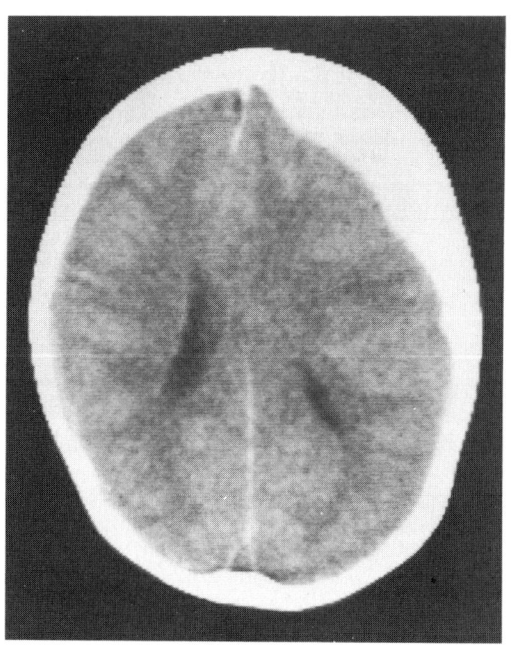

Acute subdural hemorrhages form a layer of high attenuation closely applied to the calvarium or dura. The subdural space is easily dissected by hematomas, which spread over a wide area while remaining relatively thin. This crescentic shape contrasts with the thick, biconvex morphology of epidural hematomas, as seen in Cases 206 and 207. Small subdural hematomas may blend with the skull and can be overlooked if scans are viewed only at narrow window widths.

Subdural hematomas may appear thin on single sections while surrounding large portions of a hemisphere. Such extensive hematomas can cause more significant cerebral compression and herniations than might be expected from their narrow diameter. Mass effect is often compounded by associated cerebral contusion and edema.

Many acute subdural hematomas are caused by injured cortical arteries rather than by torn bridging veins, as has been traditionally taught.

Case 191

30-year-old man. Acute subdural hematoma (and subarachnoid hemorrhage) on the superior surface of the tentorium (postcontrast scan).

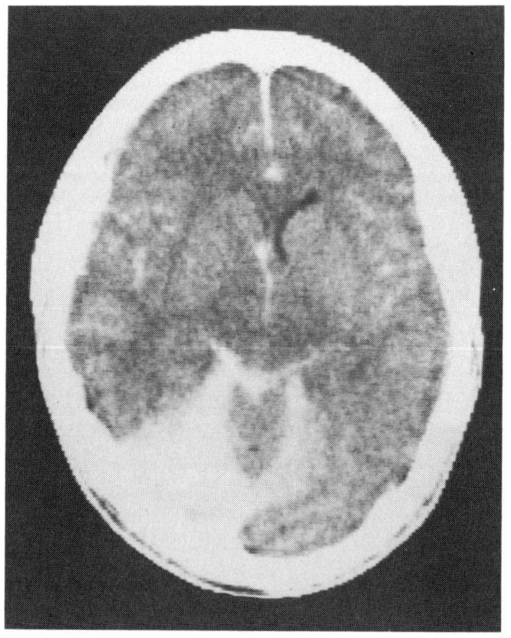

Although most subdural hematomas are found adjacent to the calvarium, they may also occur along the tentorium or falx. In this case, a thin layer of subdural and subarachnoid hemorrhage outlines the superior surface of the tentorium. A coronal scan of this hematoma would resemble the thickened tentorium in Case 162.

The lateral margin of the tentorial density continues the 45° angle of the petrous ridge, while the medial margins form a chalice or "Y" configuration enclosing the midline cerebellar vermis. Compare the location of this hematoma with the subdural empyema seen along the inferior surface of the tentorium in Case 165.

INTERHEMISPHERIC SUBDURAL HEMATOMAS

Case 192

43-year-old man.

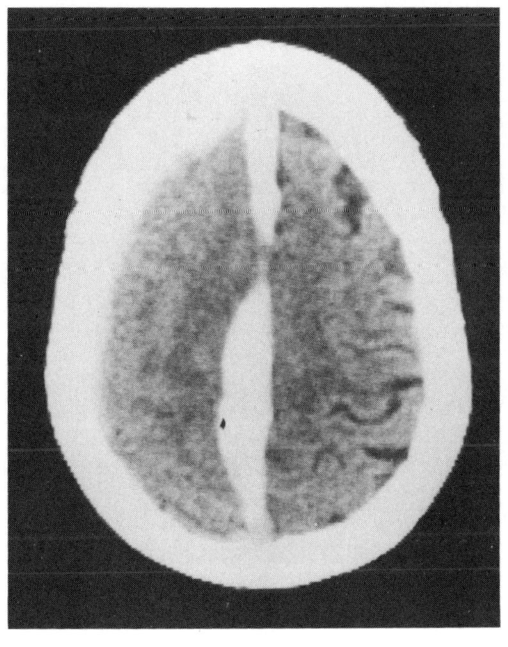

Interhemispheric subdural hematomas may accompany convexity accumulations or occur as isolated lesions. Interhemispheric clot demonstrates a flat medial margin along the falx and a variably thick lateral extension.

In this case, a thin convexity subdural hematoma merges with the inner table. Mass effect effaces sulci of the involved hemisphere.

Posterior interhemispheric subdural hematomas (near the tentorium) are commonly seen in children subjected to shaking injuries. Such hematomas are an important hallmark of the "battered child syndrome." Their discovery should lead to careful assessment of the patient and family. (Subhyaloid retinal hemorrhages are a confirmatory clue to child abuse.)

Case 193

33-year-old man.

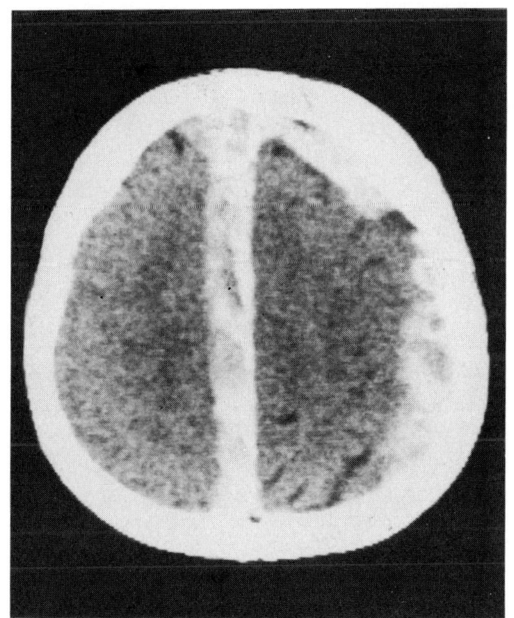

In this case a large interhemispheric subdural hematoma is associated with a contralateral convexity hematoma. Although both hematomas are acute, they are inhomogeneous and contain areas of relative isodensity (see discussion of Case 194).

ACUTE SUBDURAL HEMATOMAS: LOW-ATTENUATION COMPONENTS AND COMPARTMENTALIZATION

Case 194

83-year-old man.

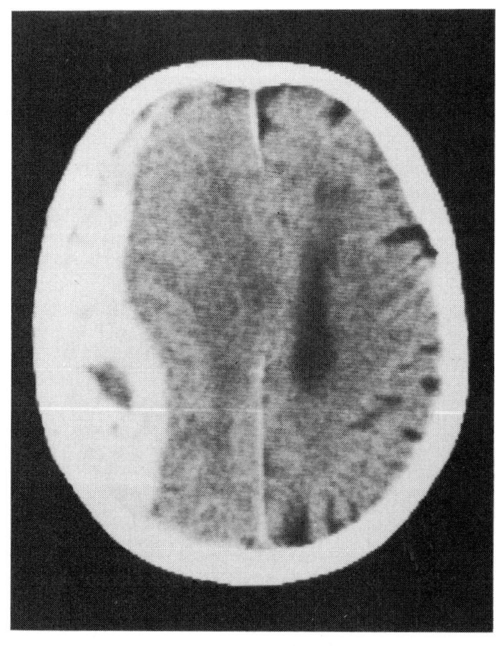

Low-attenuation pockets are occasionally found within acute subdural (and epidural) hematomas. These areas may represent older clot surrounded by fresh blood, loculated plasma that has separated from red cells, or encysted spinal fluid from an associated arachnoid tear. The diagnostic features of the hematoma (configuration and overall density) are rarely obscured.

Case 195

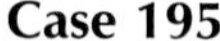

60-year-old man.

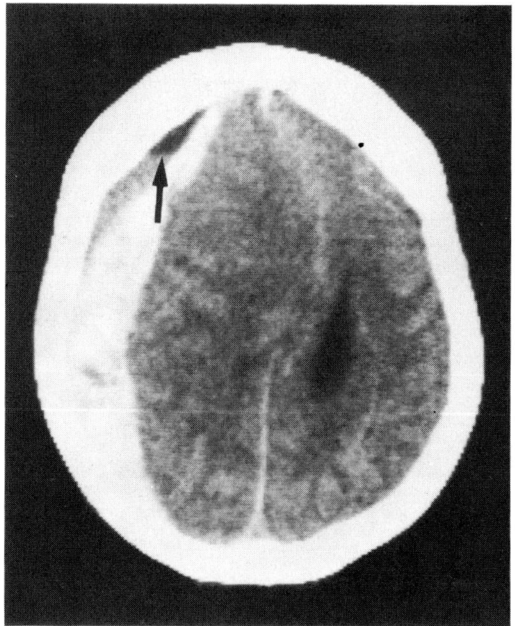

Some subdural hematomas demonstrate layers of varying attenuation. Such compartmentalization suggests that the acute hematoma is superimposed on preceding subacute or chronic collections.

In this case, a small subacute hematoma with a sedimentation level *(arrow)* is seen between the acute hematoma and the frontal bone. The sharpness of a "hematocrit" or sedimentation level within a subdural hematoma depends on the amount of mixing by patient motion prior to the scan.

Case 196

75-year-old woman.

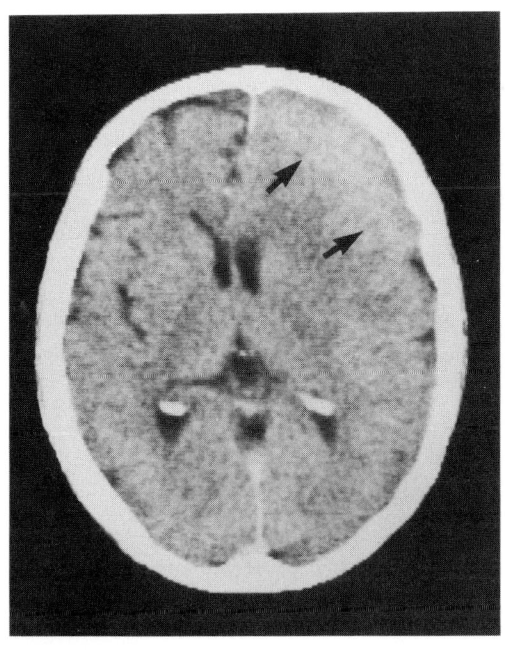

The attenuation values of subdural hematomas decrease over time, passing through an isodense period in a matter of weeks. The hematoma may be poorly defined on noncontrast scans performed at this time.

True isodensity is rare; high-resolution images will usually show slightly abnormal attenuation within the subdural collection, as in this case *(arrows)*. Even poorly visualized hematomas are evidenced by the associated mass effect (ventricular compression, effacement of cortical gyri, and medial bowing or "buckling" of the gray-white matter interface).

Isodense subdural hematomas may be seen acutely in anemic patients, or in situations such as that in Case 197.

Case 197

49-year-old man.

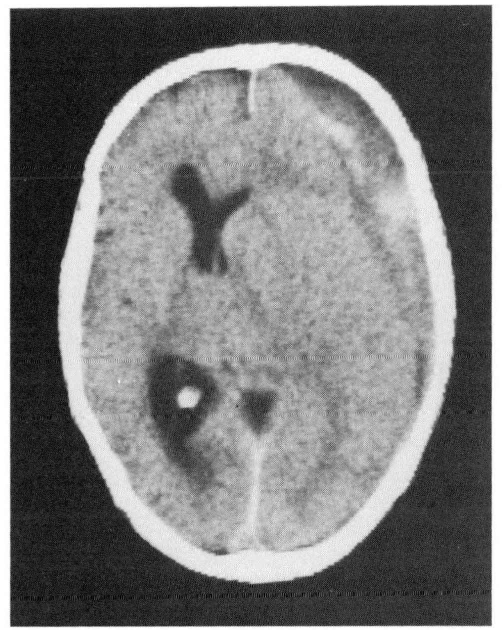

Recurrent hemorrhage may develop within an aging subdural hematoma, as seen here. The resulting mixture of high and low attenuation is occasionally isodense.

Recurrence of bleeding from the original source or from vascular membranes is probably an important mechanism in the growth of subdural hematomas.

A pseudo-"empty triangle sign" is present on this scan (see Case 278).

BILATERAL SUBDURAL HEMATOMAS

Case 198

65-year-old woman.

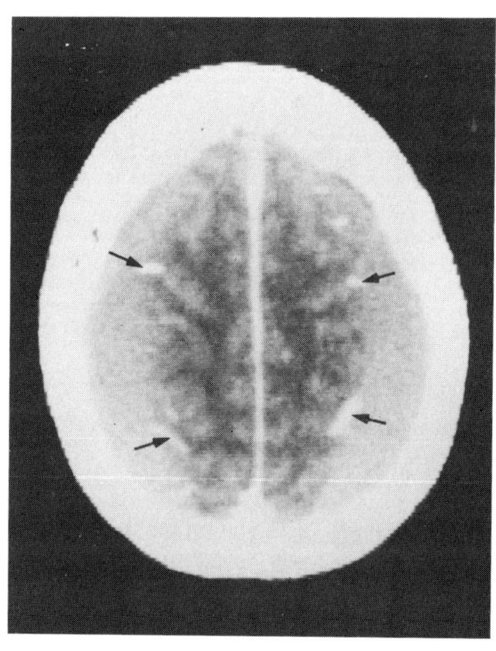

Approximately 25% of subacute and chronic subdural hematomas are bilateral. Bilateral hematomas of approximately equal size may cause symmetrical distortions of anatomy. If the hematomas themselves are nearly isodense, the presence of balancing mass effect may be overlooked.

In this case, a noncontrast scan had demonstrated an abnormal absence of vertex sulci. A follow-up scan with contrast infusion clearly shows the slightly dense, bilateral subdural hematomas. The interface between the hematomas and compressed cortex is further defined by several large cortical veins *(arrows)*.

Case 199

72-year-old man.

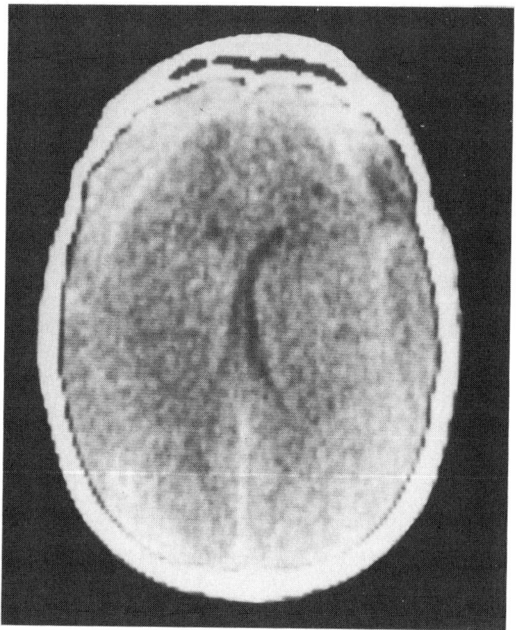

An important clue to the presence of balanced mass effect from bilateral subdural hematomas is the typical deformity of the lateral ventricles. Compression and medial displacement of the ventricular bodies change their shape to elongated slits. The narrowed and straightened ventricles are abnormally close to the midline and parallel to the sagittal plane.

These "parasagittal parentheses" are characteristic of bilateral subdural hematomas. They should suggest the diagnosis even when the hematomas are obscured by artifact or isodensity.

Extension of the patient's head will cause normal ventricles to appear elongated on axial scans. However, the ventricular bodies are not straightened and flattened as illustrated in this case.

CHRONIC SUBDURAL HEMATOMAS

Case 200

79-year-old man with history of multiple falls.

The density and morphology of subdural hematomas are time-dependent. Attenuation values decrease as the hematoma ages, so that chronic collections are well-defined as low-density regions. The initially thin and crescentic shape of a subdural hematoma usually widens over time, with the medial margin becoming straight or even convex.

As mentioned in Case 197, the mechanism of enlargement may include recurrent hemorrhage. Possibly reflecting this process (and the liquefaction that usually occurs by 2 to 3 weeks of age), chronic subdural hematomas may contain high-attenuation sediment *(black arrows)*. If the sedimenting component is isodense, the size of the hematoma may be underestimated as representing only the low-attenuation region.

A well-organized subdural membrane usually develops by three to four weeks. The membrane typically demonstrates linear enhancement adjacent to the cortical surface *(white arrows)*. Loculation of enhancing membranes may present a confusing appearance (see Case 229).

Case 201

77-year-old man with dense hemiparesis and lethargy, thought to have had a cerebrovascular accident.

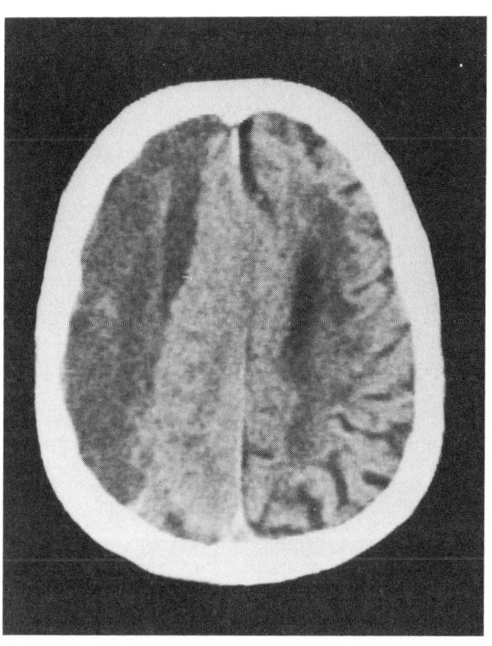

Chronic subdural hematomas may become very large as they gradually displace spinal fluid from the subarachnoid spaces of an atrophic hemisphere. Here, the subdural collection occupies more of the hemicranium than the compressed brain.

Symptoms may develop acutely when the expanding mass exceeds the buffering capacity of large ventricles and sulci. For this reason, chronic subdural hematomas are occasionally discovered in elderly patients being evaluated for "strokes." (Compare with the presentation in Cases 10 and 37.)

Hemiparesis may be contralateral or ipsilateral to the hematoma. The latter occurrence reflects brain stem displacement causing pressure on the contralateral cerebral peduncle.

Case 202

74-year-old man with head trauma three days before the scan.

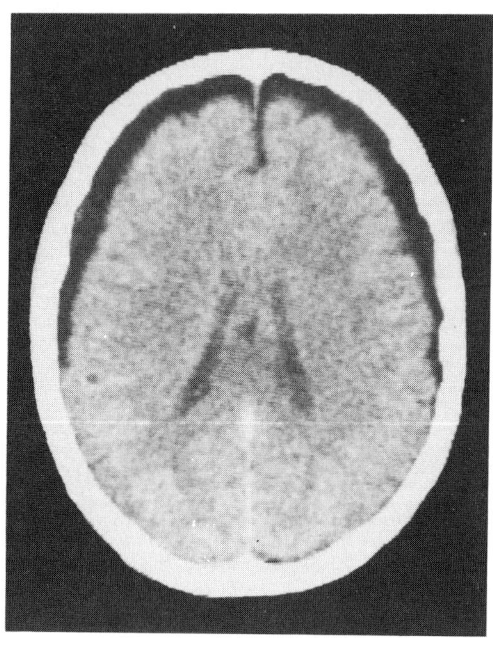

Some patients develop acute low-density subdural collections following head trauma. These accumulations have been termed "subdural hygromas" because they usually contain clear spinal fluid. The fluid apparently gains access to the subdural space through an arachnoid tear. Subdural hygromas are most often seen in elderly persons and young children. Most of these collections remain small and resolve spontaneously.

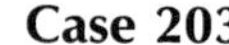

Case 203

79-year-old man.

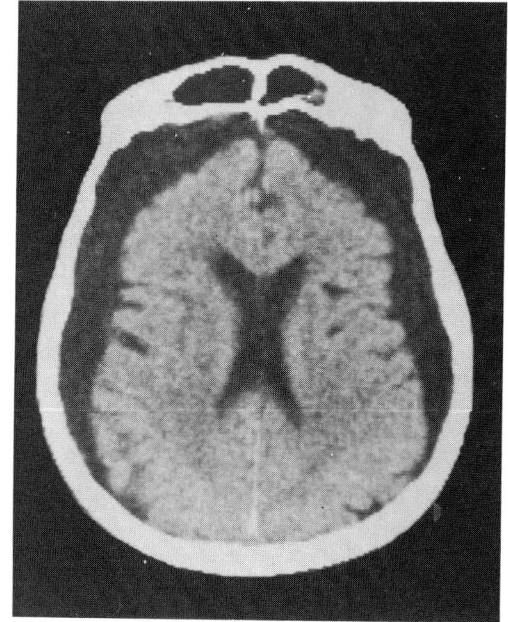

Occasional subdural hygromas enlarge and exert significant mass effect. The mechanism of enlargement is unclear but presumably involves a one-way valve for entrance of spinal fluid.

In this case, the scan suggests bilateral chronic subdural hematomas with characteristic ventricular morphology (see Case 199). However, the history indicated rapid deterioration after recent trauma, and surgery demonstrated the clear fluid of hygromas.

DIFFERENTIAL DIAGNOSIS: WIDE EXTRACEREBRAL FLUID SPACES IN AN ELDERLY PATIENT

Case 204

72-year-old man suffering recent head trauma.

Case 205

70-year-old man.

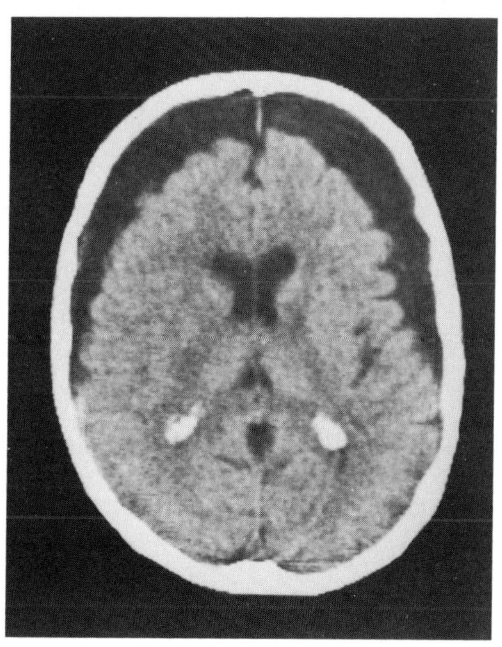

Subdural Hygromas.

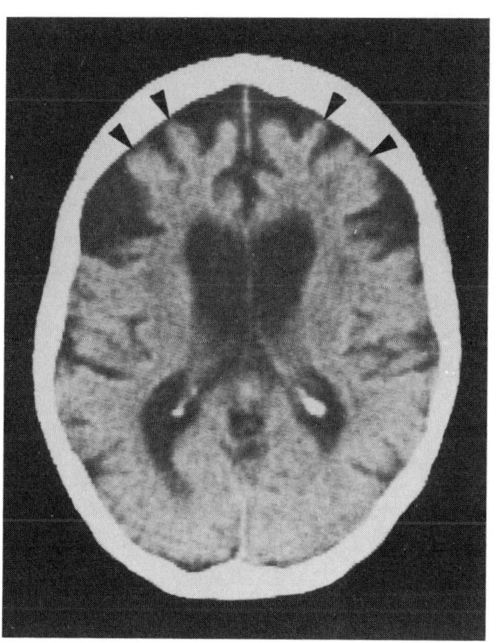

Atrophy.

Low-attenuation subdural collections (hygromas or chronic hematomas) are sometimes confused with widened subarachnoid spaces due to cerebral atrophy. The two processes are usually distinguishable on the basis of cortical contour and gyral position.

The margin of compressed cortex beneath a subdural collection is abnormally smooth, while the outline of atrophic cortex is irregular due to widened sulci. The tips of cortical gyri seldom retract significantly from the inner table even in the presence of marked atrophy (see *arrows,* Case 205). In contrast, the gyral fronds are unequivocally displaced from the calvarium by subdural collections.

A distinction between chronic subdural hematoma and subdural hygroma may be impossible on a single scan. In Case 204, the low-density collections had been observed to triple in size over a one-week period, implying predominant hygroma fluid. (A small amount of blood is present posteriorly on the right.)

Case 206

28-year-old man found in an unresponsive state.

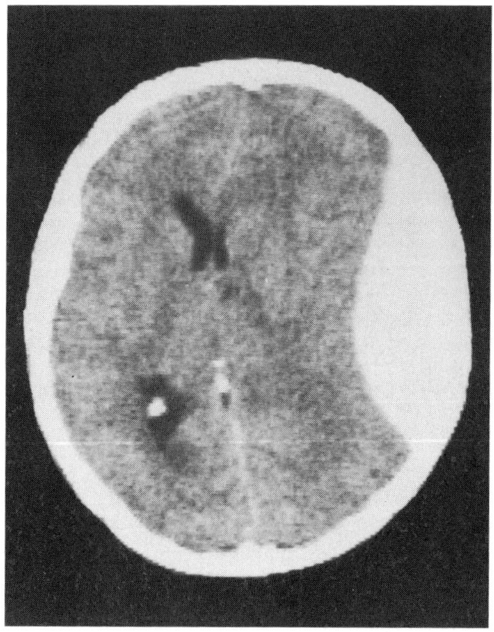

The dura functions as periosteum for the inner table and is tightly adherent to the skull. For this reason, hemorrhage accumulating between the calvarium and the dura remains relatively confined. An epidural hematoma acquires a thick "waist" with a medially convex margin before sufficient pressure has developed to strip the dura for further expansion. This biconvex or lentiform shape contrasts with the thin crescent of acute subdural hematomas (see Case 190).

Supratentorial epidural hematomas may enlarge rapidly and are considered a surgical emergency. Most are due to lacerations of branches from the middle meningeal artery at the point of skull fracture, as in this case.

Case 207

12-year-old girl with an occipital skull fracture after being struck by a car.

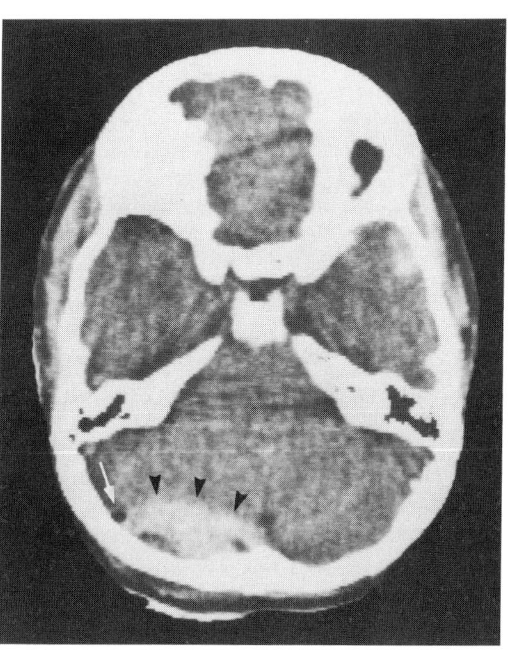

Posterior fossa epidural hematomas are usually caused by venous bleeding from torn dural sinuses. They present less acutely and may have less characteristic morphology than supratentorial epidurals. Regardless of shape, an extracerebral hematoma is established as epidural if it crosses the plane of the tentorium (or falx).

In this case the posterior fossa appears "tight," with poor visualization of the fourth ventricle. The biconvex hematoma continued superiorly across the plane of the tentorium. Other findings include an air bubble *(arrow)* of pneumocephalus adjacent to the hematoma and contusion of the contralateral temporal lobe.

OTHER DENSE EPIDURAL LESIONS

Case 208

76-year-old woman. Multiple myeloma (postcontrast scan).

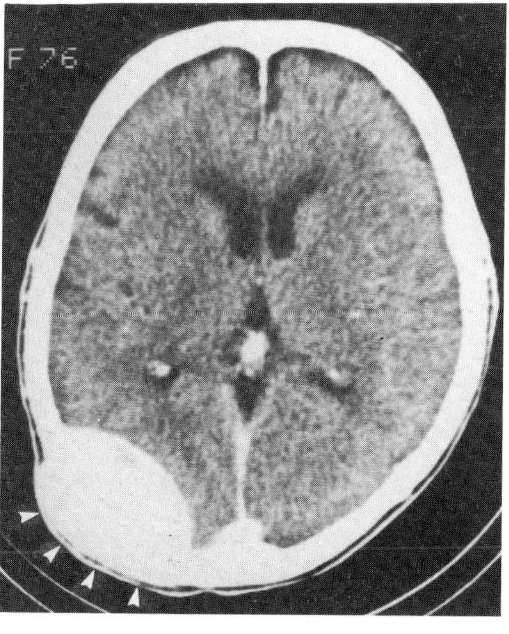

The familiar biconvex configuration of epidural hematomas may also be seen with epidural masses. Epidural tumors usually represent extension of calvarial metastases, as in this case. An identical appearance may be seen in children with metastatic neuroblastoma (and, rarely, leukemia).

Clues to the correct diagnosis include contrast enhancement, destruction of the calvarium (which would be more apparent at wider window settings), and the extracranial extent of the mass *(arrows)*.

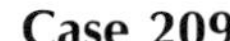

Case 209

57-year-old woman. Multiple myeloma (coronal scan postcontrast).

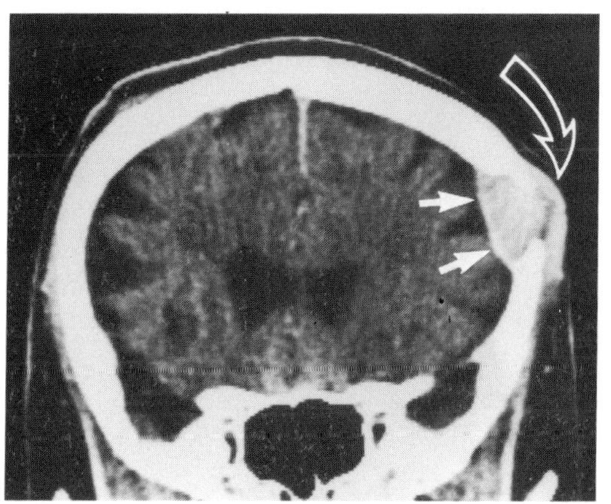

Coronal scans are often helpful in assessing the intracranial extent of a calvarial lesion. Here the enhancing dura *(straight arrows)* is medially displaced by the mass expanding from the diploic space. An associated "lump" of extracranial extension *(curved arrow)* had caused the patient to see her physician.

Epidural extension of calvarial disease is most commonly seen in metastatic lesions (e.g., carcinomas of the breast and prostate), but occasionally occurs with primary tumors (e.g., calvarial epidermoids, eosinophilic granuloma).

CT is an excellent means of obtaining a cross-sectional display of skull lesions. The extent of table involvement is well demonstrated along with the adjacent soft-tissue masses and other diagnostic features (e.g., calcification or "button sequestra").

Case 210

36-year-old achondroplastic dwarf noted to be somnolent after a beating.

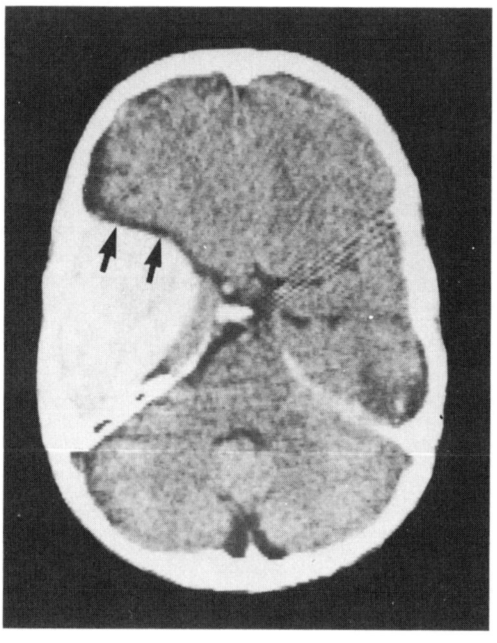

The dura in achondroplasia is abnormally adherent to the skull. As a result, the very thick morphology of this epidural hematoma represents an exaggeration of the normal restraining mechanism dicussed in Case 206.

The anterior margin of the hematoma *(arrows)* is shaped like the sphenoid wing, suggesting confinement by dura tethered along the sphenoid ridge. These findings were confirmed surgically. (The patient recovered completely.)

Case 211

27-year-old man, one day after head trauma and negative admission CT scan.

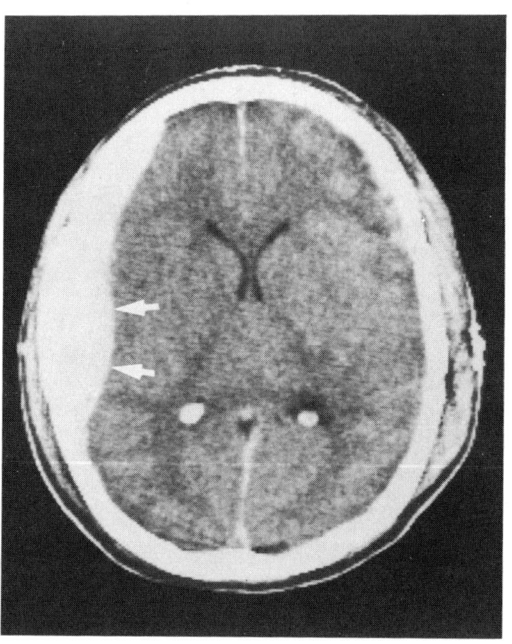

Delayed post-traumatic epidural hematomas are much less common than delayed intracerebral hemorrhages (see Case 218).

A second unusual feature of this case is the relatively thin and elongated shape of the hemorrhage. The configuration resembles an acute subdural hematoma, but the biconvex posterior component *(arrows)* establishes the correct diagnosis.

ISODENSE COMPONENTS IN EPIDURAL HEMATOMAS

Case 212

26-year-old man.

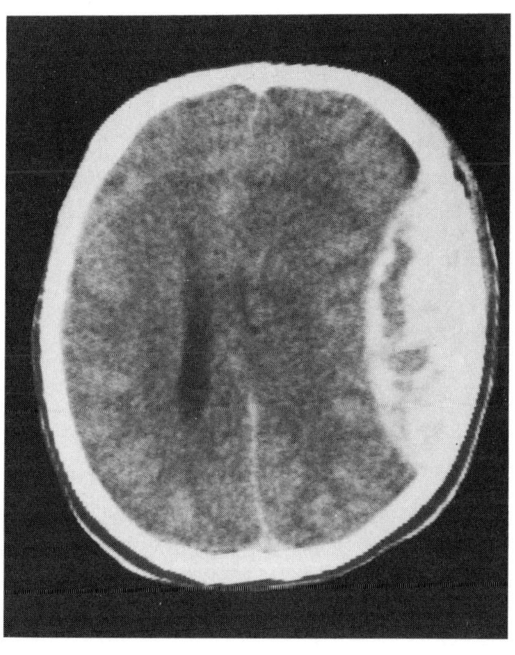

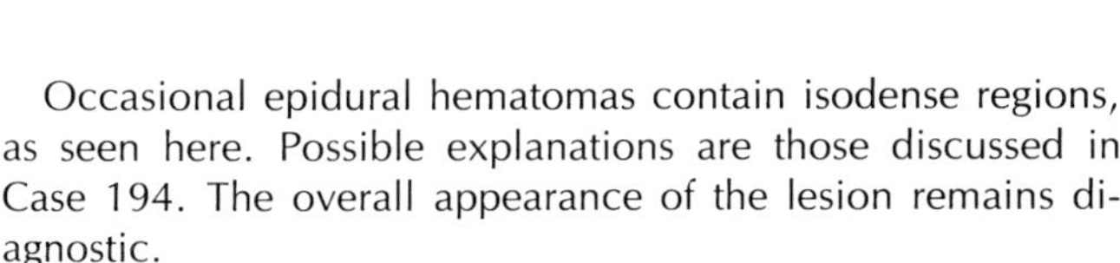

Occasional epidural hematomas contain isodense regions, as seen here. Possible explanations are those discussed in Case 194. The overall appearance of the lesion remains diagnostic.

Case 213

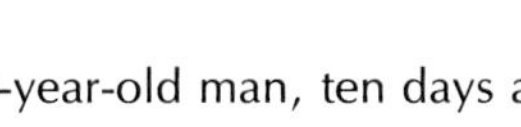

29-year-old man, ten days after ventriculostomy and craniotomy for a colloid cyst.

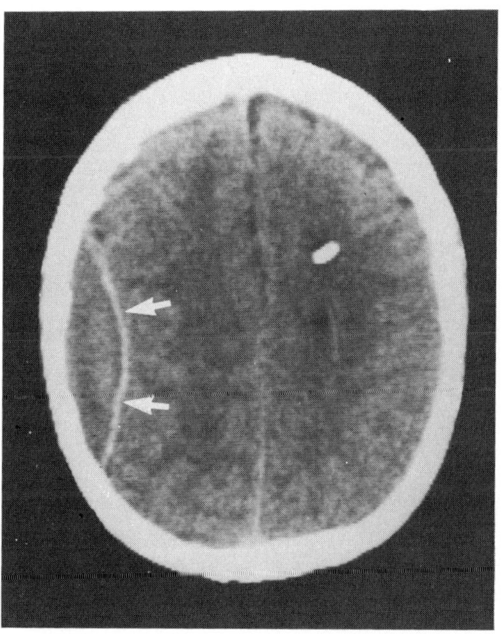

Few patients tolerate epidural hematomas long enough to allow the development of subacute attenuation changes. This epidural collection had been denser initially, appearing to contain a mixutre of blood and spinal fluid. The dense line along the medial margin of the hematoma represents the displaced dura. (Compare with the enhancing membrane of a chronic subdural hematoma, as seen in Case 200, and to the displaced dura in Case 209.)

Case 214

61-year-old man who fell, striking the back of his head.

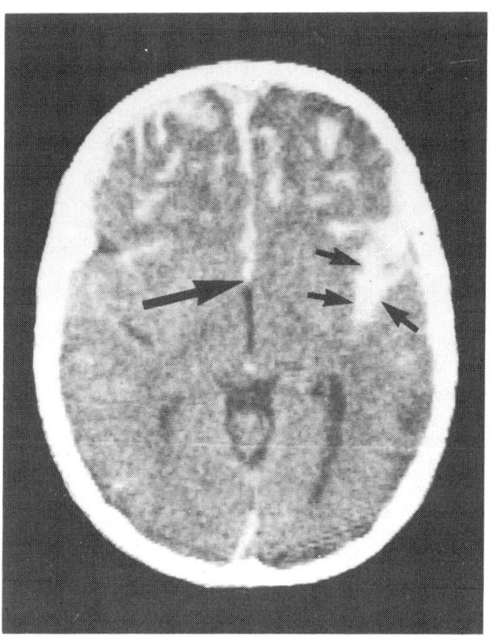

Post-traumatic intracerebral hematomas vary widely in size and number. In some cases, a region of injured brain is filled with many small hemorrhages, as seen here in the frontal lobes. This contusion pattern is soon accompanied by adjacent edema and corresponds to the surgical findings of "pulped brain."

Subarachnoid blood has accumulated in the anterior interhemispheric fissure, outlining its interface with the third ventricle at the lamina terminalis *(large arrow)*. Sufficient subarachnoid blood to fill the left sylvian cistern *(small arrows)* is unusual following trauma. Primary subarachnoid hemorrhage might be considered if the pattern of frontal contusion were less characteristic.

Case 215

34-year-old man admitted after three days in a detoxification center when his unintelligible speech failed to improve.

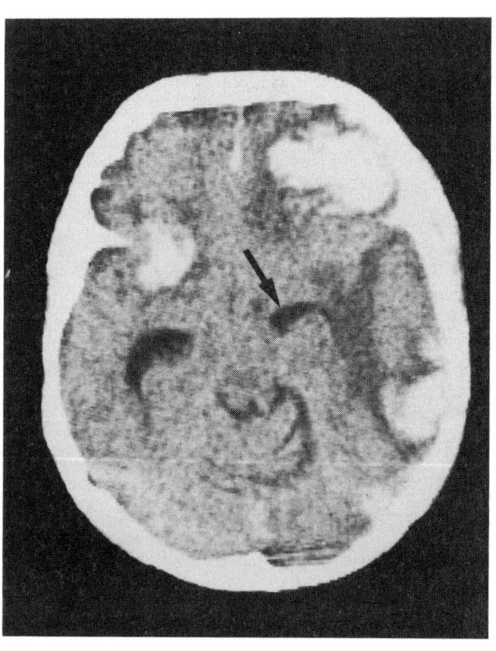

Many patients with head trauma suffer large, localized intracerebral hemorrhages. Hematomas often develop in regions initially demonstrating scattered contusion (see Case 218).

Marked edema may exacerbate the mass effect of post-traumatic hemorrhage. Here, the left temporal horn *(arrow)* is displaced medially, with uncal herniation obliterating the suprasellar cistern and compressing the brain stem.

Clues to the traumatic origin of these intracerebral hemorrhages include multiplicity and characteristic location (see Cases 216 and 217).

Case 216

79-year-old man who fell backward and sustained an occipital skull fracture.

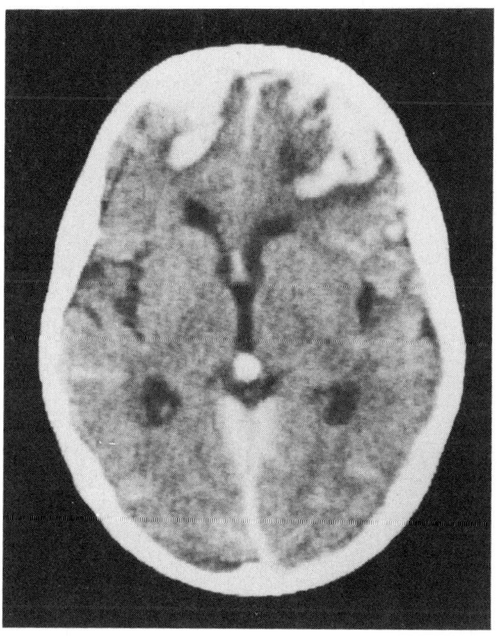

Cerebral injury may be located directly across from the site of head trauma. These "contra-coup" contusions are probably caused when the brain recoils within the calvarium, moving away from the impact region and striking the opposite side of the skull.

The pattern of bifrontal hematomas in patients with occipital skull fractures (as in this case) is a common illustration of this phenomenon. Another common site of cerebral contusion is the anterior temporal lobe, which is easily bruised against the bony margins of the middle cranial fossa.

Case 216 also demonstrates interhemispheric subdural hematomas and scattered subarachnoid blood. A simple fall from the standing position can cause this extensive intracranial hemorrhage in elderly patients (see also Case 214).

Case 217

29-year-old man.

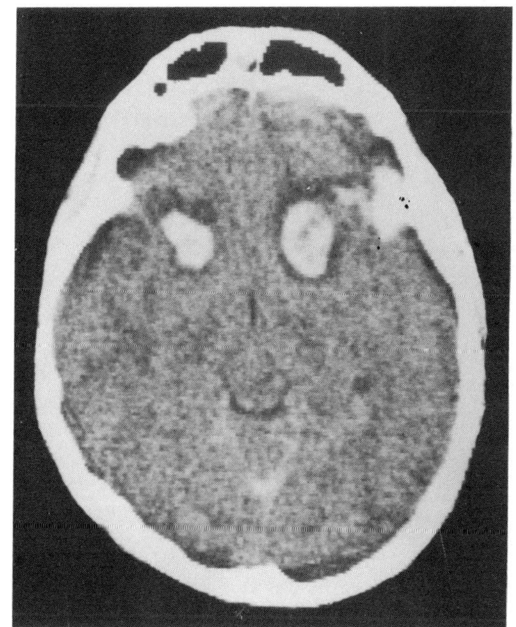

An unusual but characteristic location for post-traumatic intracerebral hemorrhage is the inferior frontotemporal region. Contusion of the brain in this area may occur against the underlying sphenoid ridge, with hemorrhages sometimes resembling imprints of the anterior clinoid processes (as in this case).

Such characteristic hematomas may establish the cause of intracerebral hemorrhage in an otherwise ambiguous context.

Case 218A

2-year-old girl struck by a car. Scan on day 1.

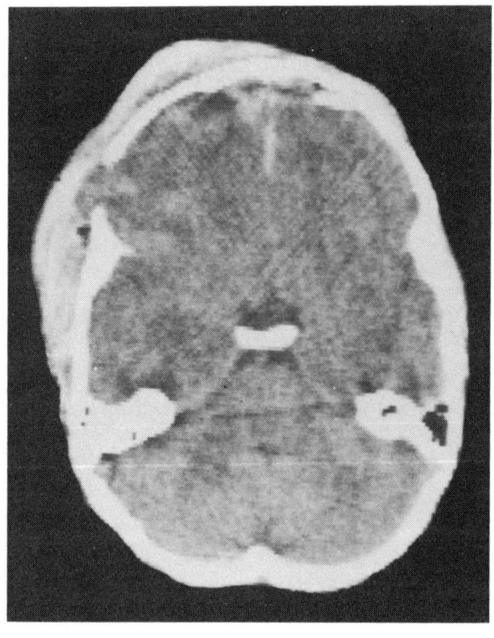

Computed tomographic scans often demonstrate the development or marked enlargement of post-traumatic intracerebral hemorrhages occurring hours or days after injury. Delayed post-traumatic extracerebral hematomas have also been noted (see Case 211).

This phenomenon should be suspected in any trauma patient whose condition deteriorates or fails to improve as expected. The appearance of widespread contusion, as seen in the right frontal lobe in this case, is often the precursor of significant delayed hemorrhage.

Case 218B

Same patient. Scan on day 2.

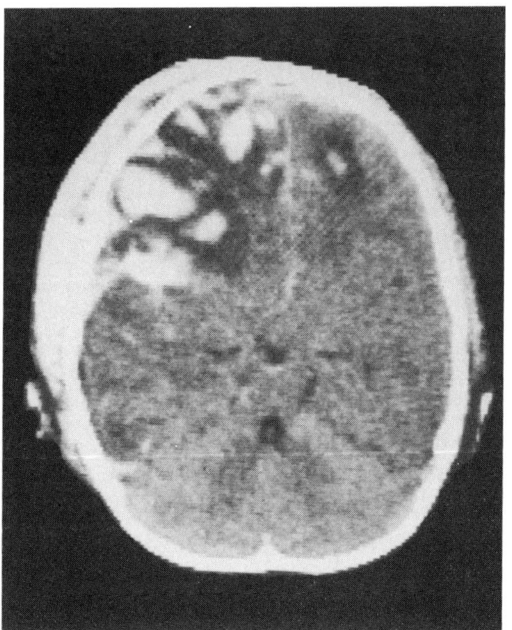

Within 20 hours, the contused right frontal lobe has developed multinodular hematomas and marked edema. A small hematoma is seen on the contralateral side.

In some cases, the development of delayed post-traumatic intracerebral hemorrhages may be facilitated by evacuation of tamponading subdural or epidural hematomas. In other instances (including this case) delayed hemorrhage occurs without surgical intervention.

POST-TRAUMATIC CEREBRAL SWELLING

Case 219

24-year-old man injured in a motorcycle accident.
Generalized swelling.

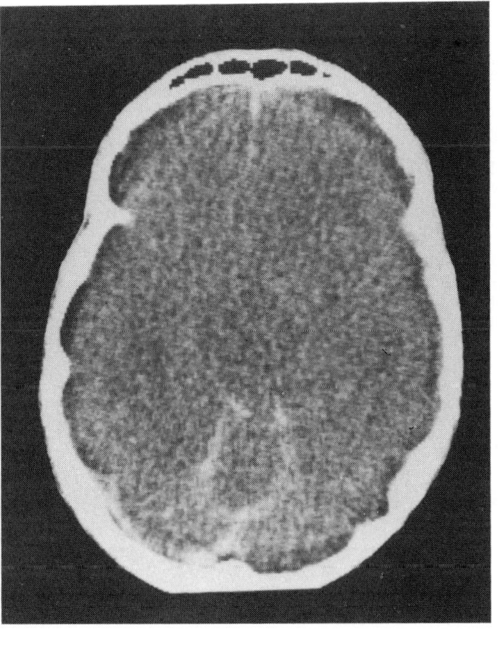

Another dangerous consequence of head trauma is nonhemorrhagic cerebral swelling. The swelling often includes a component of increased cerebral blood volume due to loss of vasomotor tone. Cerebral attenuation values may be little changed or prominently decreased, and involvement may be local or generalized.

In this case the cerebral hemispheres are diffusely swollen, with extensive edema causing uniformly decreased attenuation. Widespread mass effect has completely effaced the subarachnoid spaces, including cisterns at the tentorial hiatus. Elevated intracranial pressure and brain stem compression may be assumed when this appearance is encountered.

The relative density of the falx and tentorium (and basal vessels) in these cases probably represents a combination of margination by adjacent low-density tissue and vascular stasis due to high intracranial pressure.

Case 220

31-year-old man scanned nine days after head trauma.
Localized swelling with secondary infarction.

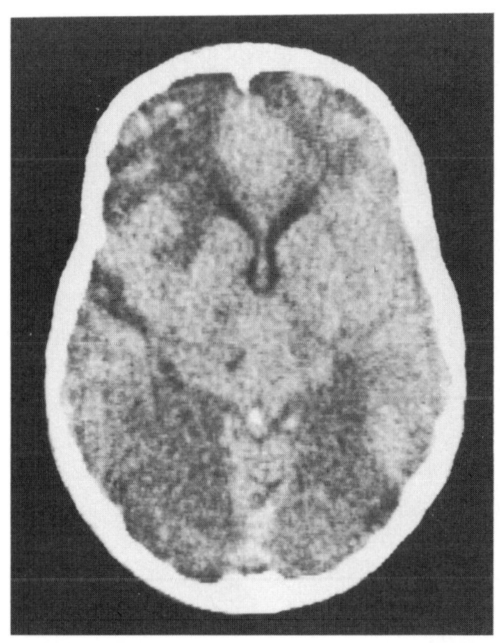

Localized post-traumatic cerebral edema can act as a mass lesion in the absence of hemorrhage. In this case, malignant bifrontal edema led to bilateral uncal herniation. The large low-density regions in the occipital lobes represent secondary infarction of the posterior cerebral artery distributions (due to compression of the arteries at the tentorial margin by the herniation process).

This scan demonstrates the contrast between the frond-like, cortical-sparing configuration of cerebral edema (frontal lobes) and the smooth, uniform involvement of gray and white matter seen in cerebral infarction (occipital lobes).

Case 221

28-year-old woman who was severely beaten.
Depressed skull fracture.

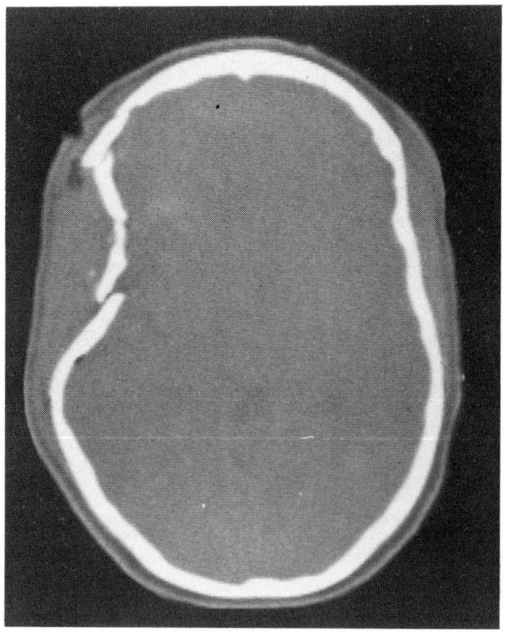

Depressed skull fractures are well evaluated in the axial plane of CT scans. These fractures are usually comminuted and are often compound. Scans demonstrate the degree of depression and localize fragments of bone for surgical debridement.

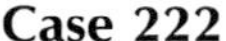

Case 222

22-year-old man injured in a motorcycle accident.
Basal skull fracture.

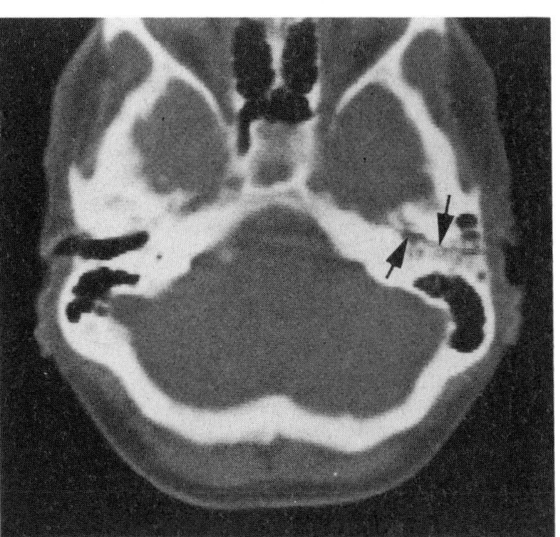

Basal skull fractures are difficult to define by standard radiographic techniques. The axial display of the skull base on CT scans aids in this evaluation.

Here a longitudinal fracture of the petrous bone is clearly seen *(arrows),* with opacification of adjacent mastoid air cells. Opacification of the sphenoid sinus suggests blood or spinal fluid within the sinus and is a secondary sign of basal fracture. (However, trauma patients who have been supine for long periods may have pooled secretions in the sphenoid sinus with no adjacent fracture.)

Case 223

56-year-old man who suffered head trauma one month earlier, now presenting with meningitis and watery nasal discharge (coronal scan, wide window width).

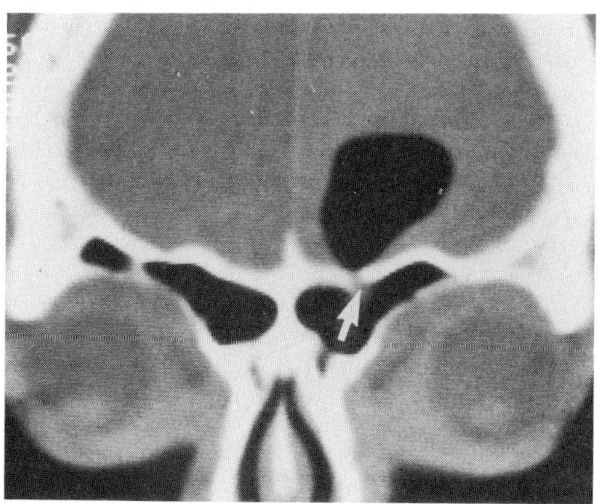

Fractures of the cribriform plate and ethmoid sinus are a common source of post-traumatic meningitis and CSF rhinorrhea. Other causes include frontal sinus fracture, parasellar fractures into the sphenoid sinus, and petrous bone fractures communicating with the middle ear and eustachian tube.

In this case, the coronal scan clearly demonstrates a fracture in the roof of the frontoethmoid sinus *(arrow)*. An unusual pocket of intracranial air arises from this site. Surgery demonstrated communication of the sinus with a cavitated hematoma in the frontal lobe. (No abscess was found.)

Case 224

45-year-old man presenting with a third episode of meningitis in five years (prone coronal scan with metrizamide, wide window width).

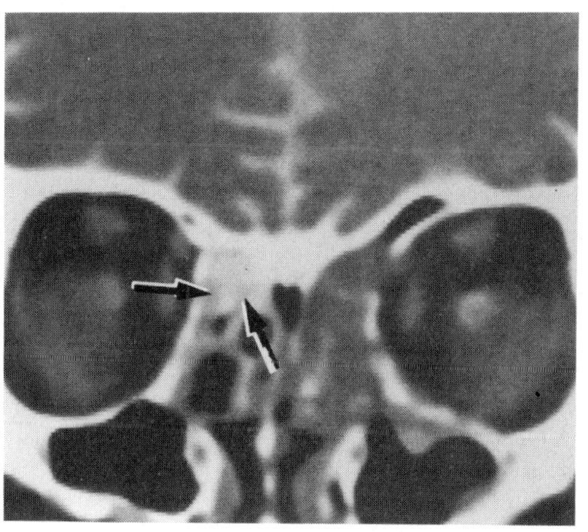

The location of a fracture causing recurrent meningitis and CSF rhinorrhea is rarely as apparent as in Case 223. Most patients require special studies to demonstrate the site of a CSF leak.

One useful technique combines CT with the injection of subarachnoid contrast material. Scans are performed in coronal and/or axial planes in an effort to detect the presence of contrast within a sinus, thereby identifying the site of CSF communication.

In this case, a posterior ethmoid air cell is filled with contrast material *(arrows)*, directing the surgeon to this site. A fracture was found in the roof of the sinus, and the dural laceration was repaired.

Case 225

20-year-old woman.

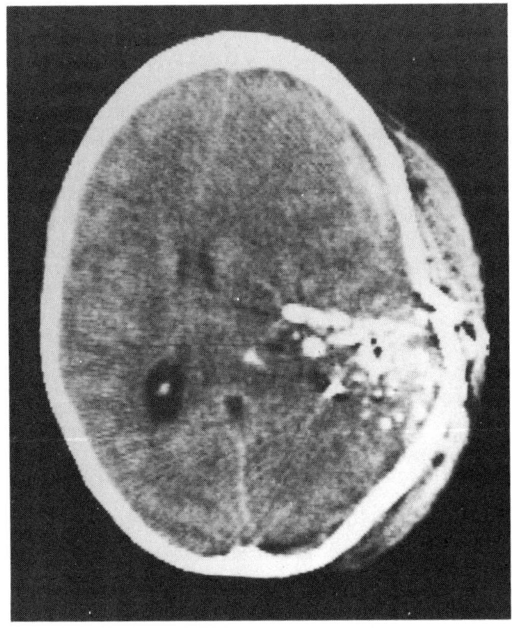

Scans may disclose multiple intracerebral densities in patients with cranial gunshot wounds. These foreign bodies include metal fragments and pieces of embedded calvarium. Bullet fragments may be relatively inert and are often left in place, while bony fragments are a common source of infection and are usually removed if possible. The distinction between metal and bone may be difficult at normal display settings, but is usually apparent at wide window widths.

In this case, a comminuted skull fracture is present. Instead of being depressed as in Case 221, the fracture region has been elevated by the blast injury and underlying subdural and intracerebral hemorrhage.

Case 226

24-year-old man.

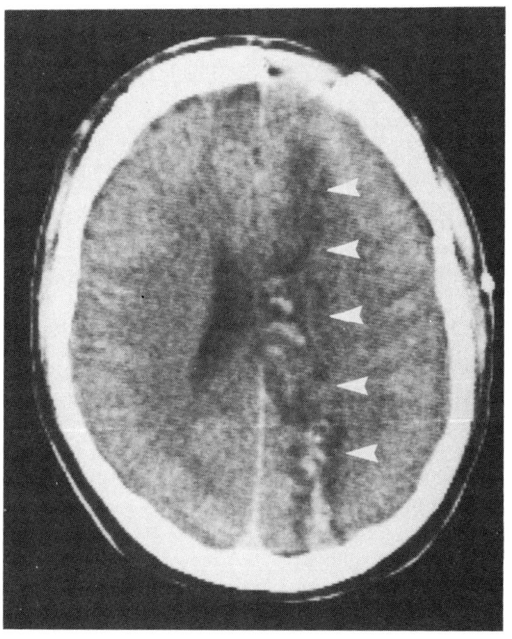

A projective passing through the brain may leave a trail of small hemorrhages or a track of hypodensity. This path indicates the extent and nature of cerebral injury more accurately than the final location of the bullet. In this case, the parasagittal track of the bullet *(arrows)* correlated with an excellent clinical recovery.

Case 227

60-year-old man 12 hours after evacuation of left frontal acute subdural hematoma. Unilateral tension pneumocephalus (wide window width).

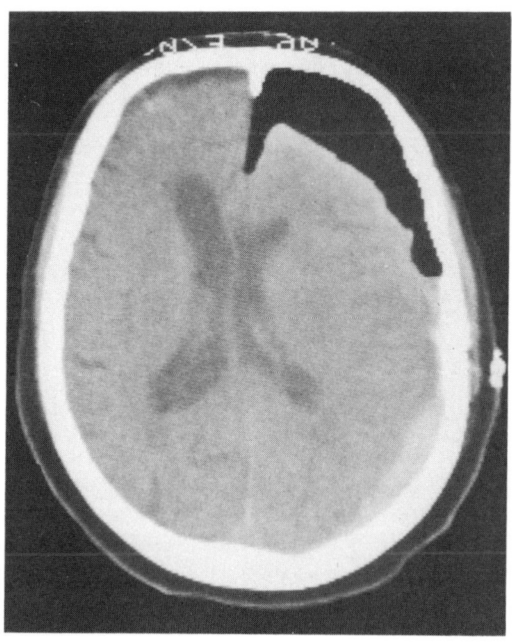

Intracranial air may be introduced at the time of surgery, particularly when large ventricles or cysts are decompressed, when extracerebral hematomas are evacuated, and when posterior fossa operations are performed with the patient in a sitting position. Postsurgical pneumocephalus is usually incidental and quickly resorbed. However, large amounts of intracranial air can act as a mass lesion causing pressure on the adjacent brain.

In this case, the mass effect of the subdural air depresses the underlying cortex and markedly deforms the left lateral ventricle. (A small acute subdural hematoma remains more posteriorly.)

Case 228

82-year-old man six hours after evacuation of bilateral chronic subdural hematomas; anesthesia included nitrous oxide. Bilateral tension pneumocephalus (wide window width).

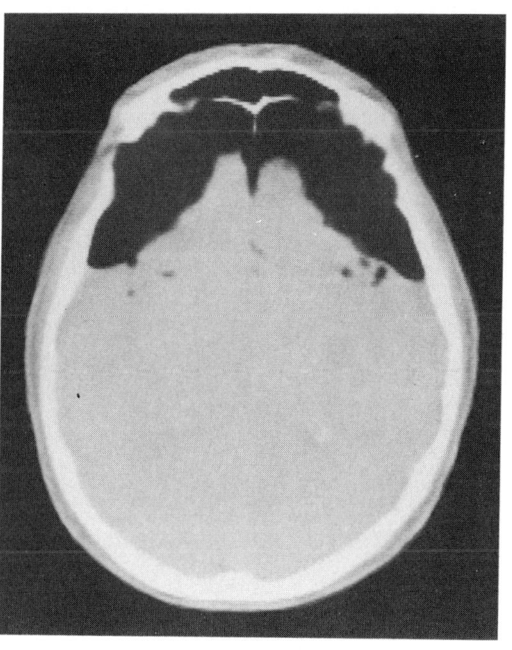

Tension within intracranial air spaces may be increased following nitrous oxide anesthesia. Nitrous oxide is more soluble than nitrogen in blood, causing postanesthesia equilibration of partial pressures to expand any collection of intracranial air

The "twin-peak" configuration of the frontal lobes illustrated here is characteristic of bilateral subdural pneumocephalus. The morphology apparently represents tethering of the frontal poles to the dura by vascular and fibrous bridges. Scattered bubbles of subarachnoid air are also seen in this case.

DIFFERENTIAL DIAGNOSIS: MULTILOCULAR, SUPERFICIAL ENHANCING MASS

Case 229

93-year-old man.

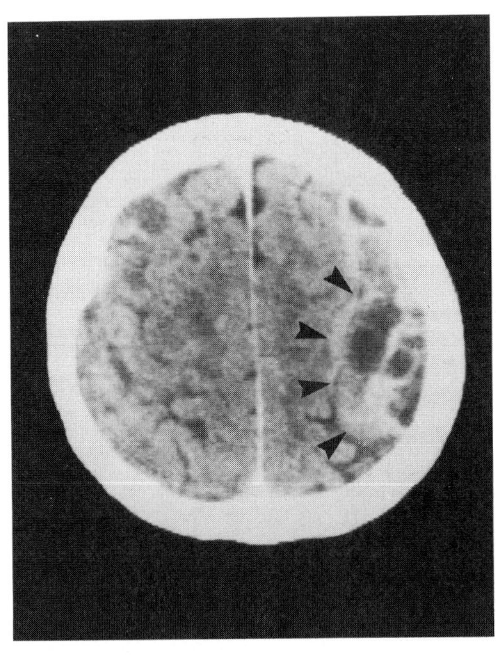

Chronic Subdural Hematoma.

Case 230

13-year-old girl.

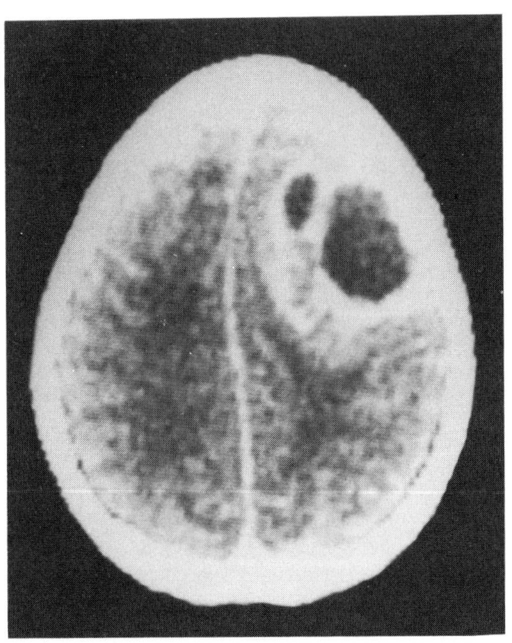

Cystic Glioblastoma Multiforme.

Some chronic subdural hematomas present an unusual appearance due to the combination of loculation and thick, enhancing membranes. The lesion in Case 229 resembles a neoplasm (or thick-walled abscess). The differential diagnosis would include unusual metastasis or atypical meningioma (see Case 15) in addition to malignant glioma (see also Case 333.)

Case 230 is unusual because of the patient's age. However, the thick-walled, multicystic morphology strongly suggests the correct diagnosis.

REFERENCES

1. Bergstrom M., Ericson K., Levander B., et al.: Computed tomography of cranial subdural and epidural hematomas: Variation of attenuation related to time and clinical events such as rebleeding. *J. Comput. Assist. Tomogr.* 1:449–455, 1977.
2. Bruce D.A., Alavi A., Bilaniuk L.T., et al.: Diffuse cerebral swelling following head injuries in children: the syndrome of "malignant brain edema." *J. Neurosurg.* 54:170–178, 1981.
3. Clifton G.L., Grossman R.G., Makela M.E., et al.: Neurological course and correlated computerized tomography findings after severe closed head injury. *J. Neurosurg.* 52:611–624, 1980.
4. Cornell S.H., Chiu L.C., Christie J.H.: Diagnosis of extracerebral fluid collections by computed tomography. *A.J.R.* 131:107–110, 1978.
5. Diaz F.G., Yock D.H. Jr., Larson D., et al.: Early diagnosis of delayed post-traumatic intracerebral hematomas. *J. Neurosurg.* 50:217–223, 1979.
6. Forbes G.S., Sheedy P.F., Piepgras D.G., et al.: Computed tomography in the evaluation of subdural hematomas. *Radiology* 126:143–148, 1978.
7. Johnson D.W., Hasso A.N., Stewart C.E., et al.: Temporal bone trauma: High resolution computed tomographic evaluation. *Radiology* 151:411–415, 1984.
8. Kim K.S., Hemmati M., Weinberg P.E.: Computed tomography in isodense subdural hematoma. *Radiology* 128:71–74, 1978.
9. Lipper M.H., Kishore P.R., Girevendulis A.K., et al.: Delayed intracranial hematoma in patients with severe head injury. *Radiology* 133:645–649, 1979.
10. Manelfe C., Cellerier P., Sobel D., et al.: Cerebrospinal fluid rhinorrhea: Evaluation with metrizamide cisternography. *A.J.N.R.* 3:25–30, 1982.
11. Markwalder T.M.: Chronic subdural hematomas: A review. *J. Neurosurg.* 54:637–645, 1981.
12. Monajati A., Cotanch W.W.: Subdural tension pneumocephalus following surgery. *J. Comput. Assist. Tomogr.* 6:902–906, 1982.
13. Naidich T.P., Leeds N.E., Kricheff I.I., et al.: The tentorium in axial section. I. Normal CT appearance and non-neoplastic pathology. *Radiology* 123:631–638, 1977.
14. Naidich T.P., Leeds N.E., Kricheff I.I., et al.: The tentorium in axial section. II. Lesion localization. *Radiology* 123:639–648, 1977.
15. Nelson A.T., Kishore P.R., Lee S.H.: Development of delayed epidural hematoma. *A.J.N.R.* 3:583–585, 1982.
16. Pop P.M., Thompson J.R., Zinke D.E., et al.: Tension pneumocephalus. *J. Comput. Assist. Tomogr.* 6:894–901, 1982.
17. Reith K.G., Davis D.O.: Subdural hematomas: An unusual appearance on CT. *J. Comput. Assist. Tomogr.* 3:331–334, 1979.
18. Shalen P.R., Handel S.F.: Diagnostic challenges in closed head trauma. *Radiol. Clin. North. Am.* 19:53–68, 1981.
19. Shalen P.R., Handel S.F.: Trauma to the skull and brain, in Haaga J.R., Alfidi R.J. (eds.): *Computed Tomography of the Whole Body*. St. Louis, C.V. Mosby Co., 1983, pp. 170–224.
20. Smith W.P., Batnitzky S., Rengachary S.S.: Acute isodense subdural hematomas. *A.J.N.R.* 2:37–40, 1981.
21. Stone J.L., Schaffer L., Ramsey R.G.: Epidural hematomas of the posterior fossa. *Surg. Neurol.* 11:419–424, 1979.
22. Tsai F.Y., Huprich J.E., Segall H.D., et al.: The contrast-enhanced CT scan in the diagnosis of isodense subdural hematoma. *J. Neurosurg.* 50:64–69, 1979.
23. Tsai F.Y., Teal J.S., Itabashi H.H., et al.: Computed tomography of posterior fossa trauma. *J. Comput. Assist. Tomogr.* 4:291–305, 1980.
24. Tsai F.Y., Teal J.S., Quinn M.F., et al.: CT of brainstem injury. *A.J.N.R.* 1:23–29, 1980.
25. Zimmerman R.A., Bilaniuk L.T.: Computed tomographic staging of traumatic epidural bleeding. *Radiology* 144:809–812, 1982.
26. Zimmerman R.A., Bilaniuk L.T., Bruce D., et al.: Computed tomography of pediatric head trauma: acute general cerebral swelling. *Radiology* 126:403–408, 1978.
27. Zimmerman R.A., Bilaniuk L.T., Bruce D., et al.: Computed tomography of craniocerebral injury in the abused child. *Radiology* 130:687–690, 1979.
28. Zimmerman R.A., Bilaniuk L.T., Gennarelli T., et al.: Cranial computed tomogrpahy in diagnosis and management of acute head trauma. *A.J.R.* 131:27–34, 1978.
29. Zimmerman R.D., Danziger A.: Extracerebral trauma. *Radiol. Clin. North. Am.* 20:105–121, 1982.
30. Zimmerman R.D., Russell E.J., Yurberg E., et al.: Falx and interhemispheric fissure on axial CT. II. Recognition and differentiation of interhemispheric subarachnoid and subdural hemorrhage. *A.J.N.R.* 3:635–642, 1982.

CHAPTER 9

INFARCTION AND ANOXIA

EVOLUTION OF SCAN FINDINGS IN CEREBRAL INFARCTION

Case 231A

73-year-old woman. Scan 12 hours after cerebrovascular accident.

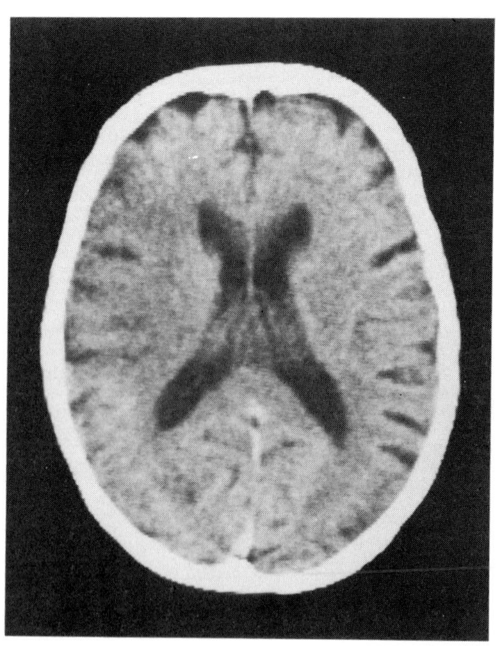

The CT appearance of cerebral infarction is highly time-dependent. The rate and nature of these changes are characteristic and may be used to identify an initially ambiguous lesion.

Scans are usually normal within the first few hours of infarction. The earliest CT changes include mildly decreased attenuation values, loss of gray-white matter discrimination, and subtle mass effect.

In this case, the definition of cortical gray matter has become indistinct in the mid-right hemisphere, and early mass effect blurs sulcal margins (compare with the contralateral side). A trapezoidal wedge of low attenuation is faintly seen.

Case 231B

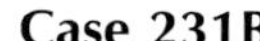

Same patient. Scan four days after CVA.

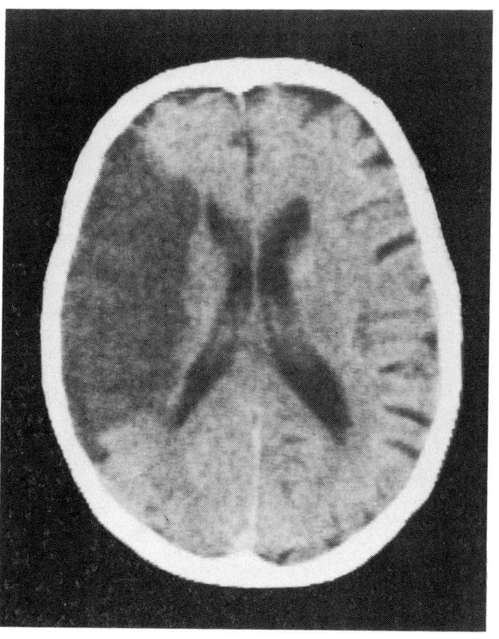

Low attenuation within an area of infarction is well defined by the second or third day. As in this case, the low density is usually homogeneous and often wedge-shaped, with widening margins reaching a broad base against the inner table. No cortical sparing is seen, in contrast to the low-density pattern of edema (see Case 220). The trapezoidal shape of this lesion is typical for occlusions involving the main trunk of the middle cerebral artery distal to the lenticulostriate artery origins.

Mass effect develops concurrently, usually reaching a maximum by the second to fourth day (see Case 233). Here the midline shift is minimal, but mass effect is indicated by effacement of ipsilateral sulci and compression of the lateral ventricle.

Case 231C

Same patient as in Cases 231A and 231B.
Scan ten days after CVA.

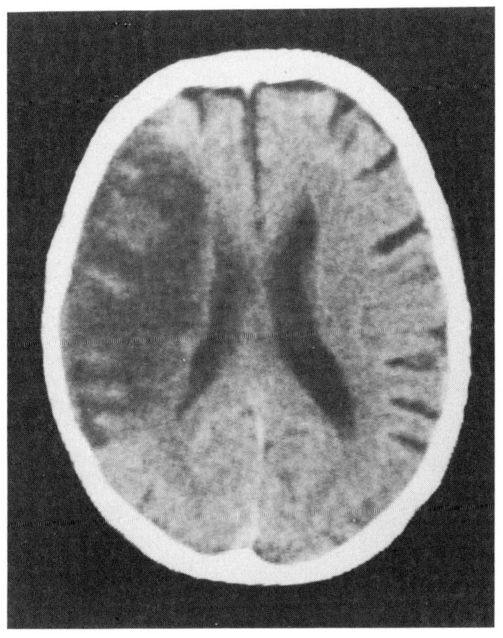

Mass effect begins to decrease by the end of the first week after infarction. In this case a few sulci are reappearing on the affected side.

The low attenuation of an infarct becomes less homogeneous in the second week, and islands of isodensity may appear (as seen above). Occasionally, the entire infarction will increase in attenuation, becoming isodense and transiently invisible on a noncontrast scan ("fogging phenomenon").

Contrast scans often show intense enhancement in the isodense regions at this stage of evolution (see Cases 234 and 235). This finding suggests that the precontrast isodensity may represent the averaging of underlying low attenuation with developing hyperemia and/or blood-brain barrier breakdown.

The mixed density pattern illustrated on this scan superficially resembles the frond-like interdigitations of cerebral edema and could possibly be mistaken for a neoplasm.

Case 232

71-year-old woman. Old infarction in the distribution of the middle cerebral artery.

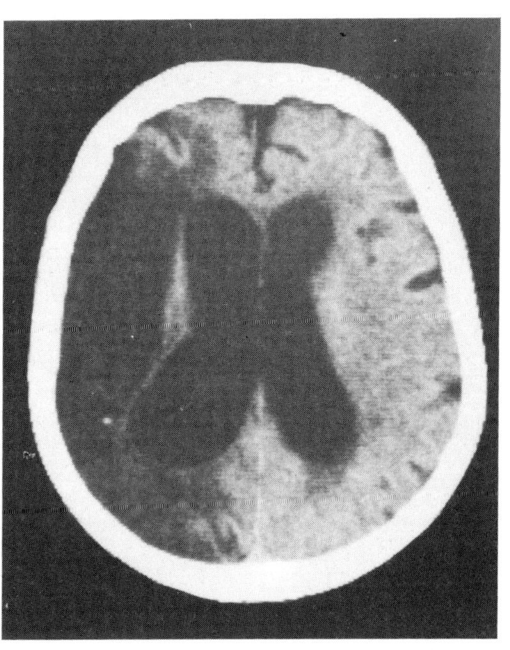

Old infarctions are seen as sharply marginated regions of low attenuation associated with parenchymal loss. The attenuation values may be as low as spinal fluid or somewhat less "black," depending on the mixture of spared and destroyed tissue. Expansion of adjacent ventricles is characteristic, as in this case, and may lead to frank porencephaly (see Cases 371 and 372).

Case 233A

68-year-old woman. One-day-old infarction.

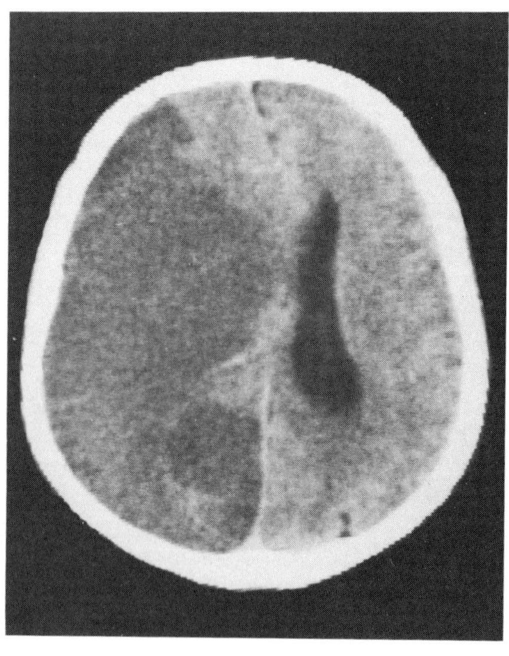

Mass effect develops during the first week of cerebral infarction, most commonly after a few days have elapsed.

This lesion is only a day old, but substantial ischemic edema is already apparent. Subfalcial herniation is present and the right lateral ventricle is effaced.

The involved region includes the territories of the middle and posterior cerebral arteries. This combination of vascular distributions suggests occlusion of the internal carotid artery with carotid origin of the posterior cerebral artery and a patent anterior communicating artery.

Case 233B

Same patient.

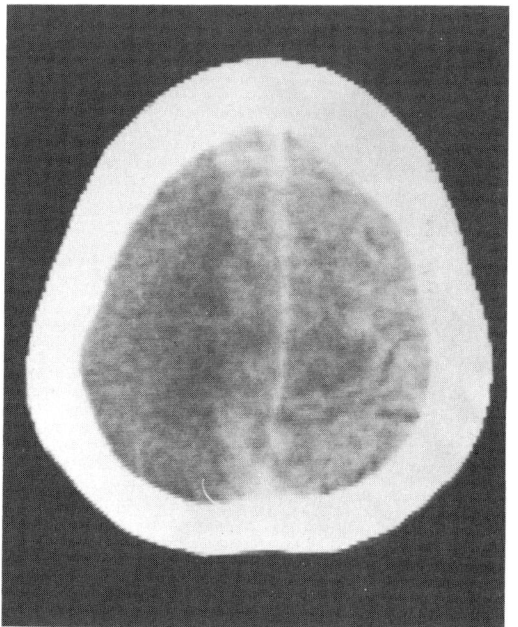

A vertex scan demonstrates compression of the spared parasagittal tissue by the homogeneous region of infarction. The parasagittal sparing represents the distribution of the anterior cerebral artery and illustrates the watershed between the anterior and middle cerebral territories. Compare the involved and spared regions in Case 233 with those in Cases 240 and 241.

CONTRAST ENHANCEMENT IN INFARCTION: GENERALIZED

Case 234

56-year-old woman with subacute bacterial endocarditis. Eleven-day-old infarction.

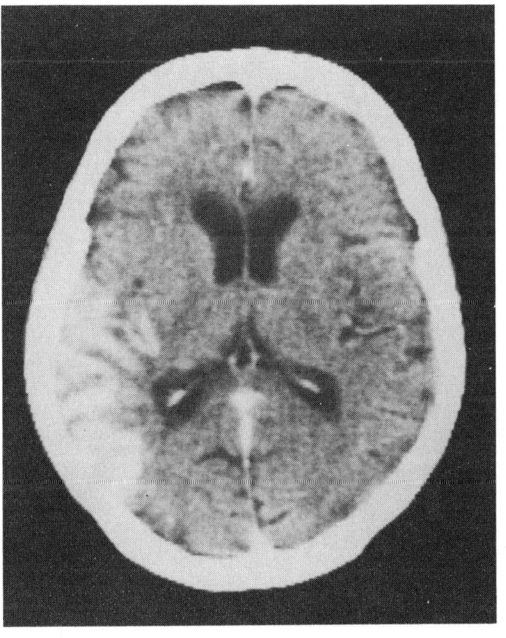

Contrast enhancement may be seen in cerebral infarctions from the end of week 1 through week 3 or 4. Reactive "luxury perfusion" (hyperperfusion with loss of autoregulation) and breakdown of the blood-brain barrier both contribute to this phenomenon.

Enhancement is usually confined to gray matter but may demonstrate variable morphology. The most characteristic pattern is band-like, tubular, or gyriform enhancement, as seen in this case.

Solid enhancement sometimes fills the region of infarction (see Case 256), particularly when deep nuclei are involved. Ring-enhancing appearances may also be found (see Case 239).

In most cases, the enhancing lesion retains the peripherally based shape typical of large infarctions (see also Case 258).

Case 235

70-year-old woman. Ten-day-old infarction.

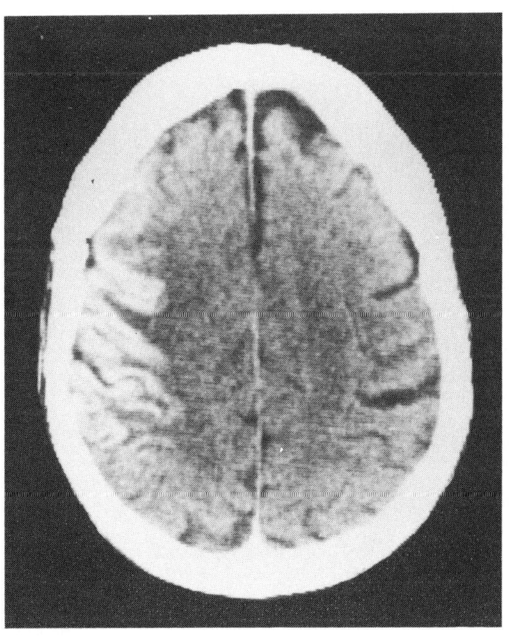

Gyriform enhancement in a subacute infarction is seen here as a thin ribbon following the cortical convolutions.

The period of prominent contrast enhancement in infarction usually follows the period of mass effect, reducing the potential resemblance to neoplasm (but see Cases 238 and 239). Even without mass effect, the serpentine enhancement pattern of a subacute infarction may closely mimic that of a vascular malformation (see Cases 258, 293, and 294).

The significance of contrast enhancement as an indicator of adverse prognosis in cerebral infarction is controversial.

Case 236

66-year-old man with multiple neurologic deficits following cardiac surgery two weeks earlier. Multifocal infarction at watershed sites.

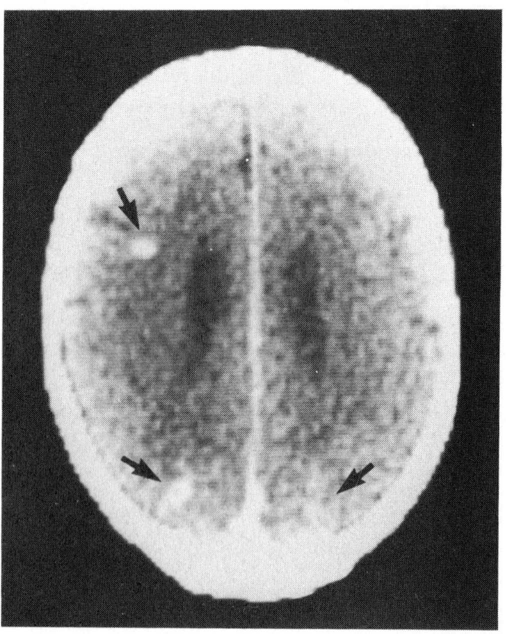

Small areas of infarction often demonstrate focal enhancement, as seen in this case. The appearance is nonspecific and by itself could suggest inflammatory or metastatic lesions. Here, the clinical context and the distribution along vascular watersheds (see Cases 233, 240, 241, 243, and 244) aid in the diagnosis.

Multifocal infarction may be caused by hypoperfusion, multiple emboli, cerebral vasculitis (e.g., systemic lupus erythematosus), meningitis, or cortical venous thrombosis.

Case 237

35-year-old woman found to have the syndrome of multiple progressive intracranial arterial occlusions ("moyamoya"). One-week-old infarct.

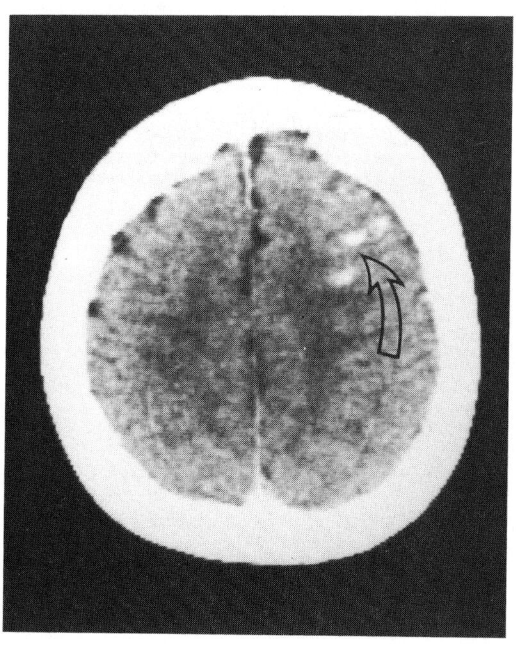

A small area of patchy enhancement is seen in the left frontal cortex. A similar appearance could be caused by a small arteriovenous malformation, focal cerebritis, a seizure focus, or an area of cortical venous infarction.

In "moyamoya," CT scans may demonstrate infarction, hemorrhage from rupture of telangiectatic vessels, or strikingly abnormal enhancement representing the hypertrophied collateral channels.

DIFFERENTIAL DIAGNOSIS: CEREBRAL LESION WITH COMPLEX BANDS AND RIMS OF CONTRAST ENHANCEMENT

Case 238

60-year-old man.

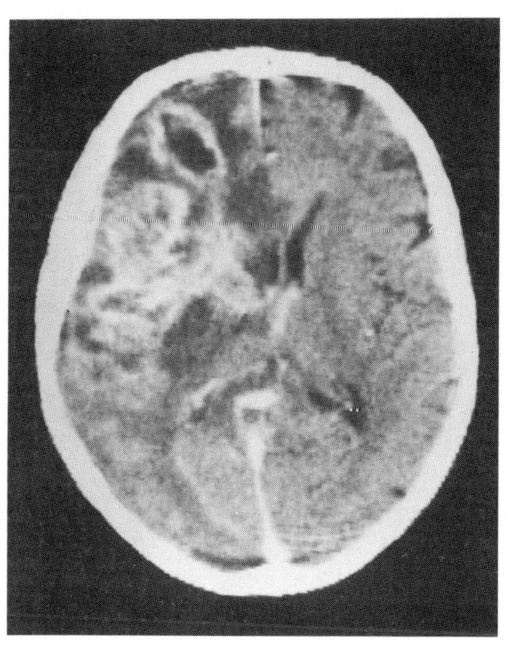

Glioblastoma Multiforme.

Case 239

72-year-old woman.

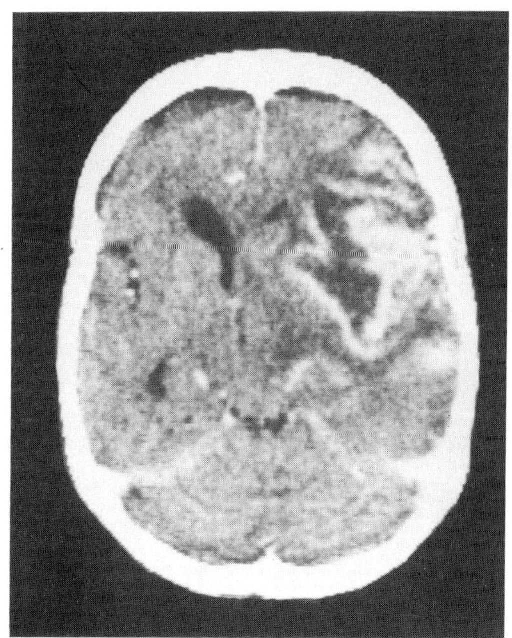

Infarction (19 Days After CVA).

The disorganized contrast enhancement of Case 238 is within the spectrum seen in high-grade gliomas, while Case 239 illustrates the wide-ranging appearance of cerebral infarction. Rim-enhancing components are occasionally found in subacute infarcts, causing the lesions to resemble malignant neoplasms.

Clues to the diagnosis in Case 239 include the gyriform pattern of superficial enhancement and the location of the lesion within the middle cerebral artery distribution. However, a good history, serial scans, or biopsy are necessary for definitive diagnosis in a lesion of this type.

Case 240

69-year-old woman.

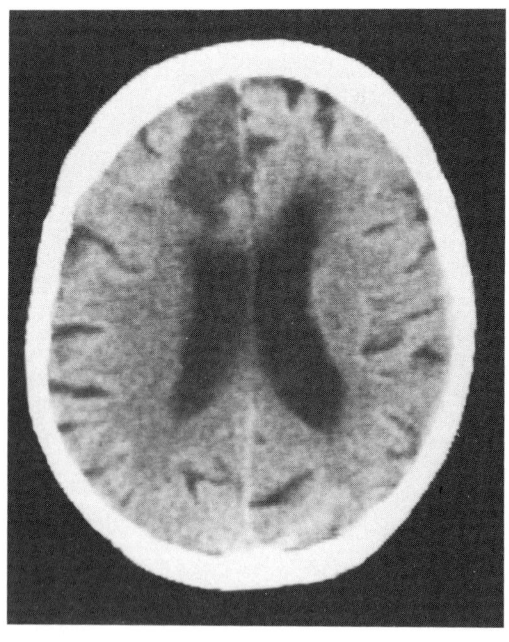

The anterior cerebral artery (ACA) supplies a parasagittal band of tissue extending from the medial frontal lobe to the parietal vertex. Uniform low attenuation in this distribution indicates obstruction of the vessel. Causes include embolization (confirmed angiographically in this case), spasm (see Case 246), compression by a subfrontal mass or infection (see Case 147), and marked subfalcial herniation (see Case 137).

The infarcted region in this case outlines the proximal distribution of the ACA and corresponds to the spared territory in Case 233A.

Case 241

64-year-old man.

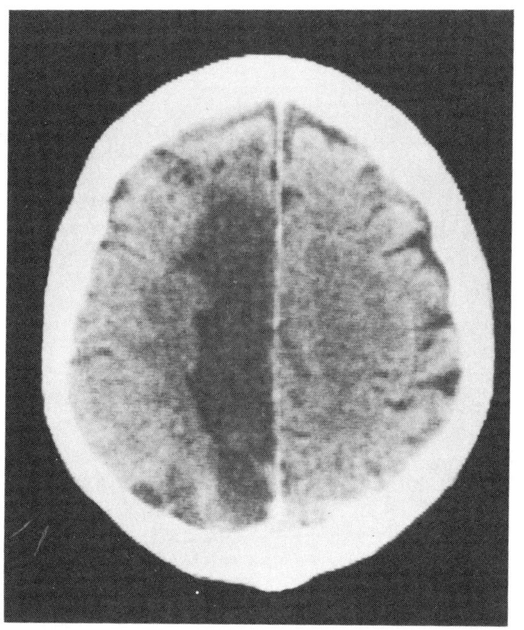

This scan illustrates infarction of the distal ACA distribution (and a portion of the posterior cerebral artery territory). The well-defined, homogeneous, low-attenuation region uniformly obliterates cortical morphology. A diagnosis of recent infarction is highly reliable when these features correspond to a vascular territory.

The parasagittal band of infarcted tissue in this case matches the spared territory in Case 233B, again illustrating the watershed between the anterior and middle cerebral arteries.

INFARCTION IN THE DISTRIBUTION OF THE POSTERIOR CEREBRAL ARTERY

Case 242A

56-year-old man.

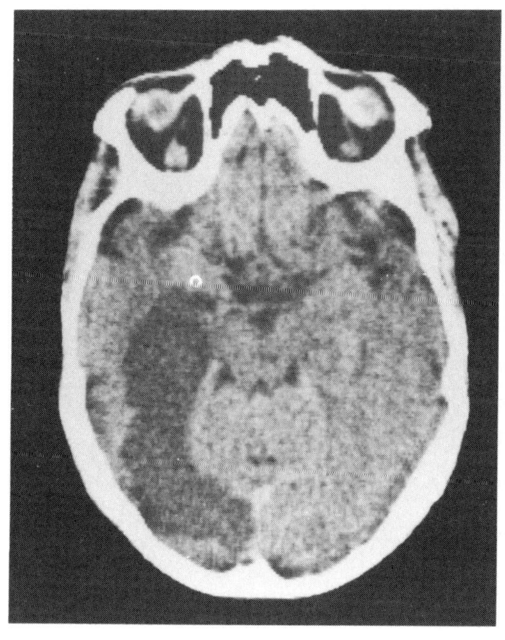

The posterior cerebral artery (PCA) supplies the medial temporal lobe, the tentorial surface of the temporal and occipital lobes, the occipital pole, and a variably extensive band of parasagittal parieto-occipital lobes.

Acute infarction in this case outlines the inferior portion of this distribution, bounded medially by the tentorial margin and laterally by the watershed with the middle cerebral artery. (Extended head position causes this scan to be parallel to the axis of the temporal lobe.)

Case 242B

Same patient.

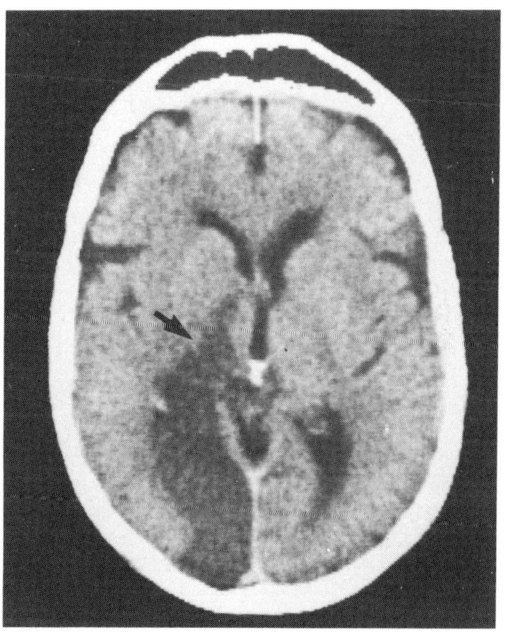

The supply of the PCA to the medial portion of the occipital lobe is illustrated here. The superior and lateral extent of this distribution is variable and reflects reciprocal variations in size of the anterior and middle cerebral arteries.

Thalamoperforating branches arise from the proximal posterior cerebral artery (as well as from the posterior communicating artery). For this reason, thalamic infarction *(arrow)* is often associated with infarctions of the medial temporal and occipital lobes.

See Cases 220 and 254 for other examples of infarction involving the PCA distribution.

LOCATION OF THE POSTERIOR CORTICAL WATERSHED

Case 243

68-year-old woman.

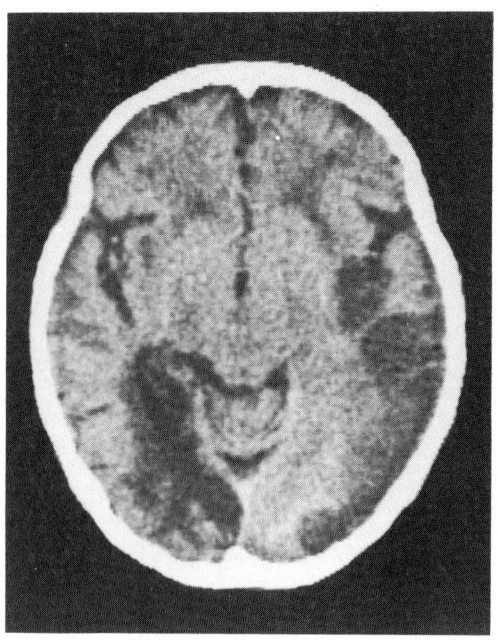
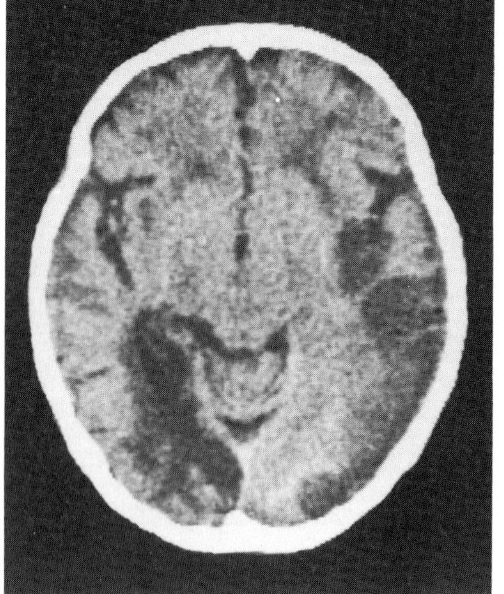

This case demonstrates an old right-sided infarction in the distribution of the posterior cerebral artery. On the left is a recent infarction involving the posterior division of the middle cerebral artery. The margin between the involved and spared regions in each hemisphere represents the watershed between the middle and posterior cerebral arteries.

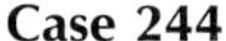

Case 244

74-year-old woman who was studied shortly after subclavian angiography at a referring hospital.

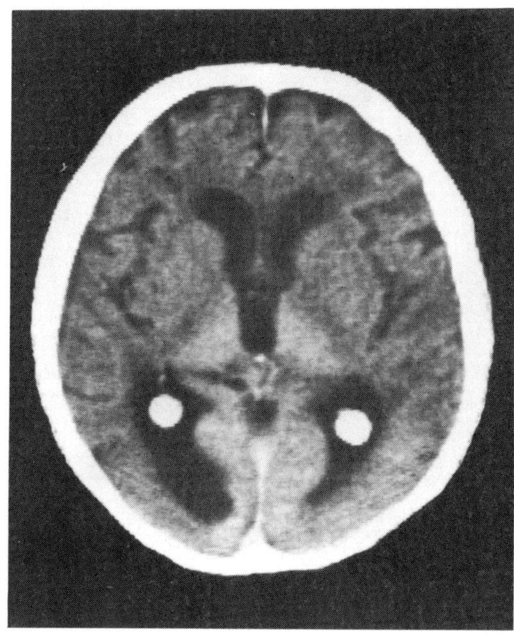

Uniformly increased attenuation is seen throughout the distribution of the posterior cerebral arteries, including the thalami. The margin of density indicates the watershed with supply from the middle cerebral arteries.

High attenuation values were also seen throughout the posterior fossa in this case, suggesting parenchymal penetrance of angiographic contrast material in the territory of the basilar artery. The subclavian angiogram had demonstrated embolic occlusion a short distance beyond the vertebral artery, which therefore received the bulk of the injected contrast. It is important to consider the subclavian origin of the vertebral artery when patients are evaluated for upper-extremity symptoms.

DIFFERENTIAL DIAGNOSIS: PARASAGITTAL LOW-ATTENUATION LESION

Case 245

39-year-old woman.

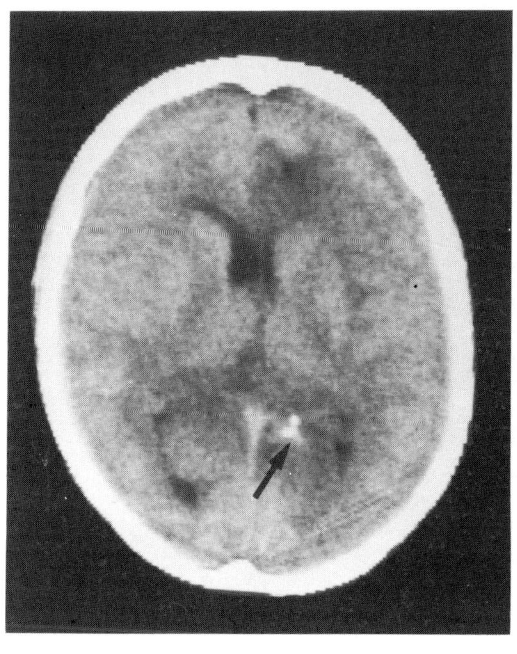

Low-grade Glioma.

Case 246

64-year-old man.

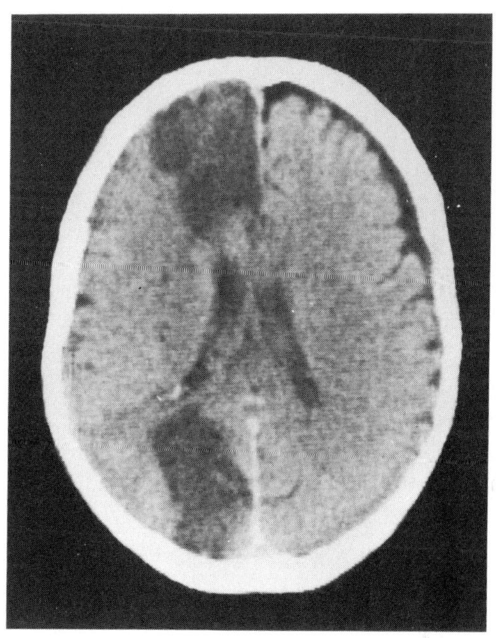

Infarction Involving The Anterior And Posterior Cerebral Arteries (Due To Spasm Following Subarachnoid Hemorrhage).

The area involved by a low-grade glioma may approximate a vascular distribution. This is most commonly seen with midhemisphere tumors occupying the territory of the middle cerebral artery. Such lesions may mimic recent infarction, especially if the tumors extend to a cortical surface (as seen medially in the frontal lobe in Case 245).

Several CT features aid in differential diagnosis. Tumors rarely involve the entire distribution of a potentially occluded vessel. Vague margins and cortical sparing (seen anteriorly and laterally in Case 245) argue against infarction. Associated calcification (*arrow,* Case 245) suggests a low-grade neoplasm. (See Case 36 for another scan of this patient.)

Conversely, the poorly defined low attenuation of an early infarction may initially mimic a low-grade glioma, particularly in the middle cerebral artery distribution (see Case 262). The clinical setting usually clarifies the diagnosis in such cases, and follow-up scans provide confirmation.

DEEP HEMISPHERE INFARCTION

Case 247

76-year-old woman, four days after cerebrovascular accident.

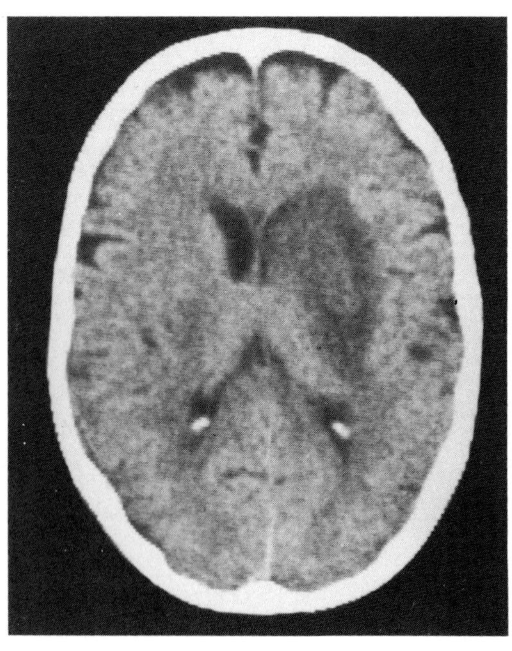

Deep hemisphere infarction may accompany large cortical infarctions or occur as an isolated event. Infarctions may involve large segments of the basal ganglia, as seen in this case, or be limited to very focal areas (see Case 250).

The basal ganglia and internal capsule are largely supplied by lenticulostriate branches arising from the horizontal portion of the middle cerebral artery. (Other contributions include medial lenticulostriate branches from the anterior cerebral artery, the anterior choroidal artery, and thalamoperforating branches of the posterior cerebral artery.)

Infarction in this region is often due to local disease of the lenticulostriate arteries. Pathologic conditions involving the proximal portion of the middle cerebral artery (e.g., plaque, embolus, or dissection) may also cause deep hemisphere infarction by compromising the origins of the penetrating branches. Deep hemisphere infarction may also occur in cases of internal carotid artery occlusion with collateral flow sparing cortical tissue.

This four-day-old infarction demonstrates typical well-defined low attenuation, with mass effect compressing the adjacent frontal horn.

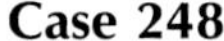

Case 248

80-year-old man with dementia ("lacunar state").

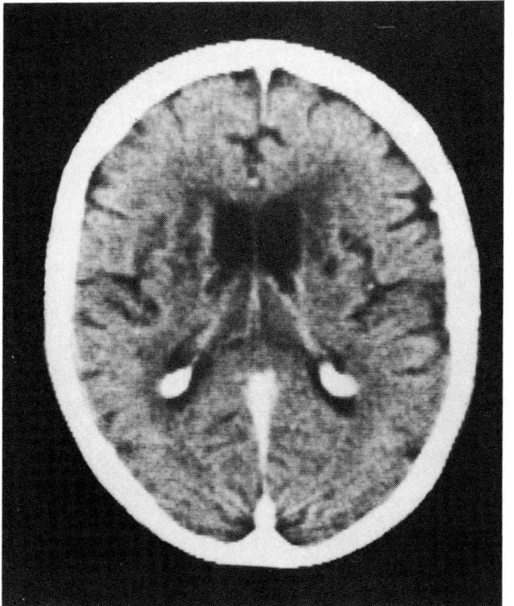

Multiple focal infarctions are present in the periventricular regions and corona radiata. Such multifocal lesions suggest diffuse small arterial disease, frequently seen in patients with diabetes and/or hypertension (see also Case 175).

Small infarctions in the basal ganglia are often called "lacunar infarcts," using the name that pathologists have given to tiny lesions found in the lenticulostriate artery distributions at autopsy.

Deep hemisphere infarctions as seen in this case may resemble the demyelinating plaques of multiple sclerosis (compare with Case 169).

DIFFERENTIAL DIAGNOSIS: LOW-ATTENUATION LESIONS IN THE BASAL GANGLIA

Case 249

44-year-old man.

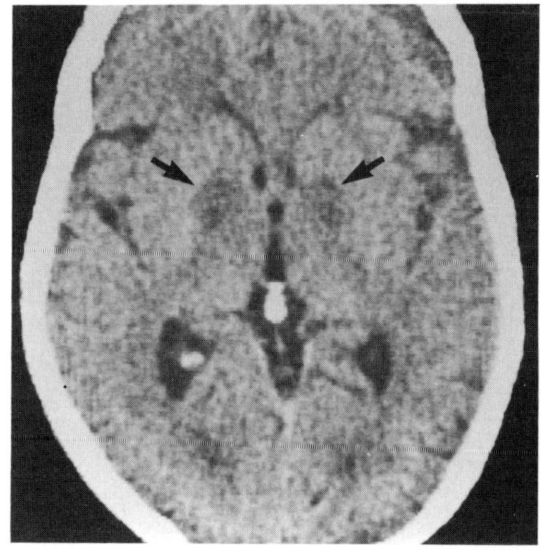

Carbon Monoxide Poisoning.

Case 250

83-year-old man.

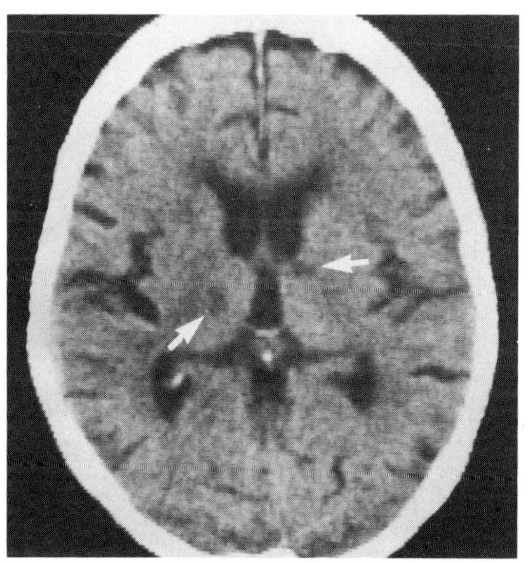

"Lacunar" Infarction.

Carbon monoxide poisoning leads to necrosis of the globus pallidus. Pallidal necrosis may be seen on CT scans as symmetrical areas of abnormal low attenuation, illustrated in Case 249 *(arrows)*. This finding is associated with a poor prognosis for recovery.

Other processes that may cause pallidal necrosis include barbiturate intoxication, cyanide poisoning, hydrogen sulfide poisoning, hypoglycemia, hypoxia, and hypotension. Wilson's disease may be associated with pallidal lucency despite the deposition of metals. The scan findings of methanol intoxication are usually seen more laterally, with hemorrhagic necrosis of the putamen.

The symmetry of involvement in Case 249 suggests a toxic or systemic cause.

Case 251

63-year-old woman.

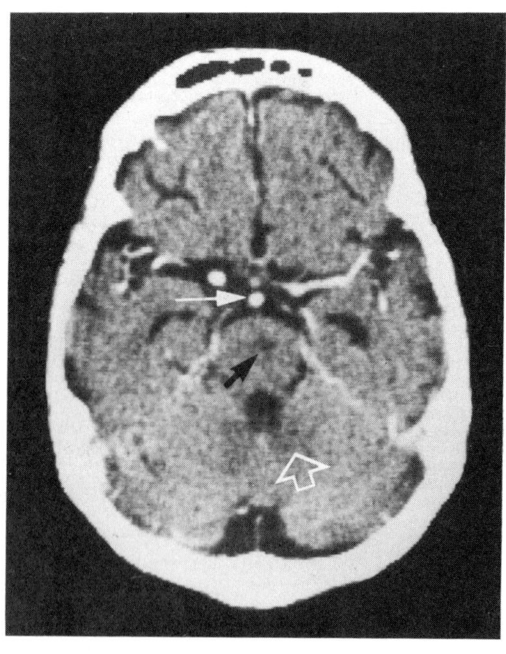

Brain stem infarctions may present as focal low-attenuation areas *(black arrow),* most common in the midbrain or pons.

The precontrast and postcontrast appearance of the basilar artery is of interest in such cases. Calcification, reduced lumen size, and even intraluminal thrombus (see Case 269) may be noted. Here, the basilar artery enhances normally *(white arrow).*

The normal low attenuation of cerebellar white matter is seen posterolateral to the fourth ventricle *(open arrow)* and should not be mistaken for ischemia.

Case 252

74-year-old man.

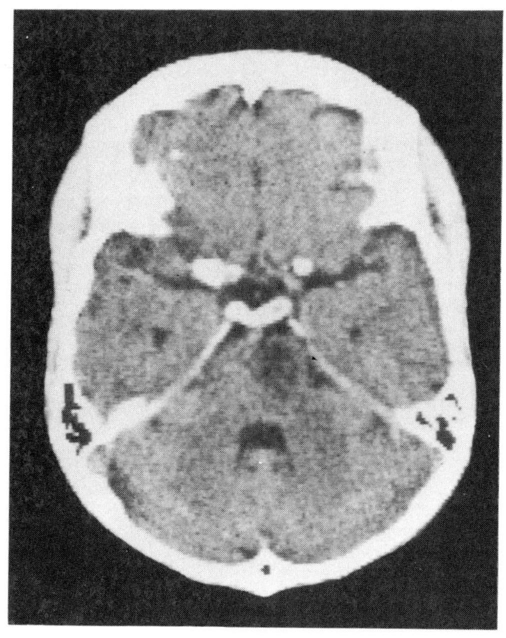

This patient was densely hemiparetic. A large hemispheric infarction was suspected, but the lesion was instead found to involve the left cerebral peduncle.

High-resolution CT scanners routinely demonstrate a midline region of low attenuation near the center of the midbrain (see Case 369 for an example). This area represents the normal decussation of the superior cerebellar peduncles. The central, symmetrical appearance high in the brain stem usually distinguishes this finding from infarction. Brain stem infarctions tend to occur at more caudal levels and are often eccentric, as in Case 252.

DIFFERENTIAL DIAGNOSIS: LOW-ATTENUATION BRAIN STEM LESION

Case 253

70-year-old man.

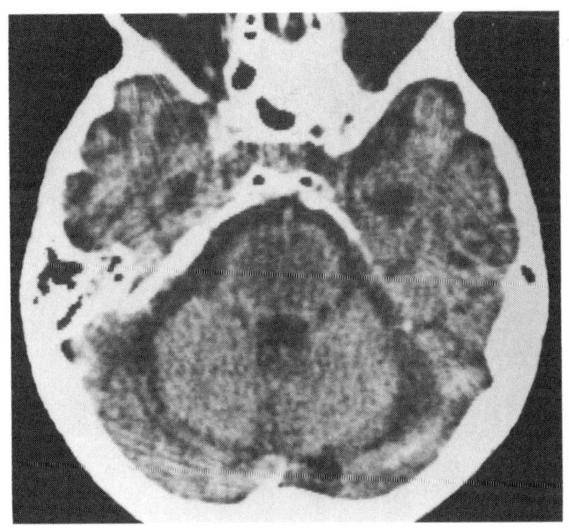

Central Pontine Myelinolysis.

Case 254

71-year-old woman.

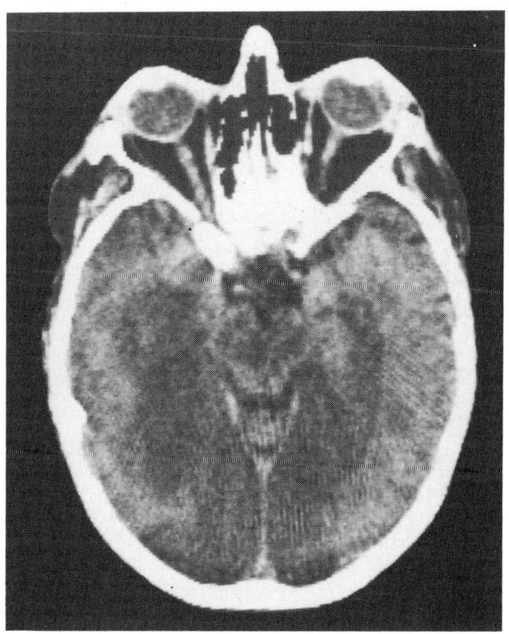

Brain Stem Infarction (Basilar Artery Occlusion).

Central pontine myelinolysis is an acute demyelinating process affecting the brain stem. It is incompletely understood but may correlate with the rapid correction (or overcorrection) of severe electrolyte abnormalities. Other factors (e.g., nutritional) may contribute.

The characteristic CT appearance of central pontine myelinolysis is illustrated in Case 253, with abnormal low attenuation developing throughout the pons. This patient had been admitted with a serum sodium concentration of 117 mEq/L, which had been rapidly overcorrected.

Case 254 is an example of extensive brain stem infarction in a patient with presumed basilar artery occlusion. Bilateral posterior cerebral artery infarctions accompany the brain stem ischemia.

INFARCTION IN THE DISTRIBUTION OF THE POSTERIOR INFERIOR CEREBELLAR ARTERY (PICA)

Case 255

75-year-old woman.

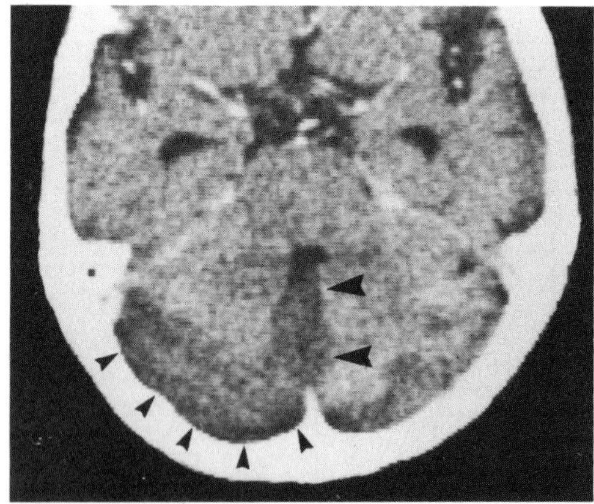

Infarction of the cerebellum may cause confusing low-attenuation changes in the posterior fossa. In many cases the diagnosis can be made by recognizing the distribution of a major cerebellar artery.

The PICA usually supplies (1) a broad rim of peripheral cerebellar hemisphere along the occipital inner table *(small arrows),* and (2) a parasagittal strip of medial hemisphere and inferior vermis extending posteriorly from the fourth ventricle *(large arrows).* An infarction of the PICA should be the first diagnostic consideration when a low-attenuation cerebellar lesion with this scythe-like configuration is encountered.

Incomplete infarction in the PICA distribution may cause low attenuation in either the peripheral or parasagittal regions (as seen in the posterior portion of the contralateral hemisphere). Infarctions of cerebellar watershed regions or multifocal infarctions present less characteristic appearances.

Case 256

35-year-old man.

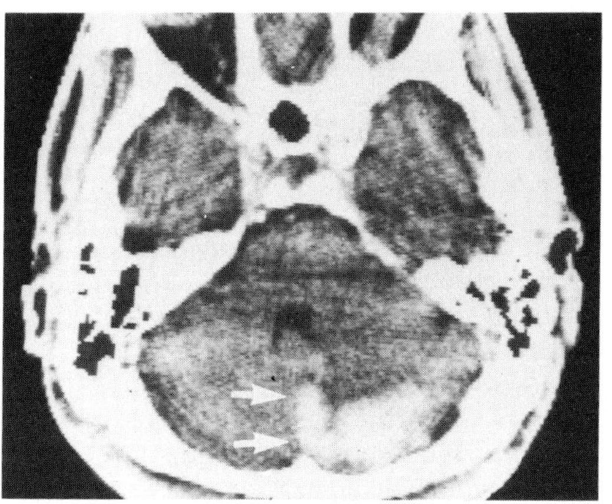

This enhancing posterior fossa lesion in a young patient could be misinterpreted as a tumor or a vascular malformation. The clue to the correct diagnosis is the scythe-like morphology of PICA infarction. A curving, peripheral crescent of involved hemisphere is linked to a straight, parasagittal band, which borders the midline. This sharp, medial margin *(arrows)* is particularly suggestive of a vascular distribution respecting an anatomical boundary.

Infarction in the PICA distribution is the most likely cause of acute cerebellar signs in a young adult.

Case 257

54-year-old man.

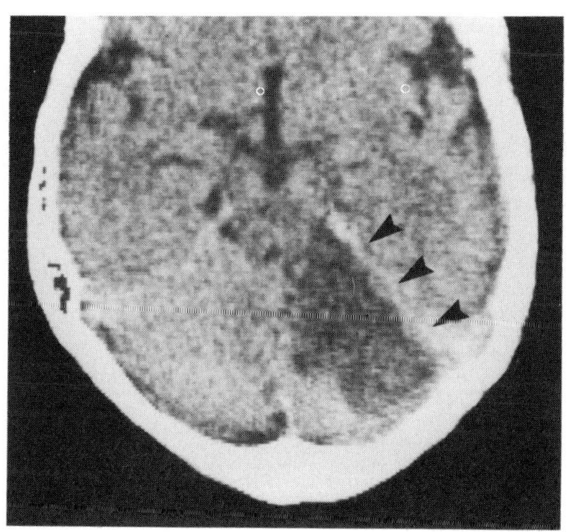

The superior cerebellar artery (SCA) supplies the superior portion of the cerebellar hemisphere and vermis. Infarction in the distribution of this vessel involves the hemisphere but may spare the vermis due to collateral circulation from the inferior vermian arteries.

As in supratentorial infarctions, the lesion demonstrates homogeneous low attenuation with a broad peripheral base. The straight, diagonal, lateral margin *(arrows)* is a hallmark of infarction in the SCA distribution, which is bounded laterally by the tentorium. The medial margin is variable and less distinct, depending on collateral flow patterns.

Associated mass effect compresses the ipsilateral quadrigeminal cistern (compare with Case 364).

Case 258

78-year-old woman.

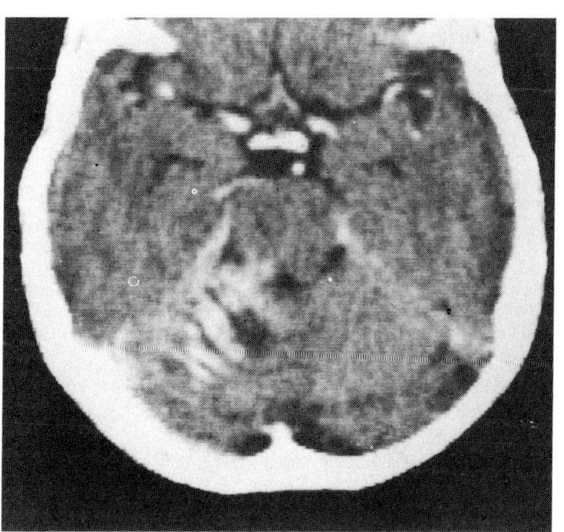

In this case, the hemispheric distribution of the superior cerebellar artery is outlined by gyriform contrast enhancement. The shape and location of the lesion are more specific than its internal appearance, which could be confused with a vascular malformation.

DIFFERENTIAL DIAGNOSIS: LOW-ATTENUATION CEREBELLAR MASS

Case 259

80-year-old man.

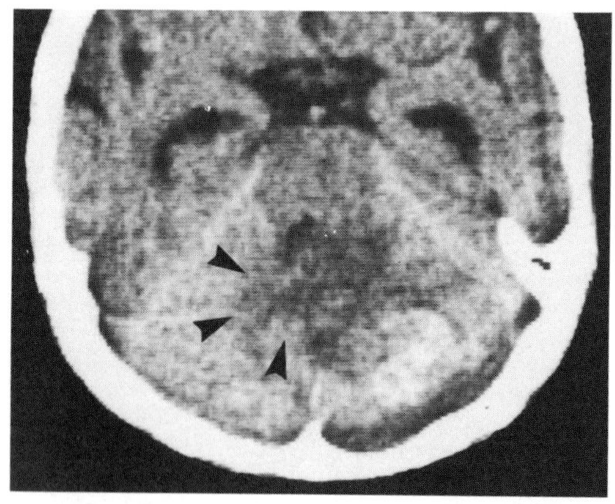

Metastatic Bronchogenic Carcinoma, Left Cerebellar Hemisphere.

Case 260

70-year-old woman.

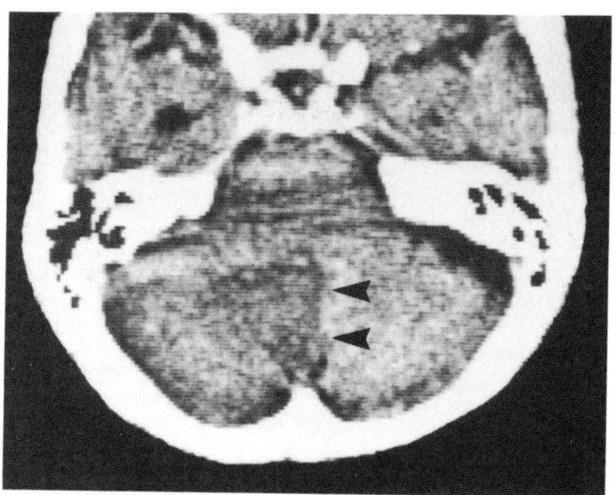

Cerebellar Infarction, Right Cerebellar Hemisphere.

Metastases are the most common cause of cerebellar masses in adults. The lesion in Case 259 is unusually poorly defined (compare with Case 7). Adjacent edema compresses the fourth ventricle and crosses the midline through the vermis *(arrows)*.

Acute cerebellar infarction may also produce extensive low attenuation and mass effect, as seen in Case 260. Swelling may compress the brain stem and require acute decompression, similar to a cerebellar hematoma.

The clue to the diagnosis in Case 260 is the very straight medial margin of the lesion *(arrows)*, which suggests a vascular boundary. This appearance contrasts with the vague medial margin of edema in Case 259.

DIFFERENTIAL DIAGNOSIS: VAGUE LOW-ATTENUATION IN THE SYLVIAN REGION

Case 261

90-year-old man.

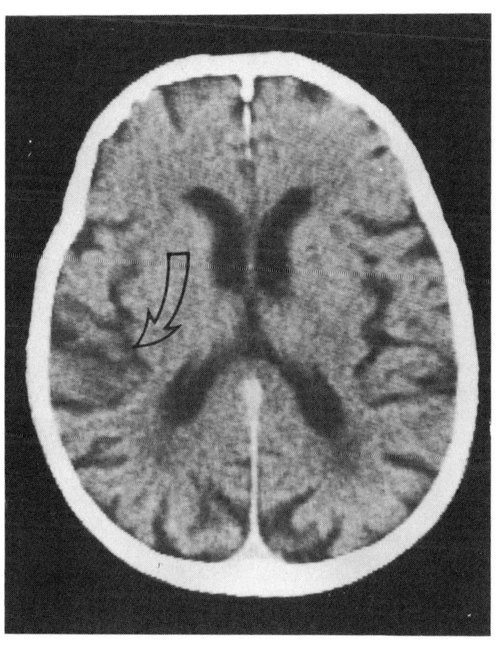

Normal (Partial Volume Of Sylvian Cistern).

Case 262

68-year-old man.

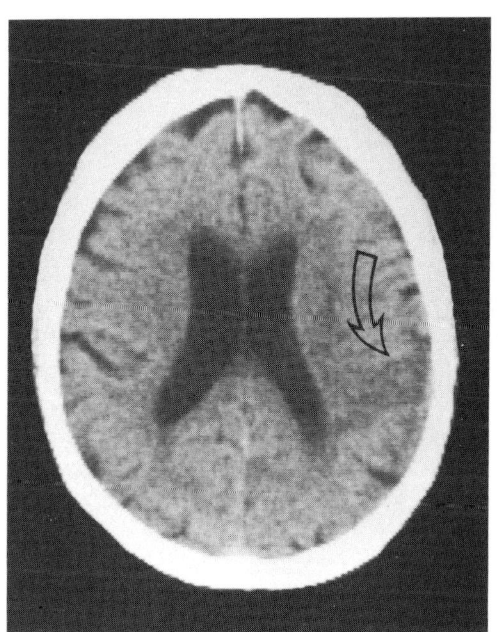

Early Infarction (Middle Cerebral Artery Distribution).

Large subarachnoid spaces are commonly found in elderly patients. When the plane of a scan passes parallel to the sulcus or cistern, a vague area of low attenuation is seen.

The posterior portion of the sylvian cistern commonly causes this appearance, as seen in Case 261 (*arrow;* see also Case 186). This poorly defined low-density region may be mistaken for early ischemic change in the middle cerebral artery distribution, as represented by Case 262.

A pseudoinfarction lacks mass effect and is usually seen at only one level. On the other hand, a true infarction involves several sections and is usually associated with loss of gray-white matter discrimination and early cerebral edema.

Other locations where partial imaging of sulci and cisterns may mimic focal infarction include the circular sulcus/external capsular area, the lateral suprasellar cistern/hypothalamic region, the calcarine sulcus/medial occipital lobe, and the horizontal fissure/posterior cerebellar hemisphere.

The poorly defined infarction in Case 262 could also be mistaken for a low-grade glioma (see Cases 33 and 34).

WATERSHED INFARCTION

Case 263

70-year-old woman.

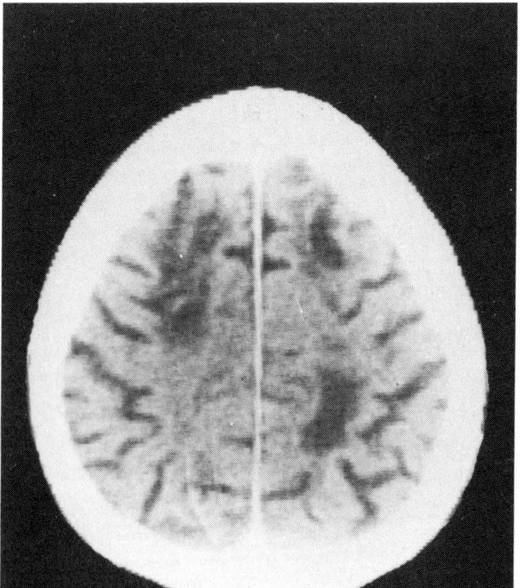

Infarction occurs along the margins of cerebral vascular territories when flow is impaired on both sides of the boundary. This circumstance may be due to generalized hypoperfusion, isolated vascular compromise, or a combination of both factors. For example, stenosis of an internal carotid artery may cause infarction along the anterior-middle cerebral artery watershed during systemic hypotension.

The location of the cortical watersheds has been illustrated in Cases 240, 241, 243, and 244. Watershed infarctions are typically small, patchy lesions, aligned along these same parasagittal boundaries.

This case illustrates typical infarctions along the anterior cortical watersheds between the anterior and middle cerebral arteries. Differential diagnosis of this parasagittal pattern includes venous infarction due to thrombosis of the superior sagittal sinus (see Case 276).

Case 264

60-year-old woman.

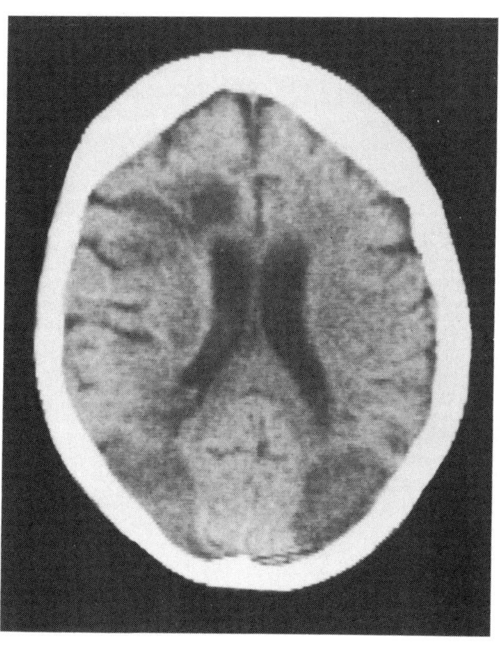

A second watershed region exists within the hemispheres. This zone occurs at the junction of the centripetal supply from cortical penetrating arteries and the centrifugal distribution of deep hemisphere perforating vessels. The superficial-deep arterial watershed falls near the margins of the lateral ventricles at the midhemisphere level.

In this case, symmetrical watershed infarctions of the posterior cortical distributions are accompanied by a superficial-deep watershed infarct in the right frontal lobe.

DIFFERENTIAL DIAGNOSIS: MULTIFOCAL INFARCTION

Case 265

72-year-old man.

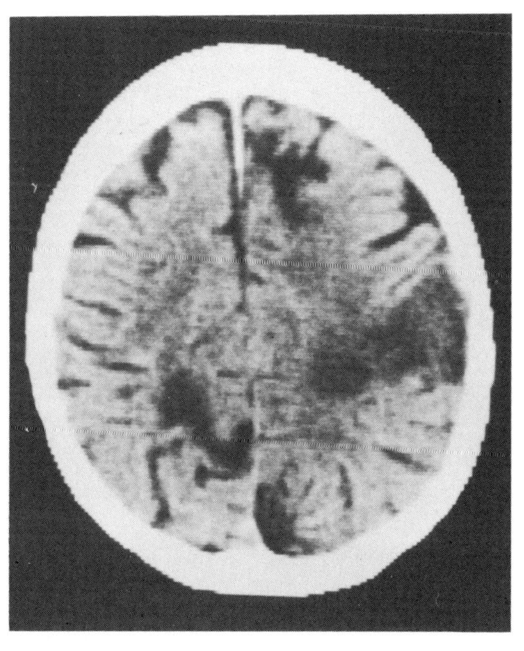

Multiple Embolic Infarctions.

Case 266

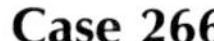

70-year-old woman.

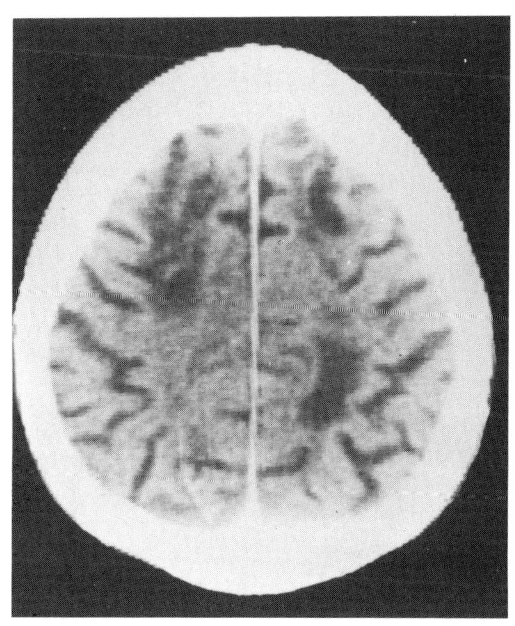

Watershed Infarctions.

The distribution of multiple cerebral infarctions may help characterize the underlying pathophysiology. In Case 265, multiple infarctions are present at scattered cortical locations, largely independent of watershed territories. The pattern suggests multifocal occlusions of distal cerebral arteries, raising the possibility of embolization, cerebral vasculitis, or coagulopathy.

By contrast, the multiple infarctions in Case 266 are aligned along watershed distributions. This pattern favors generalized hypoperfusion rather than involvement of individual cortical arteries.

HEMORRHAGE INTO ISCHEMIC INFARCTIONS

Case 267

80-year-old man receiving hemodialysis.

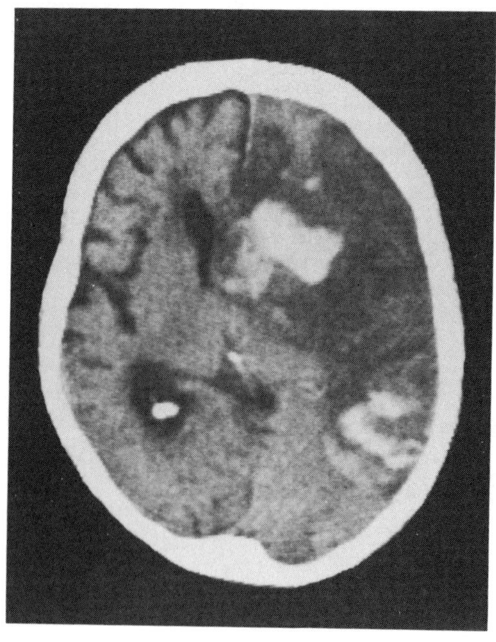

A small number of ischemic infarctions become hemorrhagic, either spontaneously or following anticoagulation therapy. The hemorrhage in these lesions may vary from tiny petechiae to frank hematomas.

Here, large areas of hemorrhage have developed at several locations within an infarction of the anterior and middle cerebral artery distributions. The patient had received anticoagulants during dialysis and probably also suffered from uremic platelet dysfunction.

Case 268

22-year-old woman who suffered a stroke shortly after severe head trauma.

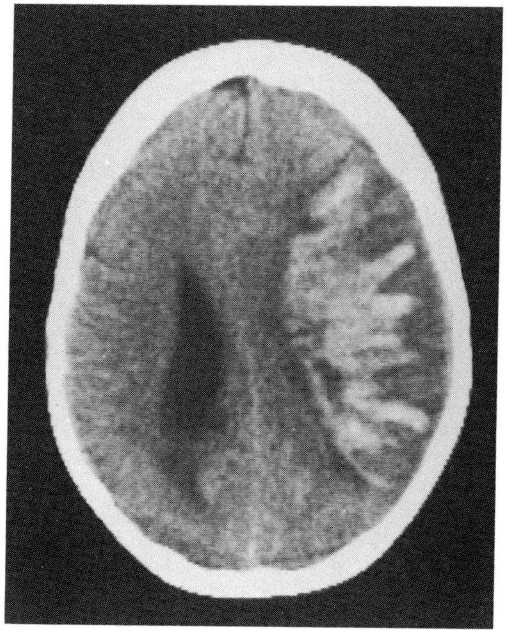

A cerebrovascular accident in a young patient should suggest the possibility of an embolic source. Leading causes include spontaneous dissection of the carotid or vertebral arteries or post-traumatic lesions of these vessels.

In this case, infarction was due to embolization from a traumatic dissection of the common carotid artery. Originally bland infarction became diffusely hemorrhagic two days after the patient began to receive anticoagulant therapy.

Dissolution of a cerebral embolus may predispose to hemorrhagic infarction by allowing reperfusion of damaged vessels.

Case 269

27-year-old man recently treated for subacute bacterial endocarditis, now presenting with acute diplopia (noncontrast scan). Saddle embolus in the basilar artery.

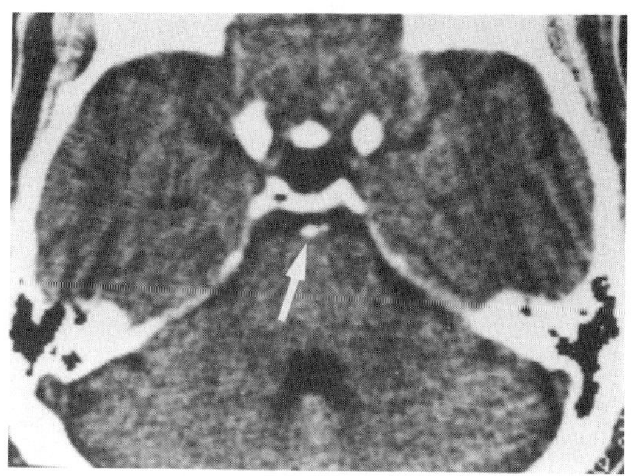

Thromboemboli can occasionally be seen as small densities within cerebral arteries. The density of an embolus may be due to calcification (e.g., a fragment of atheroma) or to the dense fibrin network within a thrombus.

Common locations for lodged emboli include the horizontal segment of the middle cerebral artery and the anterior cerebral artery bifurcation near the genu of the corpus callosum. Small densities near vessels in the subarachnoid cisterns may also be caused by calcified atherosclerotic plaque, falx calcification, and intracranial iophendylate (Pantopaque) droplets.

In this patient, an abnormal density occupies the tip of the basilar artery on the noncontrast scan *(arrow)*. The density was angiographically proved to represent a "saddle embolus" lodged at the basilar bifurcation. The patient later suffered subarachnoid hemorrhage, and autopsy confirmed a noncalcified, septic thromboembolus associated with erosion of the basilar artery tip.

Case 270

15-year-old-boy involved in a fight ten hours before the acute onset of hemiparesis. "Supernormal" occluded middle cerebral artery (noncontrast scan).

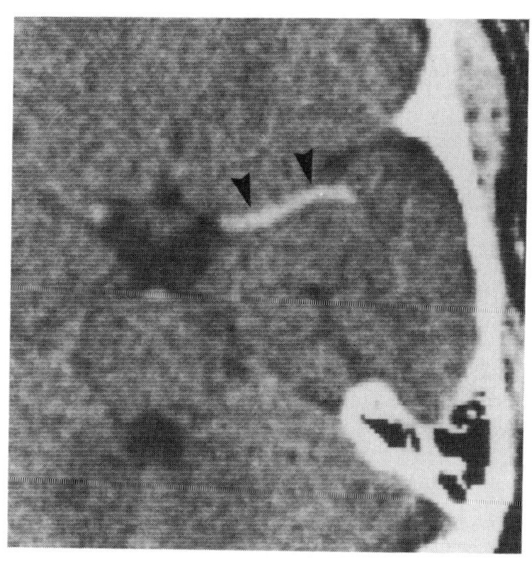

Occlusion of the middle cerebral artery (MCA) may be associated with abnormal prominence of the proximal segment on CT scans *(arrows)*. This "supernormal" horizontal segment may represent intraluminal stasis and/or thrombus. Angiograms in such cases have shown occlusion both distal and proximal to the dense arterial segment.

The "supernormal" artery may be seen before infarction is apparent and can provide the earliest clue to the diagnosis. Angiography in this case demonstrated dissection of the internal carotid artery with embolic occlusion at the MCA origin.

Case 271

2-year-old boy. Near-drowning.

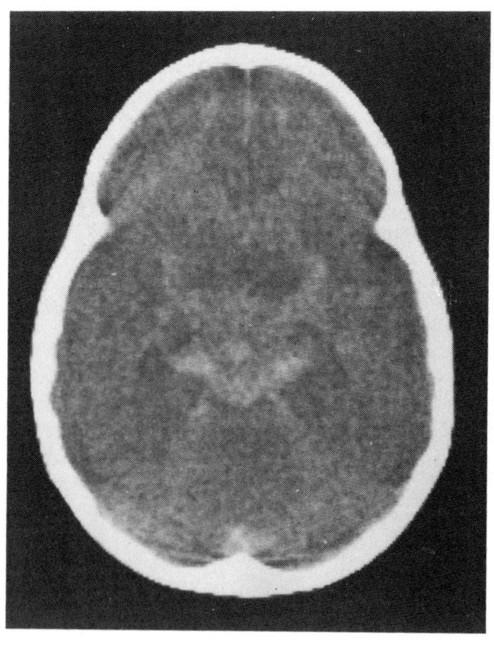

Anoxia may cause diffuse ischemic and cytotoxic edema leading to low attenuation and cerebral swelling. Gray matter is severely affected and may become lower in density than the underlying white matter. Reversal of the normal density relationship of gray and white matter can be faintly seen in the frontal lobes in this case, and is clearly demonstrated in Cases 272 and 274.

Deep-seated structures may be relatively spared, as seen here in the diencephalon and quadrigeminal plate. Diffuse cerebral and cerebellar swelling has completely effaced ventricles, cisterns, and sulci.

Case 342 illustrates the result of severe anoxia as displayed on follow-up scans.

Case 272

3-month-old boy. Sudden infant death syndrome.

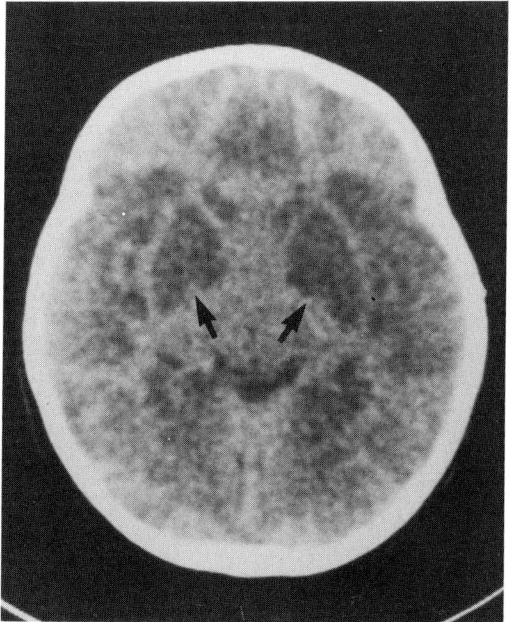

The lenticular nucleus *(arrows)* may be strikingly involved along with cortical gray matter in cases of cerebral anoxia. Here the cortical gyri and basal ganglia demonstrate equivalent and symmetrical low attenuation, while the density of white matter is relatively preserved.

The metabolic activity of gray matter increases its susceptibility to anoxic damage. The basal ganglia are perfused by "end-arteries," making them additionally vulnerable to an anoxic insult. Some cases of adult anoxia (e.g., carbon monoxide poisoning; see Case 249) show selective damage in the deep nuclei.

DIFFERENTIAL DIAGNOSIS: DIFFUSE CEREBRAL LOW ATTENUATION AND SWELLING IN AN INFANT

Case 273

10-week-old boy.

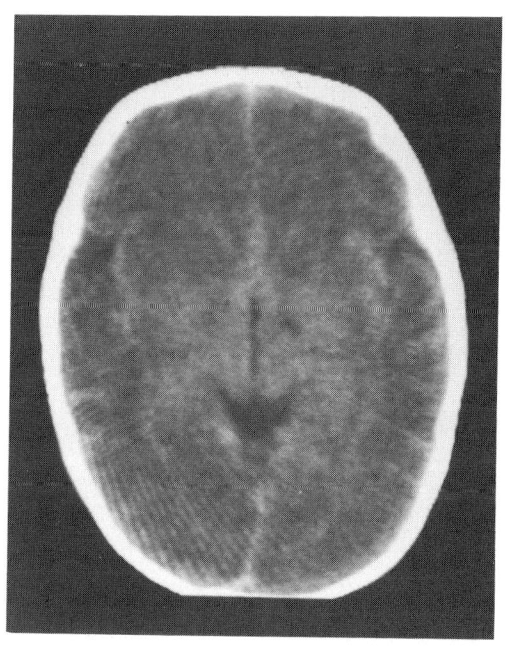

Herpes Encephalitis.

Case 274

15-month-old girl.

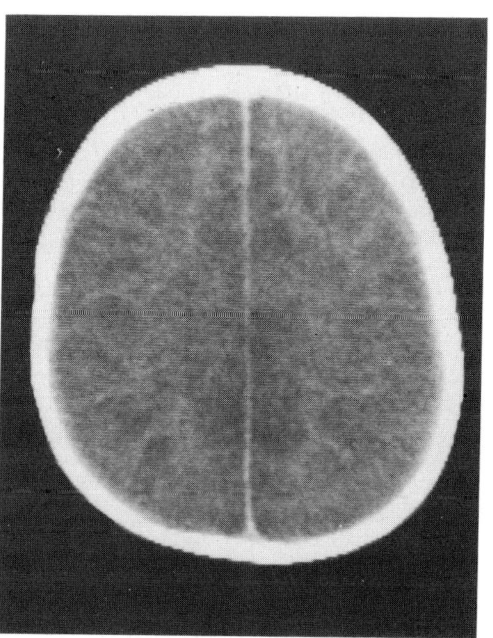

Anoxia (Cardiopulmonary Arrest Following Aspiration Of Food).

Scans in the acute phases of infantile encephalitis and anoxia may be similar. Both processes demonstrate widespread swelling and low-attenuation change.

The edema of encephalitis in Case 273 involves white matter regions and shows relative sparing of basal ganglia and some cortical areas. In contrast, the anoxia in Case 274 causes low attenuation throughout the cortex with relatively less abnormality of white matter.

Cases 152 and 153 illustrate the atrophy and calcification that commonly follow neonatal encephalitis, such as in Case 273.

SUPERIOR SAGITTAL SINUS THROMBOSIS

Case 275

10 month-old-boy who suffered a midline parietal skull fracture two days earlier, now lethargic and vomiting (noncontrast scan).

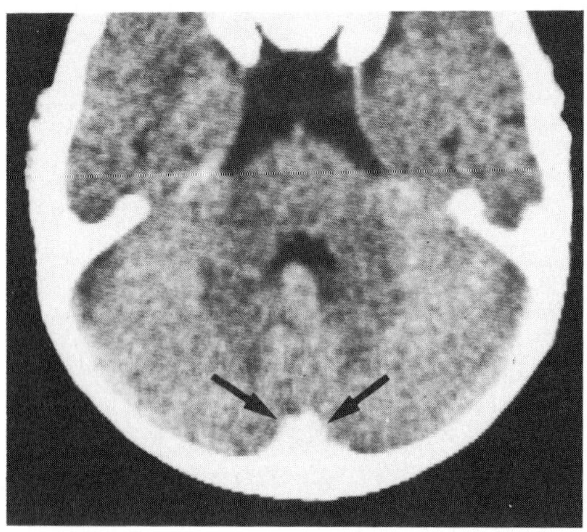

Case 276

21-year-old man injured in an automobile accident six days earlier, now presenting with impaired level of consciousness (postcontrast scan).

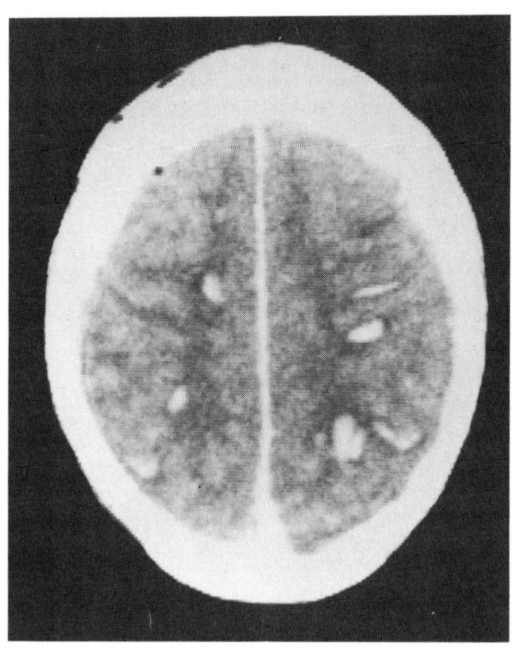

The CT findings of superior sagittal sinus thrombosis (SSST) depend on the age of the process and the presence or absence of contrast material. Acute SSST may present as an abnormally dense sinus on noncontrast scans *(arrow)*. (See Case 176 for discussion of normally dense sinuses in neonates.) The density of acute thrombosis may be masked by contrast enhancement of the sinus and adjacent dura.

Other potential clues to the diagnosis of SSST on noncontrast scans include parasagittal hemorrhages or edema (see Case 276) and cerebral swelling.

Digital subtraction angiography is an excellent procedure for assessing sinus patency in equivocal cases.

Parasagittal hemorrhages due to cortical venous infarction are a highly specific secondary finding in SSST. The parasagittal densities in this case were present on noncontrast scans, with no additional enhancement on this postcontrast study.

Patchy parasagittal edema without hemorrhage is also suggestive of SSST, although the appearance may be similar to that of arterial watershed infarction (see Cases 263 and 266). Occasional gyriform enhancement may be seen in the same parasagittal areas.

Postcontrast scans in SSST may also show abnormally intense enhancement of the tentorium, probably due to a combination of collateral venous flow and stasis.

DIFFERENTIAL DIAGNOSIS: THE "EMPTY TRIANGLE" SIGN

Case 277

21-year-old man (same patient as Case 276). Superior sagittal sinus thrombosis (contrast scan, high window level, narrow window width).

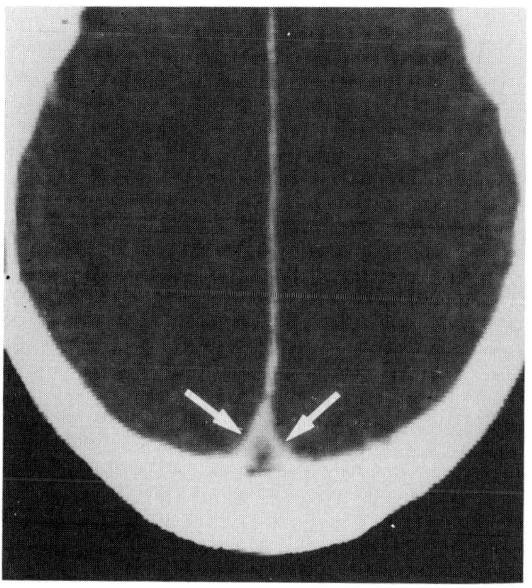

Case 278

25-year-old man suffering head trauma. Interhemispheric hemorrhage outlining a patent sagittal sinus (noncontrast scan).

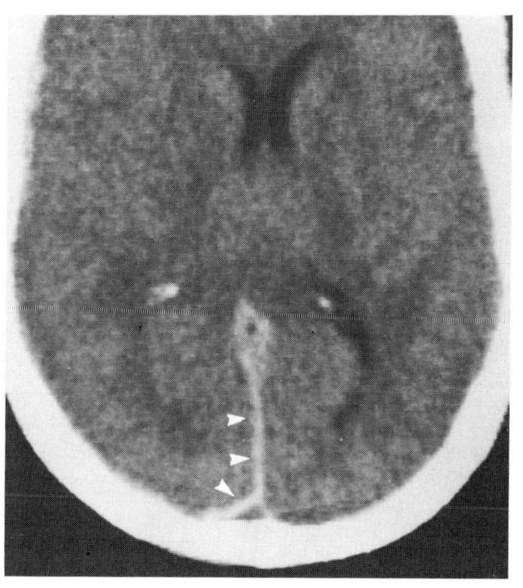

Clot within a dural sinus may be seen as a filling defect when surrounded by contrast in the residual lumen or outlined by the enhancing margins of the sinus. On axial scans, the superior sagittal sinus is viewed in cross section as a triangular structure near the occipital inner table. Thrombus filling this portion of the sinus creates the "empty triangle" sign of SSST on postcontrast images, as seen in Case 277 *(arrows)*. Optimal demonstration of the sign may require adjustment of display settings, with high window levels and narrow window widths.

The appearance of an "empty triangle" on noncontrast scans is usually due to subdural or subarachnoid blood outlining the sinus margins and does not imply thrombosis (see Cases 197, 211, and 278). As discussed in Case 275, the diagnosis of SSST on a noncontrast scan should be based on a *dense* sinus or on the characteristic secondary findings.

Another false "empty triangle" appearance may be caused by artifact crossing the posterior portion of the superior sagittal sinus on postcontrast scans. Prominent ridges of bone at the edges of the sinus groove favor this low-density band, analogous to the interpetrous ("Hounsfield") artifact in the posterior fossa.

Finally, the normal sinus may separate slightly from the occipital inner table as it nears the torcular. This variation causes a nonenhancing zone along the posterior wall of the sinus that may be misinterpreted as thrombus.

REFERENCES

1. Becker H., Desch H., Hacker H.: CT fogging effect with ischemic cerebral infarcts. *Neuroradiology* 18:185–192, 1979.
2. Berns T.F., Daniels D.L., Williams A.L.: Mesencephalic anatomy: Demonstration by computed tomography. *A.J.N.R.* 2:65–67, 1981.
3. Bradac G.B., Oberson R.: CT and angiography in cases with occlusive disease of supratentorial cerebral vessels. *Neuroradiology* 19:193–200, 1980.
4. Buonanno F.S., Moody D.M., Ball M.R., et al.: Computed cranial tomographic findings in cerebral sinovenous occlusion. *J. Comput. Assist. Tomogr.* 2:281–290, 1978.
5. Campbell J.K., Houser O.W., Stevens J.C., et al.: Computed tomography and radionuclide imaging in the evaluation of ischemic stroke. *Radiology* 126:695–702, 1978.
6. Di Chiro G., Arimitsu T., Pellock J.M., et al.: Periventricular leukomalacia related to neonatal anoxia: recognition by computed tomography. *J. Comput. Assist. Tomogr.* 2:352–355, 1978.
7. Drayer B.P., Rosenbaum A.E.: Brain edema defined by cranial computed tomography. *J. Comput. Assist. Tomogr.* 3:317–323, 1979.
8. Fieback B.J., Dabir K., Hermie P., et al.: Cerebral CT in fatal courses of resuscitated sudden infant death. *A.J.N.R.* 4:689–691, 1983.
9. Ford K., Sarwar M.: Computed tomography of dural sinus thrombosis. *A.J.N.R.* 2:539–543, 1981.
10. Goldberg H.I.: Stroke, in Lee S.H., Rao K.C. (eds.): *Cranial Computed Tomography,* New York, McGraw Hill Inc., 1983, pp. 583-657.
11. Houser O.W., Campbell J.K., Baker H.L., et al.: Radiologic evaluation of ischemic cerebrovascular syndromes with emphasis on computed tomography. *Radiol. Clin. North. Am.* 20:123–142, 1982.
12. Inoue Y., Takemoto K., Miyamoto T., et al.: Sequential computed tomography scans in acute cerebral infarction. *Radiology* 135:655–662, 1980.
13. Kendall B.E., Pullicino P.: Intravascular contrast injection in ischaemic lesions. II. Effect on prognosis. *Neuroradiology* 19:241–243, 1980.
14. Kim K.S., Weinberg P.E., Suh J.H., et al.: Acute carbon monoxide poisoning; Computed tomography of the brain. *A.J.N.R.* 1:399–402, 1980.
15. Lee K.F., Chambers R.H., Diamond C., et al.: Evaluation of cerebral infarction by computed tomography with special emphasis on microinfarction. *Neuroradiology* 16:156–158, 1978.
16. Manelfe C., Clanet M., Gigaud M., et al: Internal capsule: Normal anatomy and ischemic changes demonstrated by CT. *A.J.N.R.* 2:149–155, 1981.
17. Maravilla K.R., Pastel M.S., Kirkpatrick J.B.: White matter of the cerebellum demonstrated by CT: Normal anatomy and physical principles. *J. Comput. Assist. Tomogr.* 2:156–161, 1978.
18. Masdeu J.C.: Infarct versus neoplasm on CT: Four helpful signs. *A.J.N.R.* 4:522–524, 1983.
19. Modic M.T., Weinstein M.A.: Cerebrovascular disease of the brain, in Haaga J.R., Alfidi R.J., (eds.): *Computed Tomography of the Whole Body.* St. Louis, C.V. Mosby Co., 1983, pp. 136–169.
20. Murray R.R., Kapila A., Blanco E., et al.: Cerebral computed tomography in drowning victims. *A.J.N.R.* 5:177–179, 1984.
21. Naidich T.P., Chakera T.M.H.: Multicystic encephalomalacia: CT appearance and pathological correlation. *J. Comput. Assist. Tomogr.* 8:631–636, 1984.
22. Nelson R.F., Pullicino P., Kendall B.E., et al.: Computed tomography in patients presenting with lacunar syndromes. *Stroke* 11:256–261, 1980.
23. Norton G.A., Kishore P.R., Lin J.: CT contrast enhancement in cerebral infarction. *A.J.R.* 131:881–885, 1978.
24. Pullicino P., Kendall B.E.: Contrast enhancement in ischemic lesions. I. Relationship to prognosis. *Neuroradiology* 19:235–239, 1980.
25. Pullicino P., Nelson R.F., Kendall B.E.: Small deep infarcts diagnosed on computed tomography. *Neurology* 30:1090–1096, 1980.
26. Rao K.C., Knipp H.C., Wagner E.J.: Computed tomographic findings in cerebral sinus and venous thrombosis. *Radiology* 140:391–398, 1981.
27. Rosenbloom S., Buchholz D., Kumar A.J., et al.: Evolution of central pontine myelinolysis on CT. *A.J.N.R.* 5:110–112, 1984.
28. Swada Y., Ohashi N., Maemura K., et al.: Computed tomography as an indication of long term outcome after acute carbon monoxide poisoning. *Lancet* 1:783–784, 1980.
29. Takeuchi S., Kobayashi K., Tsuchida T., et al: Computed tomography in moyamoya disease. *J. Comput. Assist. Tomogr.* 6:24–32, 1982.
30. Taneda M., Ozaki K., Wakayama A., et al.: Cerebellar infarction with obstructive hydrocephalus. *J. Neurosurg.* 57:83–91, 1982.
31. Tsai F.Y., Teal J.S., Heishima G.B., et al.: Computed tomography in acute posterior fossa infarcts. *A.J.N.R.* 3:149–156, 1982.
32. Vonofakos D., Marcu H., Hacker H.: CT diagnosis of basilar artery occlusion. *A.J.N.R.* 4:525–528, 1983.
33. Wall S.D., Brant-Zawadzki M., Jeffry R.B., et al.: High frequency CT findings within 24 hours after cerebral infarction. *A.J.N.R.* 2:553–557, 1981.
34. Wodarz R.: Watershed infarcts and computed tomography. A topographical study in cases with stenosis or occlusion of the internal carotid artery. *Neuroradiology* 19:245–251, 1980.
35. Yagnik P., Gonzalez C.: White matter involvement in anoxic encephalopathy in adults. *J. Comput. Assist. Tomogr.* 4:788–790, 1980.
36. Yock D.H. Jr.: CT demonstration of cerebral emboli. *J. Comput. Assist. Tomogr.* 5:190–196, 1981.
37. Zimmermann R.A., Bilaniuk L.T., Packer R.J., et al.: Computed tomographic-arteriographic correlates in acute basal ganglionic infarction of childhood. *Neuroradiology* 24:241–248, 1983.

CHAPTER 10

VASCULAR LESIONS AND HEMORRHAGE

Case 279A

35-year-old woman with left hemifacial spasm.

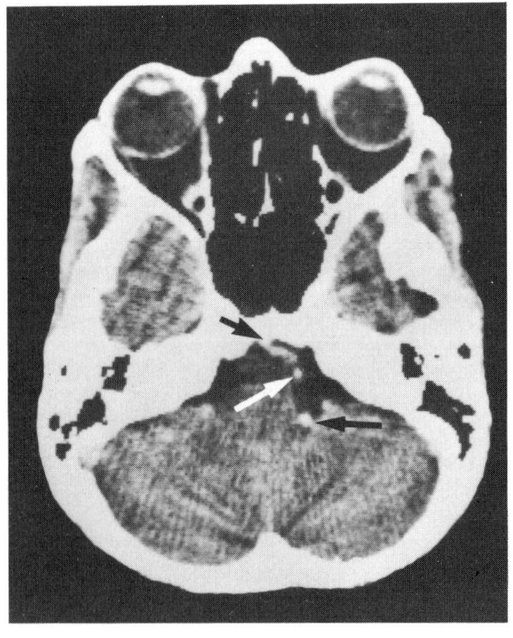

Some patients experience recurrent symptoms due to distortion of cranial nerves by adjacent vessels. Both tic douloureux (trigeminal nerve) and hemifacial spasm (facial nerve) may be caused by contact of an artery or vein with the nerve near its junction with the brain stem ("entry zone"). Although CT scans rarely give an image of the microvascular anatomical findings responsible for most cases of nerve irritation, occasional symptomatic arterial loops can be identified.

Here a prominent cephalic loop of the distal left vertebral artery is seen. The vessel ascends dorsally *(black arrow)* before descending ventrally *(white arrow)* to join the basilar artery *(short arrow)*.

Case 279B

Same patient. Higher scan.

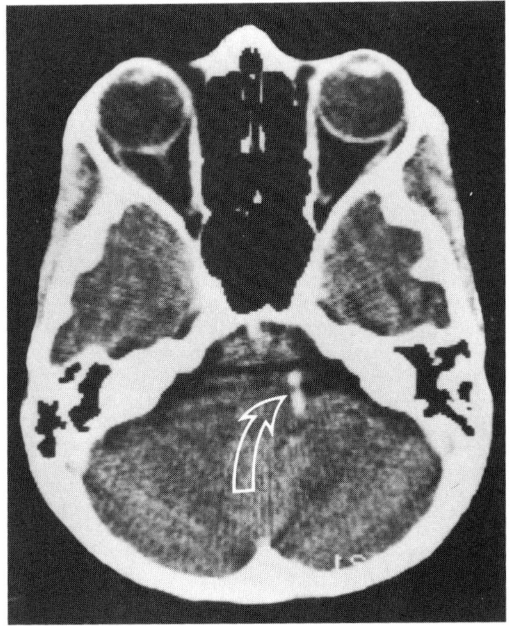

This scan passes through the top of the loop formed by the distal vertebral artery in the cerebellopontine angle. The apex of the loop lies against the brain stem near the level of the facial nerve. Surgery confirmed compression and distortion of the seventh nerve by the large arterial loop. Separation of the artery from the nerve resulted in cessation of facial spasms.

Case 280

32-year-old woman presenting with seizures.

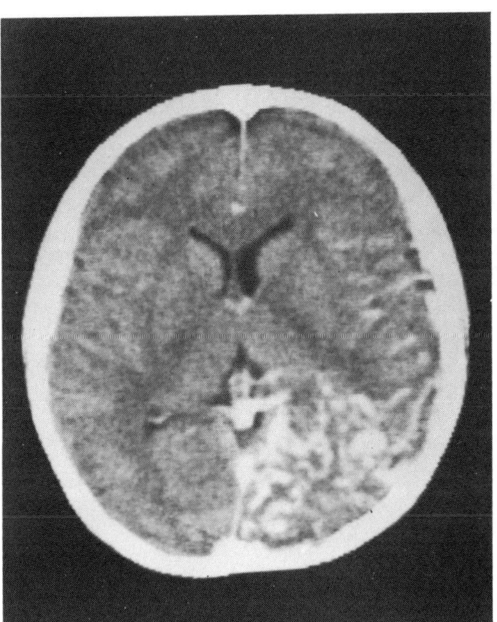

Arteriovenous malformations (AVMs) are found with a variety of CT appearances. The characteristic lesion is a closely packed tangle of serpentine, enhancing vascular channels, as seen here in the left temporal occipital lobe (see also Cases 284, 285, and 294). Large feeding arteries or draining veins may be apparent.

Mass effect is unusual in the absence of associated hemorrhage, although some large AVMs do present with bulky vascular components (see Case 281). Encephalomalacia may be present, due to old hemorrhage or to parenchymal damage from the pulsations or "steal" of the malformation.

Case 281

2-day-old boy with congestive heart failure (noncontrast scan).

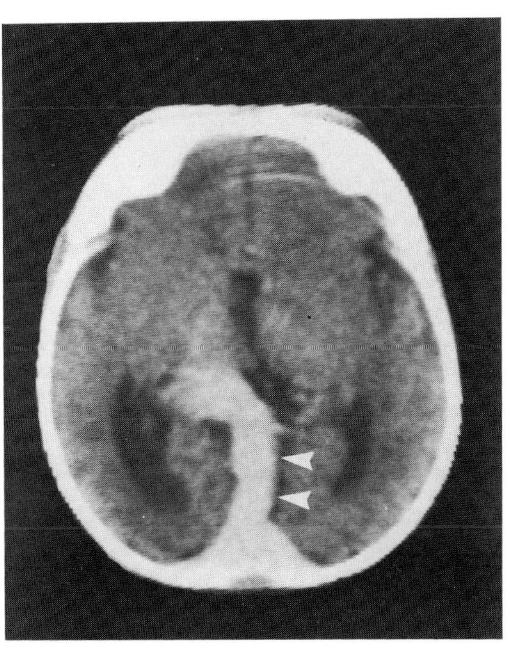

Some AVMs contain hugely dilated vascular channels. These structures may represent expansion of anatomically normal veins, as is commonly seen with malformations draining into the vein of Galen. Such malformations in this region often contain direct arteriovenous shunts. The associated high flow causes marked enlargement of the receiving veins, traditionally misnamed as a "vein of Galen 'aneurysm'."

This case demonstrates expansion of the straight sinus *(arrows)* leading from a "vein of Galen aneurysm" to the torcular. High flow through a cerebral AVM is an important cause of neonatal heart failure, as in this patient.

Cases 283 and 296 present a "vein of Galen aneurysm" in an adult.

Case 282

22-year-old woman presenting with seizures (noncontrast scan).

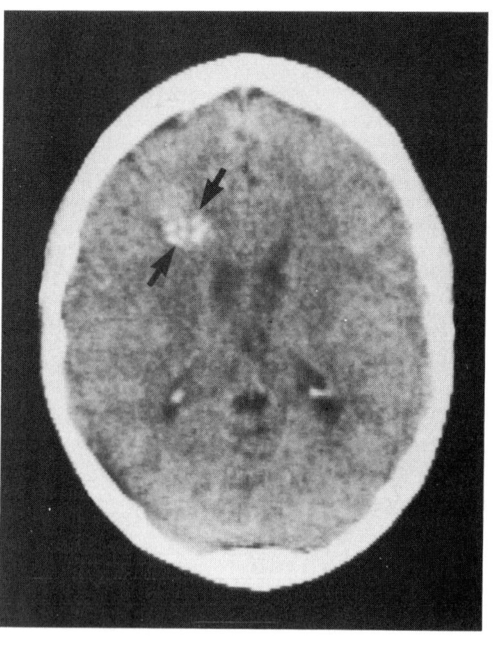

Many AVMs are associated with intracerebral calcification. The calcium may occur within the walls of vascular channels or within dystrophic cerebral parenchyma.

In this case, the cluster of deep frontal calcifications is not associated with abnormal low attenuation, as might be seen in a low-grade glioma. A contrast scan demonstrated characteristic serpentine enhancement throughout the lesion.

Some AVMs are angiographically inapparent or "cryptic" due to thrombosis and/or low flow. Such lesions are usually detected on CT scans as small, high-attenuation regions (see Case 290). Their density may be due to calcification, blood volume, and/or contrast enhancement.

Patients with AVMs commonly present with seizures, as in this case. Other presentations include hemorrhage, headache, and focal hemispheric deficits.

Case 283

33-year-old woman with a large head (noncontrast scan).

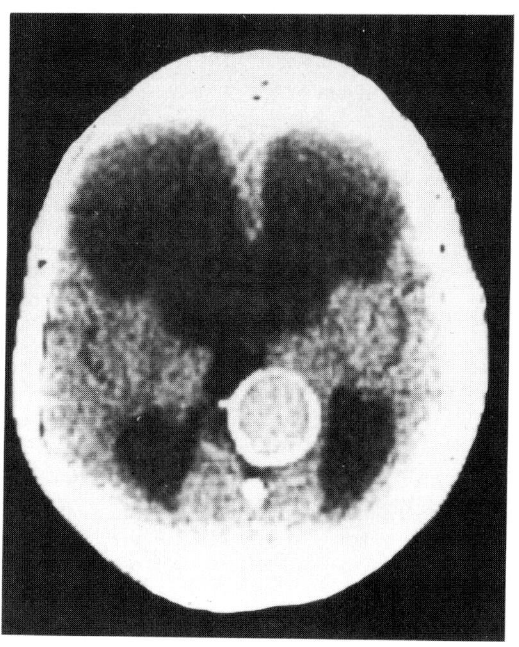

Rings or arcs of calcification may be seen in the walls of large arteries or veins within an AVM.

Here, a peripherally calcified, centrally dense mass compresses the posterior third ventricle, resembling a pineal region neoplasm. The mass was proved angiographically to be a variceal (or "aneurysmal") vein of Galen (see Case 281). The central density of the vein represents circulating blood.

Round, variceal components of AVMs may mimic the precontrast density and intense enhancement of a meningioma or a giant aneurysm (see Case 296 for a postcontrast scan on this patient; compare with Cases 319 and 320).

Case 284

81-year-old woman presenting with a cerebrovascular accident.

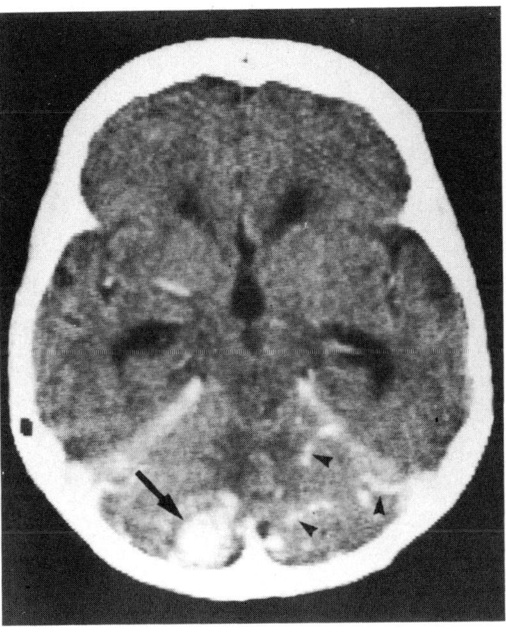

Hemorrhage is the most common presentation of AVMs, occurring in one third to two thirds of patients in most series. The majority of these hemorrhages are intracerebral rather than subarachnoid.

A CT scan usually demonstrates both the hematoma and the responsible vascular malformation. Rarely a small AVM is destroyed at the time of rupture or compressed by the resulting hematoma. In this case, a small cerebellar hematoma is seen *(large arrow)*, associated with several tortuous vascular channels *(small arrows)*.

Large veins are normally present near the tentorium (see Case 321B). These prominent vessels drain the inferior surface of the temporal and occipital lobes, passing through or near the tentorial dura to reach the transverse sinuses. Their superficial location adjacent to the tentorium distinguishes normal veins from the deeper and more scattered components of a true AVM, as seen in this case.

Case 285

72-year-old man presenting with a cerebrovascular accident.

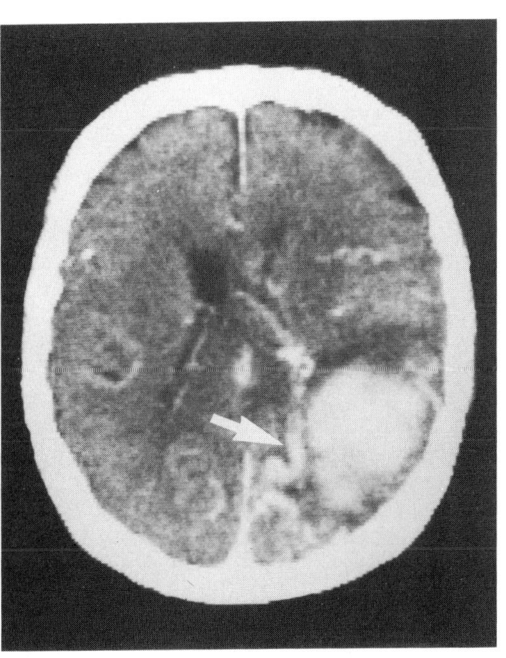

This scan shows a large supratentorial hematoma. Prominent vessels are seen anteriorly and laterally. The very large vein in the medial occipital lobe *(arrow)* leaves little doubt as to the pathologic condition responsible for the hemorrhage. (Compare with the more subtle findings in Case 331.)

VENOUS ANGIOMAS

Case 286

52-year-old man.

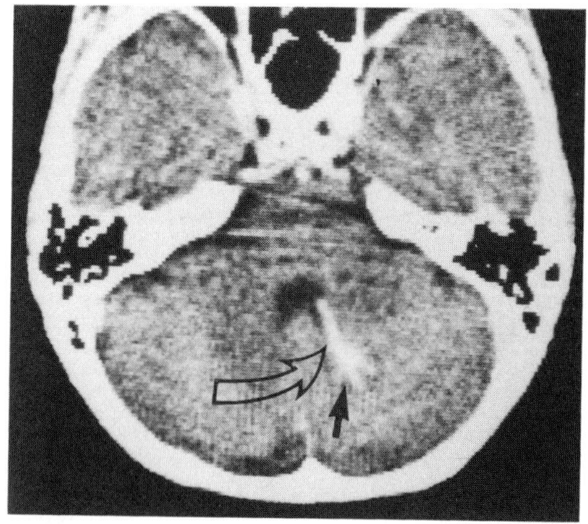

Venous angiomas have a characteristic morphology which is often recognizable on CT scans. The lesion has two components: (1) a group of radially oriented tributory veins converging like spokes of an umbrella to a central point, and (2) a single, abnormally large draining vein, formed at the confluence of the tributaries and following an aberrant route through cerebral parenchyma.

Here, the confluence of tributary channels is seen posteriorly *(solid arrow)*, with the draining vein *(open arrow)* coursing anteriorly to reach the fourth ventricle.

Case 287

65-year-old man.

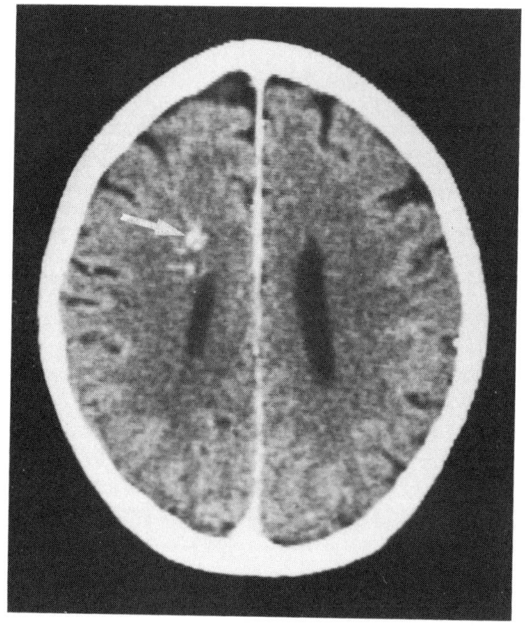

This scan demonstrates a cross section of the enlarged draining vein as it is formed deep within the cerebral hemisphere. Radially oriented tributaries are faintly visible in the adjacent parenchyma. The aberrantly located, dilated "stem" vein of a venous angioma is highly characteristic even when the tributary veins are inconspicuous.

Venous angiomas are infrequently associated with seizures. Rare hemorrhage may be most common in cerebellar lesions.

CAVERNOUS HEMANGIOMAS

Case 288A

26-year-old woman with right arm weakness (noncontrast scan).

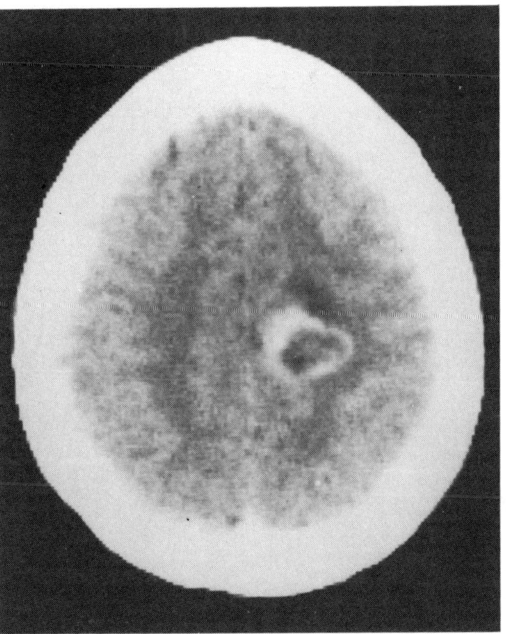

Case 288B

Same patient (noncontrast scan; higher level).

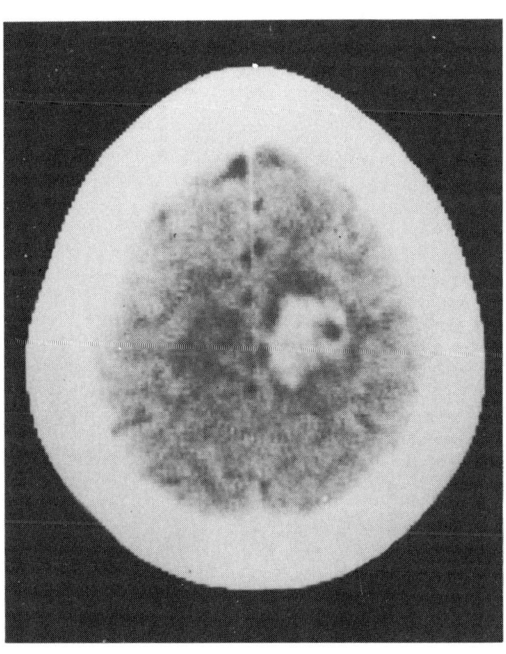

Cavernous hemangiomas are collections of sinusoidal vascular spaces without intervening neuroglial tissue. Although well recognized pathologically as one of the major categories of cerebrovascular malformations, these lesions have been difficult to diagnose prior to CT scanning. Their frequent discovery by CT requires recognition and distinction from other masses.

Noncontrast CT scans typically demonstrate a mixed- or high-attenuation mass, which may be several centimeters in diameter. The high density represents blood volume, thrombosed channels, and/or associated calcification. Low attenuation may reflect adjacent encephalomalacia or old, clotted portions of the malformation. Contrast enhancement varies from minimal to intense.

The CT appearance may resemble a neoplasm, as in this case. Precontrast density is an important clue to the benign etiology of the lesion.

Cavernous hemangiomas are often apparent on CT scans despite their lack of angiographic visualization. (The angiogram in this case showed no abnormal vascularity or stain.) They account for a substantial number of the so-called "cryptic" vascular malformations (see also Cases 282 and 290).

The walls of the cavernous channels within hemangiomas are often thickened, with calcification or even ossification. Heavily calcified lesions have been termed "hemangioma calcificans."

DIFFERENTIAL DIAGNOSIS: INTRACEREBRAL CALCIFICATION WITH ADJACENT LOW ATTENUATION

Case 289

61-year-old woman presenting with seizures.

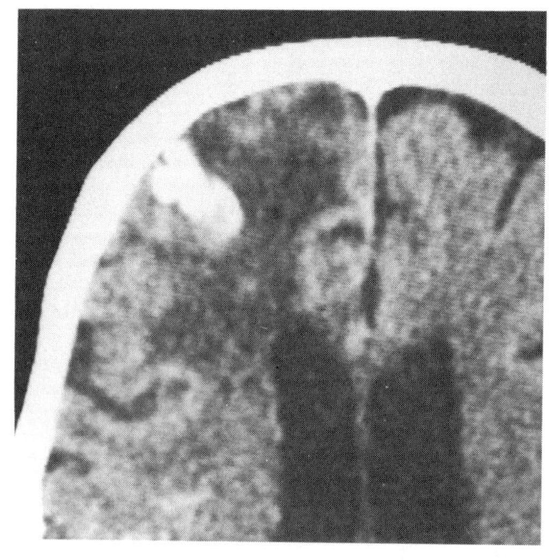

Low-Grade Astrocytoma.

Case 290

19-year-old woman presenting with seizures (postcontrast scan).

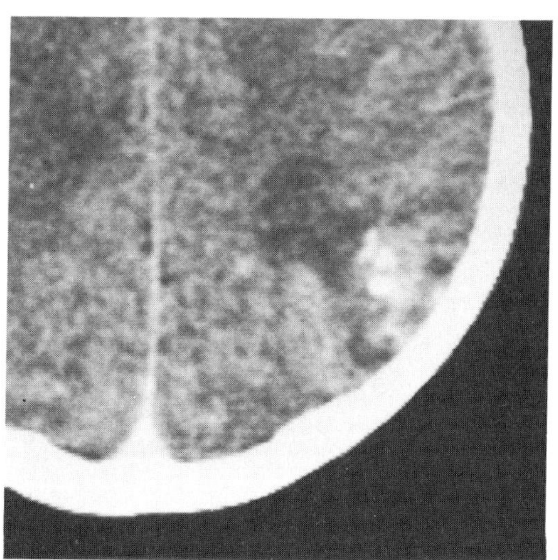

Thrombosed AVM.

The combination of cerebral calcification and low attenuation is frequently seen in low-grade gliomas, as illustrated by Case 289.

Calcification is also common in AVMs. This finding is sometimes accompanied by adjacent low density, as discussed in Case 280. When such a lesion demonstrates minimal contrast enhancement (as in Case 290), the appearance may resemble a low-grade tumor or inflammatory focus.

Angiography was nondiagnostic in Case 290. Surgery demonstrated a thrombosed AVM. (See Case 282 for discussion of "cryptic" vascular malformations.)

DIFFERENTIAL DIAGNOSIS: ENHANCING BRAIN STEM LESION

Case 291

7-year-old boy.

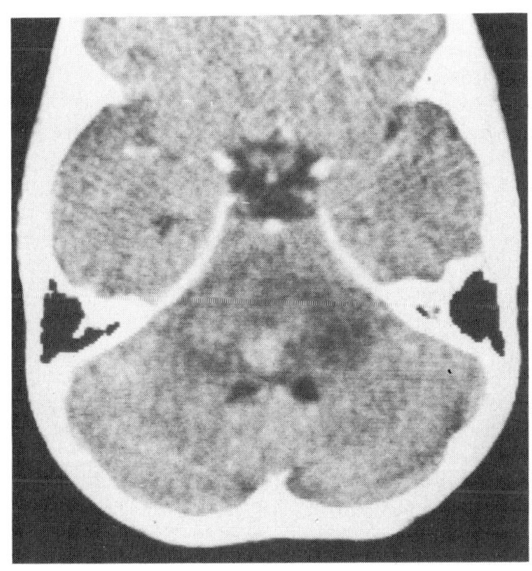

Brain Stem Glioma.

Case 292

45-year-old man.

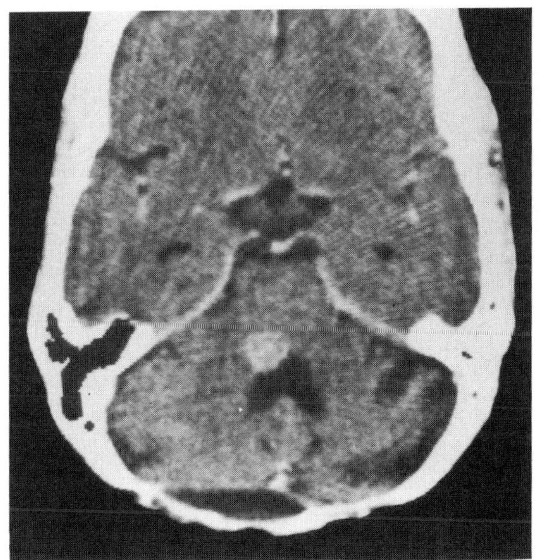

AVM (Previous Surgery At Age 16 To Evacuate A Posterior Fossa Hematoma).

Vascular malformations often involve the brain stem. The pathologically common capillary telangiectasia is rarely evident on CT scans, but may cause pontine hemorrhage. True AVMs of the brain stem may be detected because of calcification, hemorrhage, or contrast enhancement.

These lesions often border the fourth ventricle, as seen in Case 292. Bulky components of the AVM may fill the ventricle, with their prominent enhancement suggesting an intraventricular tumor.

In other cases, the poorly defined margins of a brain stem AVM may combine with nonspecific symptoms to mimic a brain stem glioma. The usual absence of mass effect favors the correct diagnosis.

DIFFERENTIAL DIAGNOSIS: CEREBRAL LESION WITH INTENSE, TUBULAR, CONTRAST ENHANCEMENT

Case 293

72-year-old woman.

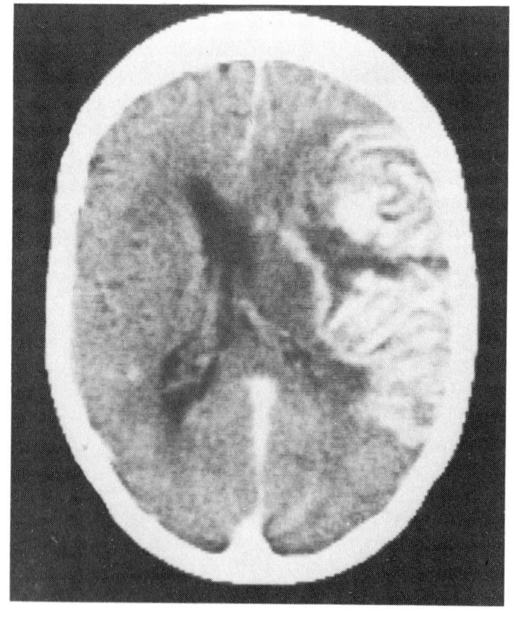

Infarction (19 Days Old).

Case 294

18-year-old man with seizures.

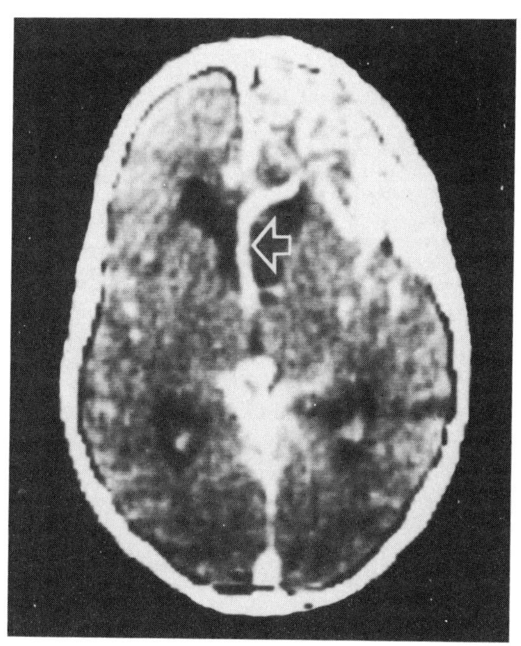

AVM.

The intense, gyriform contrast enhancement of subacute infarction may assume a tubular morphology mimicking a vascular malformation, as seen in Case 293. A clue to the correct diagnosis on this scan is the overall shape of the lesion, which conforms to the distribution of the middle cerebral artery.

The large frontal lobe AVM in Case 294 includes a prominent draining vein in the septum pellucidum *(arrows)*. The lesion spans the territories of the anterior and middle cerebral arteries.

DIFFERENTIAL DIAGNOSIS: INTENSELY ENHANCING MASS NEAR THE VEIN OF GALEN

Case 295

30-year-old woman with neurofibromatosis.

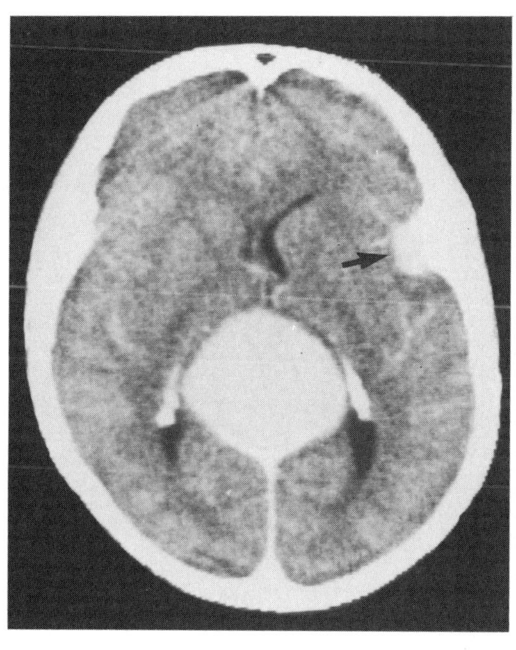

Meningiomas.

Case 296

33-year-old woman.

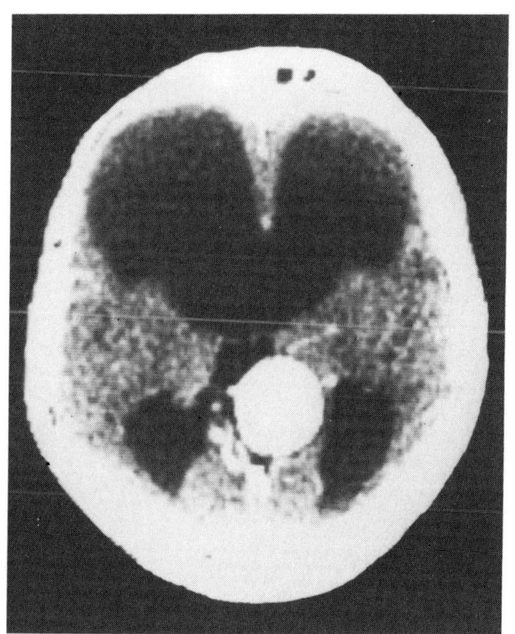

Vein of Galen Aneurysm.

Large, round aneurysms or varices demonstrate uniform density and intense contrast enhancement resembling the CT features of meningiomas. The scan in Case 296 represents the postcontrast appearance of the lesion in Case 283.

The large subsplenial meningioma in Case 295 splays the posterior bodies of the lateral ventricles. A second, small meningioma is present near the pterion *(arrow)*.

Case 297

58-year-old man with sudden headache followed by loss of consciousness. Ruptured aneurysm of the anterior communicating artery.

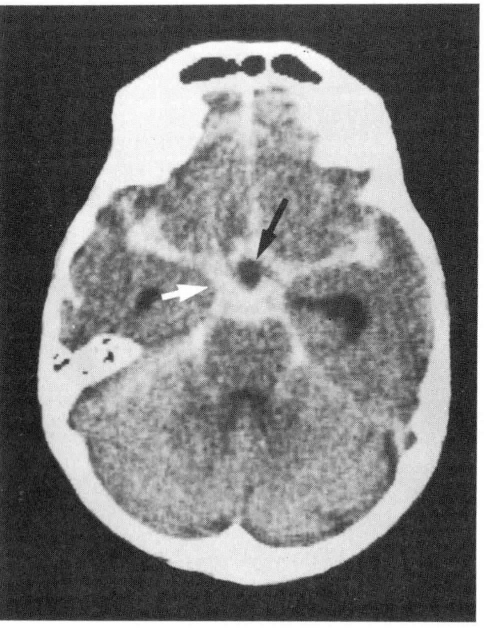

Subarachnoid hemorrhage is usually apparent on CT scans. The high attenuation of blood replaces the low density of spinal fluid, causing normally "black" CSF spaces to become "white." The hemorrhage may be symmetrical and diffuse, as in this case, or localized to a single cistern.

Blood within the spinal fluid serves as a subarachnoid contrast agent, outlining surface anatomy. Here the brain stem is well defined, as is the uncus *(white arrow)*. The filling defect in the suprasellar cistern *(black arrow)* is a combined image of the optic chiasm (anterior, transverse band) and the dilated anterior recesses of the third ventricle (circular posterior component).

Case 298

54-year-old man now comatose after the acute onset of headache. Ruptured aneurysm of the anterior communicating artery.

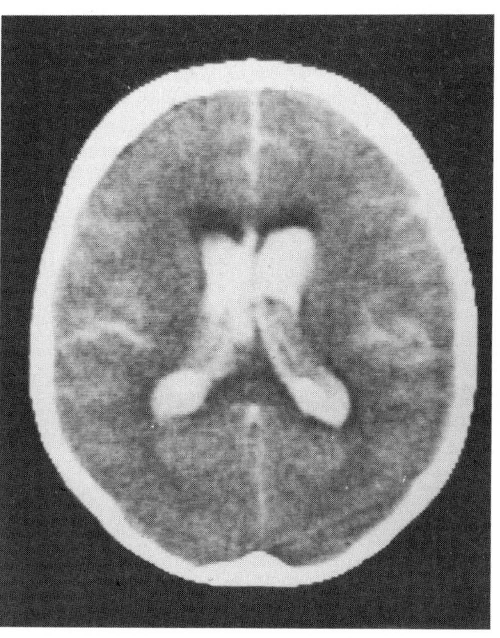

Scans above the skull base demonstrate subarachnoid blood filling the sylvian cisterns, interhemispheric fissure, and cortical sulci.

Intraventricular hemorrhage is commonly associated with subarachnoid blood, as seen in this case. An aneurysm may rupture directly into the ventricular system, or a parenchymal hematoma caused by an aneurysm may secondarily decompress into the ventricles.

In other cases no direct communication from the aneurysm site can be demonstrated, and blood appears to have flooded retrograde through the fourth ventricle and aqueduct. This occurrence is particularly common with ruptured aneurysms of the vertebral or basilar arteries.

Case 299

57-year-old man scanned six days after rupture of an aneurysm of the anterior communicating artery. Isodense subarachnoid spaces.

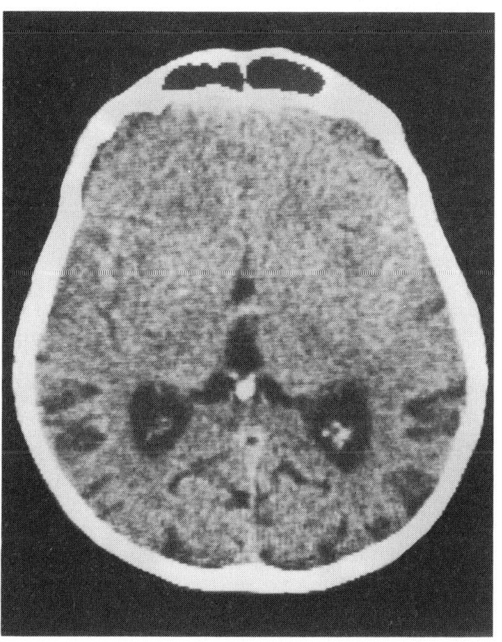

The attenuation of blood within the subarachnoid space depends on the amount and age of the hemorrhage. Cases with small or subacute hemorrhages may demonstrate isodense cisterns and sulci, as seen here in the frontal and sylvian regions. (Compare the lack of surface topography anteriorly with the normal sulcal markings posteriorly; see also Case 311.)

Other causes for isodense subarachnoid spaces include filling of the cisterns by inflammatory exudate (i.e., pyogenic meningitis) or tumor spread (e.g., CSF seeding from medulloblastoma, ependymoma, or germinoma).

Case 300

65-year-old woman presenting with headache and stiff neck. Enhancing subarachnoid spaces approximately one week after rupture of an aneurysm of the posterior communicating artery.

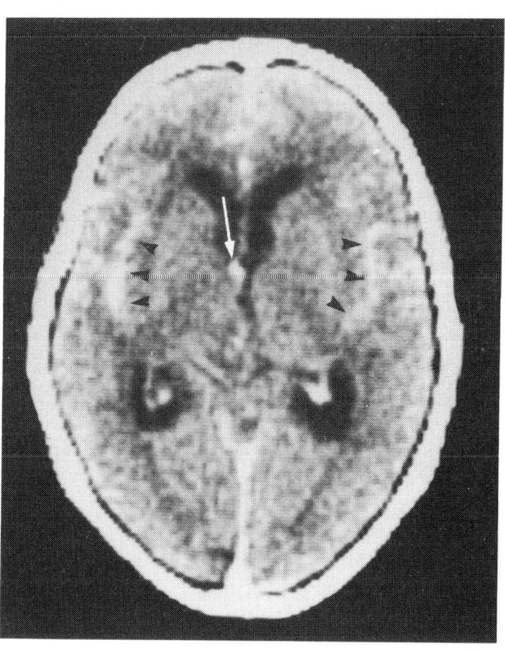

Contrast enhancement is often seen in cisterns and sulci recently exposed to subarachnoid hemorrhage. In this case, the subarachnoid spaces were isodense on a preconstrast scan. Diffuse enhancement is demonstrated, best seen in the sylvian cisterns *(black arrows)*.

The mechanism of this enhancement is unclear but may include components of contrast extravasation as well as meningeal hyperemia. Cisternal enhancement may be more apparent than the underlying subarachnoid hemorrhage, offering an important clue to the diagnosis. The differential diagnosis of enhancing subarachnoid spaces includes meningitis and meningeal tumor, as previously discussed.

A tiny clot at the foramen of Monro *(white arrow)* is occasionally an isolated clue to recent intraventricular hemorrhage.

DIFFERENTIAL DIAGNOSIS: HIGH ATTENUATION WITHIN CEREBRAL SULCI

Case 301

76-year-old woman.

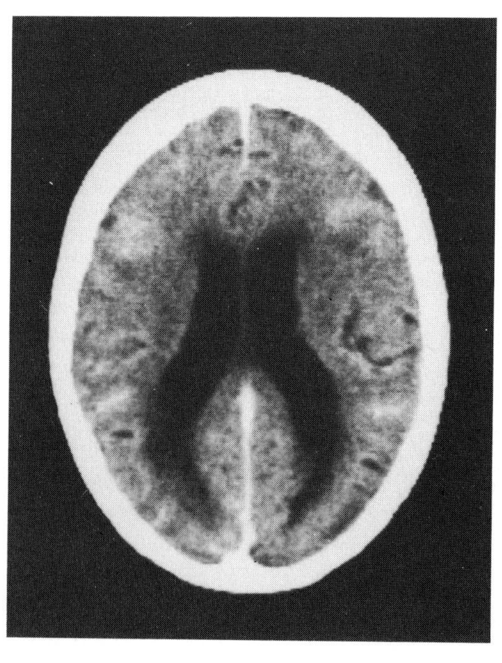

Meningeal Carcinomatosis From Metastatic Breast Carcinoma (Postcontrast Scan).

Case 302

50-year-old woman.

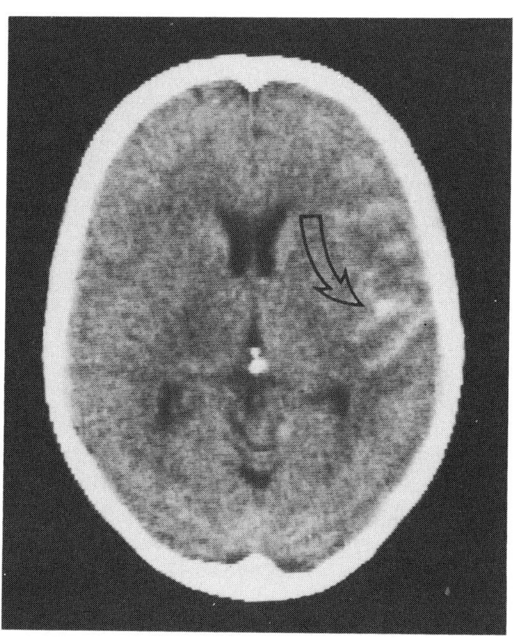

Subarachnoid Hemorrhage From A Middle Cerebral Artery Aneurysm (Noncontrast Scan).

The interpretation of abnormal density within cerebral sulci depends on the circumstances of the scan. On a noncontrast scan (e.g., Case 302) this finding strongly implies subarachnoid hemorrhage. Other meningeal processes (e.g., exudate, tumor) may raise cisternal attenuation to an isodense level, but rarely beyond.

Dense subarachnoid spaces on a postcontrast scan may be due to a variety of causes, including subarachnoid hemorrhage, meningeal spread of CNS or systemic neoplasm, and meningitis (pyogenic, fungal, tuberculous, or parasitic). In Case 301, enhancing sulci filled with meningeal tumor contrast with the normal low attenuation of adjacent uninvolved subarachnoid spaces.

The subarachnoid spaces of children may normally appear dense on postcontrast scans when enhancing vessels almost fill the small sulci. A similar finding may be seen within compressed cisterns in the presence of hydrocephalus or increased intracranial pressure (see Cases 117, 123, and 191). A component of stasis may contribute in such circumstances. When this appearance accompanies hydrocephalus due to a tumor, the possibility of CSF "seeding" may be difficult to exclude.

Case 303

79-year-old woman. Secondary hydrocephalus.

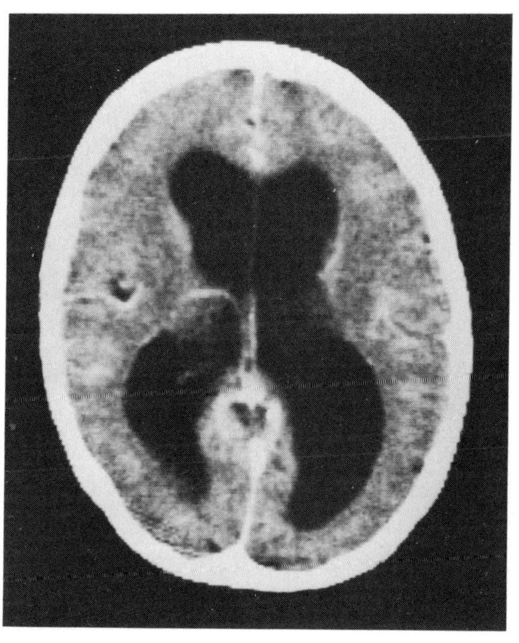

Hydrocephalus may develop at several stages following subarachnoid hemorrhage. Acute hydrocephalus (see Case 307) may be obstructive (due to clot within the ventricular system) or communicating (attributed to clogging of arachnoid granulations by erythrocytes). Delayed communicating hydrocephalus is thought to be caused by postinflammatory changes in meningeal CSF pathways, including the arachnoid granulations. Faint meningeal enhancement is seen in this case (see Case 300).

Hydrocephalus may increase intracranial pressure at a time when cerebral perfusion is marginal due to developing spasm.

Case 304

65-year-old woman. Secondary infarction.

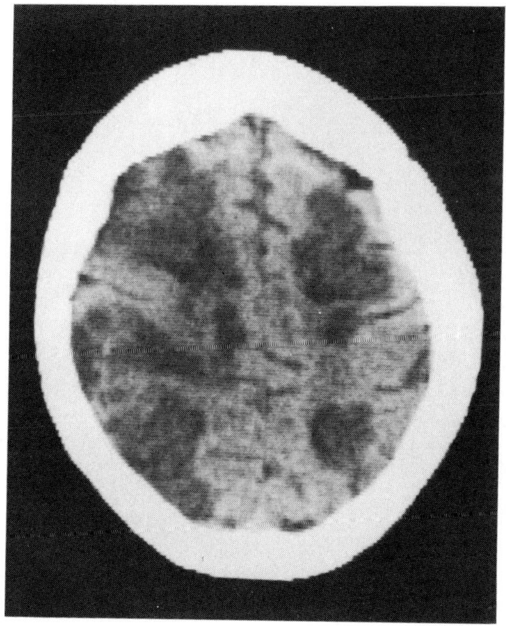

Spasm of cerebral arteries is a common and serious complication of subarachnoid hemorrhage. Spasm typically develops a few days after hemorrhage, reaching a maximum in the late first week to early second week and subsiding thereafter. The vessels most severely involved tend to be those in areas of densest subarachnoid hemorrhage.

Infarction due to spasm may present in watershed regions, as in this case, or in major arterial distributions (see Case 246).

Case 305

50-year-old man. Ruptured aneurysm of the anterior communicating artery.

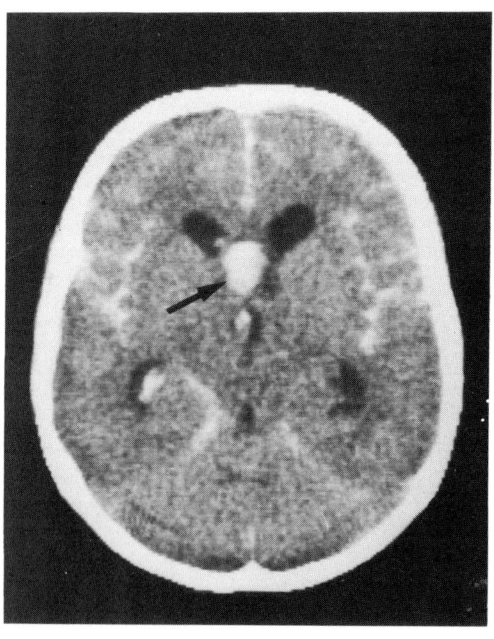

Hemorrhage from anterior communicating artery aneurysms may include subarachnoid and intracerebral components. The subarachnoid blood is often symmetrically distributed, as seen here and in Cases 297 through 299. Asymmetrical subarachnoid hemorrhage does occur and should not be thought to exclude the diagnosis.

Parenchymal hematomas from ruptured aneurysms of the anterior communicating artery often involve anterior midline structures. A hematoma within the lamina terminalis/septum pellucidum region *(arrow)* is highly specific but occurs in a minority of cases. Ruptured aneurysms of the anterior communicating artery may cause eccentric intracerebral hematomas, often demonstrating a "tail" or track leading back to the aneurysm site (see Case 330).

Case 306

64-year-old man. Ruptured aneurysm of a posterior communicating artery.

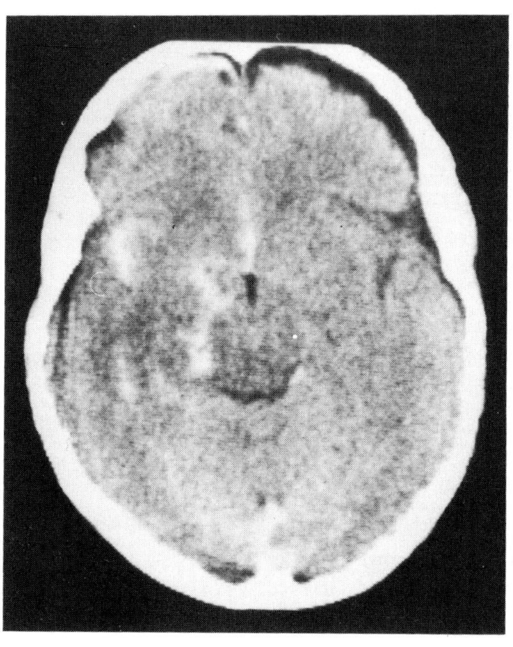

The so-called "posterior communicating artery" aneurysms arise from the supraclinoid internal carotid artery at the origin of the posterior communicating artery. Rupture of these aneurysms may produce a typical distribution of subarachnoid blood, as illustrated here.

Hemorrhage is most dense within the ipsilateral portions of the suprasellar, perimesencephalic, and proximal sylvian cisterns. A small subdural hematoma is present at the frontal pole and a small subdural hygroma is seen on the opposite side, suggesting superimposed trauma.

Rupture of aneurysms may cause acute subdural hematomas, most commonly associated with aneurysms of the internal carotid and middle cerebral arteries. On the other hand, head trauma rarely causes dense, basal subarachnoid hemorrhage. An underlying aneurysm should be suspected whenever such hemorrhage is found, even with a history of trauma.

HEMORRHAGE FROM ANEURYSMS OF THE MIDDLE CEREBRAL ARTERY

Case 307

69-year-old woman.

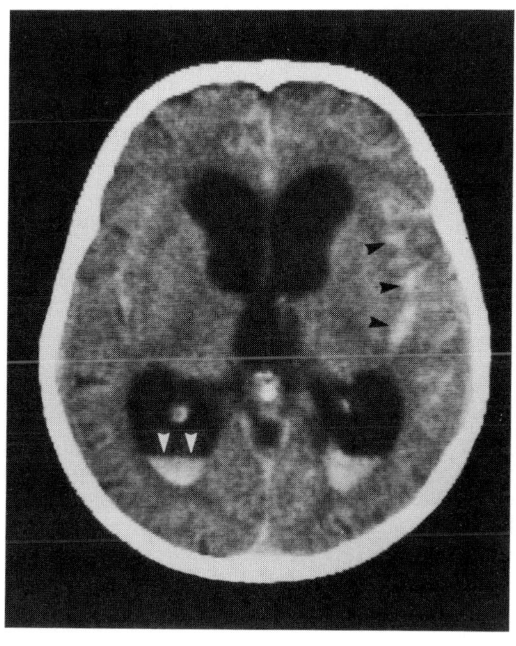

Subarachnoid hemorrhage from rupture of middle cerebral artery aneurysms often accumulates asymmetrically in the ipsilateral sylvian cistern, as seen here *(black arrows)*. Secondary hydrocephalus has developed in this case.

Small amounts of hemorrhage cause fluid levels in the dependent portions of the lateral ventricles *(white arrows)*. This sign is sometimes the only clue to recent subarachnoid hemorrhage, and the ventricular trigones should be closely examined in suspected cases.

The distribution of subarachnoid hemorrhage is not an infallible guide to the location of a responsible aneurysm. Considerable overlap occurs in the patterns of hemorrhage from different aneurysm sites. For example, ruptured aneurysms of the anterior or posterior communicating artery could produce an image identical to that in this case.

Apart from predicting aneurysm location, the amount and distribution of subarachnoid blood may be important for estimating the likelihood and location of subsequent vascular spasm.

Case 308

48-year-old woman.

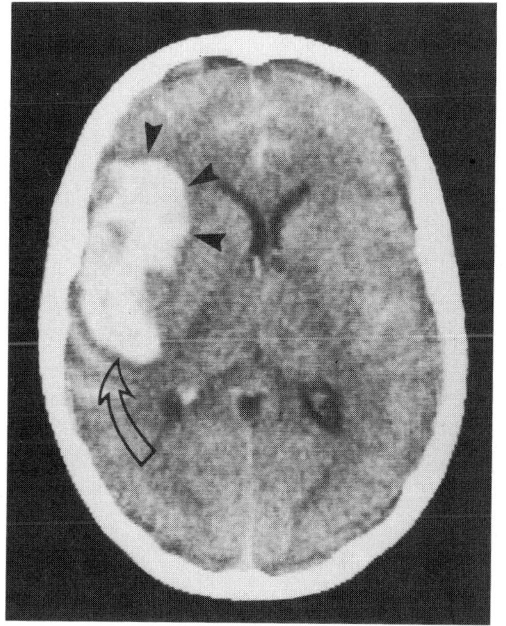

Intracerebral hemorrhage from aneurysms of the middle cerebral artery usually occurs in the inferior frontotemporal region *(solid arrows)*. A more common finding is a cisternal hematoma in the sylvian area *(open arrow)*.

Such clot represents accumulation of subarachnoid blood within the confines of the expanded sylvian cistern. The resulting subarachnoid hematoma acts like an intracerebral mass, but can be removed from the cistern without a cortical incision.

Localization of subarachnoid blood to the posterior fossa suggests rupture of an infratentorial aneurysm. The possibility of spinal subarachnoid hemorrhage should also be considered in such cases.

Case 309

82-year-old woman. Aneurysm at the genu of the middle cerebral artery (noncontrast scan).

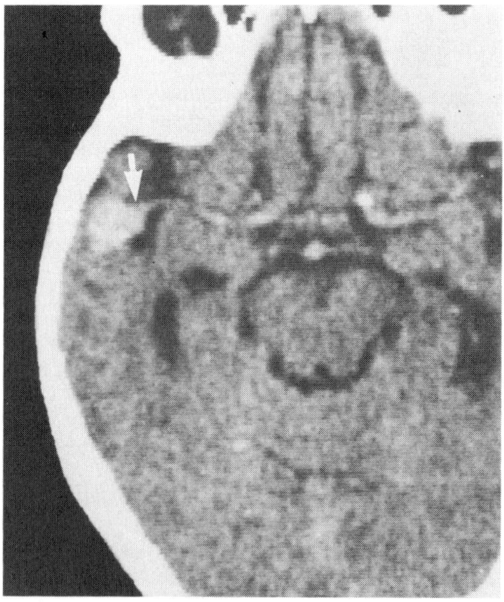

Unruptured aneurysms are sometimes discovered incidentally. They present as small, round masses with central high attenuation due to the blood they contain. A few flecks of peripheral calcification are common (see Case 84).

The relationship of the aneurysm to a parent vessel may be clearly demonstrated, as in this case (*arrow;* see also Case 312).

Case 310

72-year-old man. Posterior cerebral artery aneurysm (postcontrast scan).

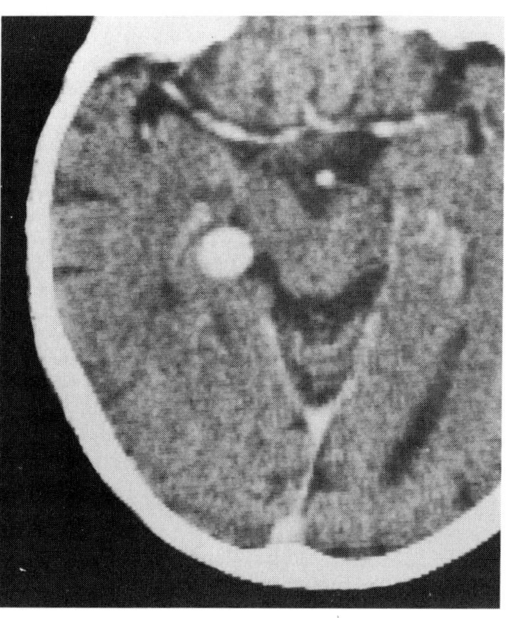

Aneurysms may be found at sites distant from the circle of Willis. Peripheral aneurysms exhibit the same characteristics of extra-axial location and intense contrast enhancement seen in conventional lesions. In this case the aneurysm is well defined as an extra-axial mass displacing the adjacent peduncle and widening the perimesencephalic cistern.

When aneurysms are found in peripheral locations, the possibility of mycotic, traumatic, or neoplastic origin should be considered. This lesion was found to be an unusual congenital aneurysm arising from the perimesencephalic portion of the posterior cerebral artery.

DIFFERENTIAL DIAGNOSIS: SMALL, MIDLINE HIGH-ATTENUATION STRUCTURE NEAR THE ANTERIOR CIRCLE OF WILLIS

Case 311

37-year-old woman.

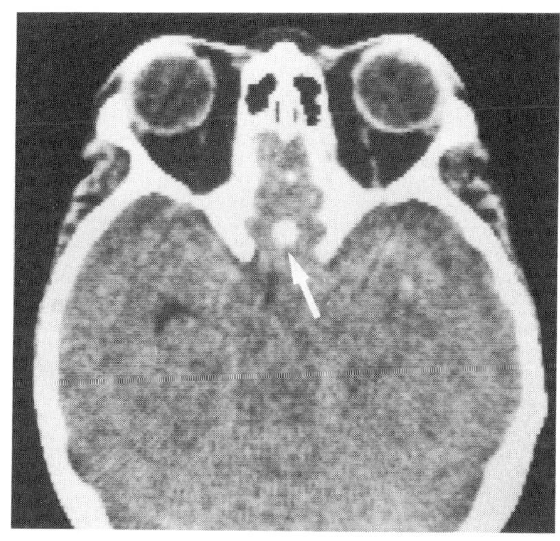

Tuberculum Sellae (With Subarachnoid Hemorrhage From A Posterior Communicating Artery Aneurysm; Noncontrast Scan).

Case 312

73-year-old man.

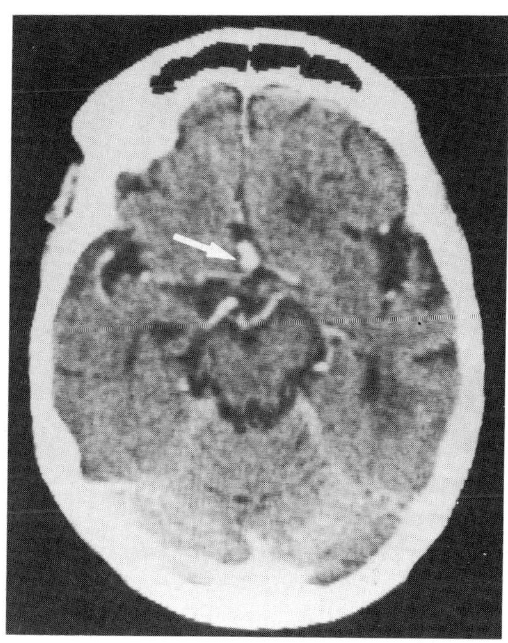

Unruptured Anterior Communicating Artery Aneurysm (Postcontrast Scan).

The superior surface of the tuberculum sellae is often imaged as a small area of high attenuation on scans passing through the circle of Willis (*arrow,* Case 311). This midline density may be mistaken for calcification, contrast, or clot within an aneurysm of the anterior communicating artery.

Partial imaging of an anterior clinoid process may produce a similar "pseudoaneurysm" near the supraclinoid internal carotid artery. These spurious "islands" of density are comparable to the partial visualization of the petrous bones in Cases 321B and 336A.

In Case 311, hemorrhage within CSF spaces causes them to appear isodense (see Case 299).

DIFFERENTIAL DIAGNOSIS: RIM-ENHANCING SUPRASELLAR MASS

Case 313

58-year-old woman presenting with bitemporal hemianopia.

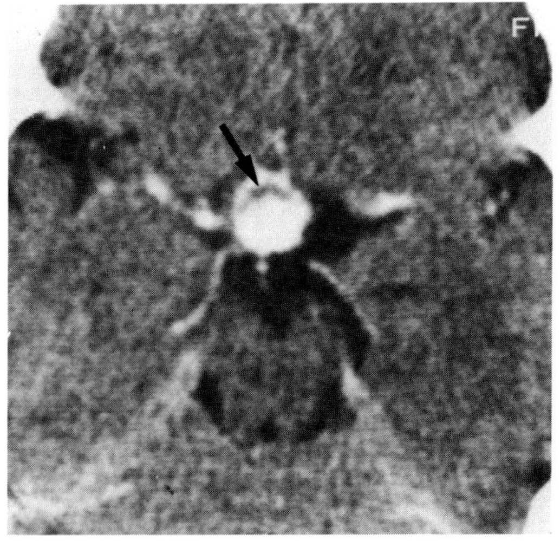

Aneurysm Of The Supraclinoid Internal Carotid Artery.

Case 314

18-year-old man presenting with bitemporal hemianopia.

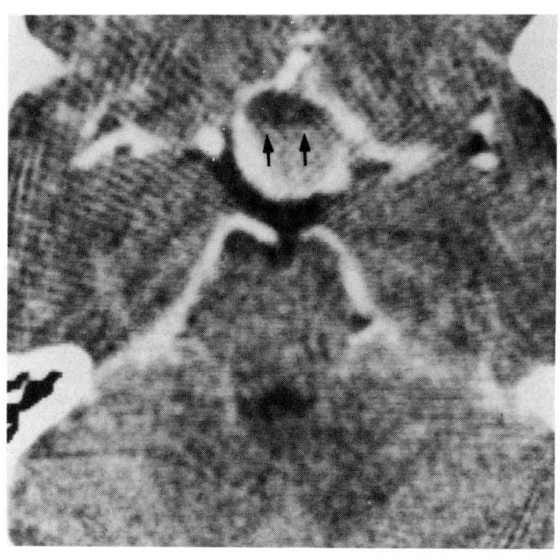

Pituitary Adenoma.

The aneurysm in Case 313 contains a small thrombus *(arrow),* causing enhancement to be inhomogeneous. Greater amounts of intraluminal clot would result in a more prominent appearance of rim enhancement. Such partially thrombosed aneurysms may mimic several other suprasellar lesions, including pituitary adenomas and craniopharyngiomas (see Cases 100 and 101).

The cystic pituitary adenoma in Case 314 demonstrates a sedimentation level *(arrows).*

Case 83 and 84 discuss the differential diagnosis of suprasellar aneurysms not containing thrombus.

DIFFERENTIAL DIAGNOSIS: CALCIFIED, ENHANCING PARASELLAR MASS

Case 315

79-year-old woman.

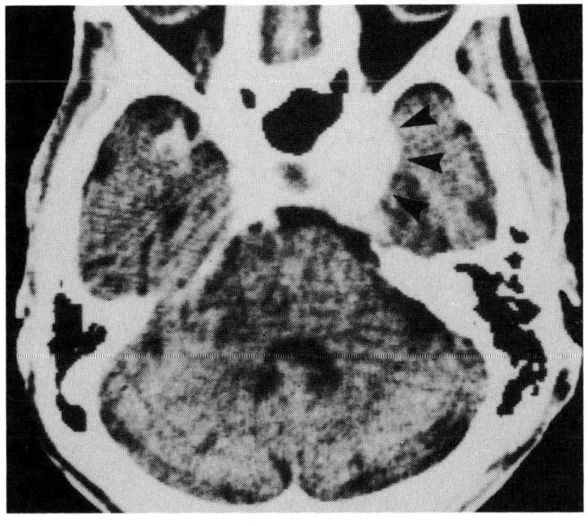

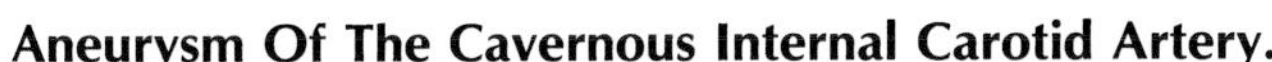

Aneurysm Of The Cavernous Internal Carotid Artery.

Case 316

24-year-old woman with neurofibromatosis.

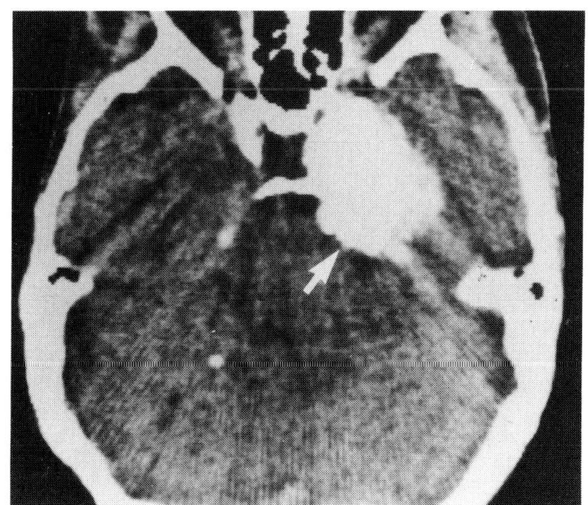

Meningioma.

Aneurysmal ectasia of the internal carotid artery is a common parasellar mass in adults. The vessel is typically calcified, with little intraluminal thrombus. The resulting precontrast density and marked contrast enhancement may closely resemble a parasellar meningioma.

In Case 315, the lateral margin of the intracavernous aneurysm *(arrows)* bulges into the medial portion of the middle cranial fossa. The meningioma in Case 316 occupies a similar location, with a tiny posterior fossa component *(arrow)*. Both of these long-standing lesions have caused erosion of the sphenoid bone.

Other enhancing parasellar masses include lateral extensions of pituitary adenomas, metastases (see Cases 111 and 112), chordomas (see Case 141), carotid-cavernous fistulas distending the cavernous sinus (see Case 381), inflammatory processes extending from the sphenoid sinus (e.g., mucocele, aspergillosis) and inflammatory disorders involving the cavernous sinus (e.g., Wegener's granulomatosis).

GIANT ANEURYSMS

Case 317

41-year-old man. Giant aneurysm of the middle cerebral artery (noncontrast scan).

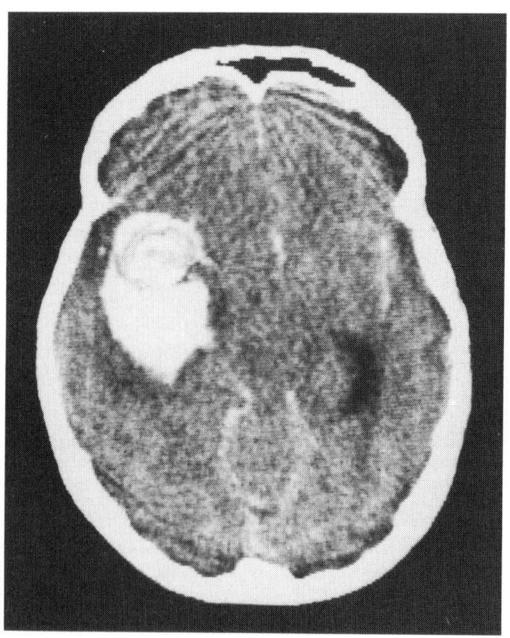

Large aneurysms have been angiographically described as "giant" when their diameter reaches 2.5 cm. Giant aneurysms most commonly arise from the supraclinoid internal carotid artery or the middle cerebral artery. They often present as mass lesions, but hemorrhage is not as rare as previously believed.

Giant aneurysms frequently demonstrate peripheral arcs or rims of calcification. Their lumens are usually at least partially occupied by thrombus, which often has a lamellar or concentric appearance, as in this case. The association of hemorrhage with a large, marble-like mass near the skull base is highly characteristic of a ruptured giant aneurysm.

When giant aneurysms occur in a suprasellar location, the combination of peripheral calcification and mixed attenuation may resemble a craniopharyngioma (see Case 95).

Case 318

64-year-old woman. Giant aneurysm of the basilar artery (postcontrast scan).

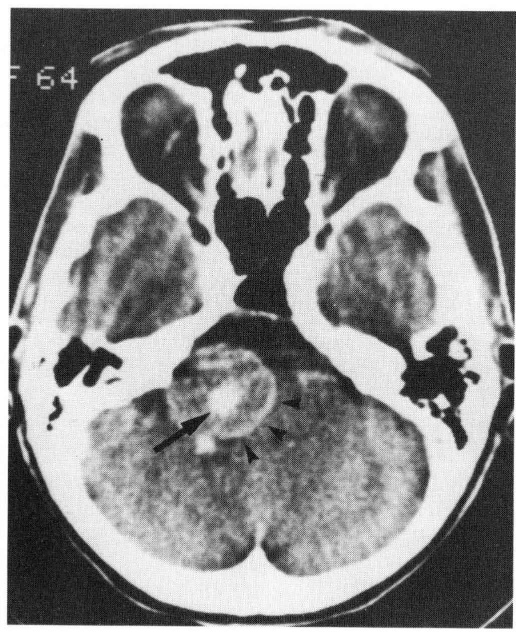

Contrast enhancement within giant aneurysms may take several forms. Patent portions of an aneurysm lumen are densely opacified. Thrombosed aneurysms typically demonstrate rim enhancement.

Many lesions present a combination or "target" appearance, as in this case. A small, slightly eccentric lumen *(arrow)* is surrounded by a large zone of nonenhancing thrombus, which is in turn bordered by a thin rim of peripheral enhancement *(small arrows)* in the adventitia or "capsule."

DIFFERENTIAL DIAGNOSIS: INTENSELY ENHANCING PREPONTINE MASS

Case 319

50-year-old woman.

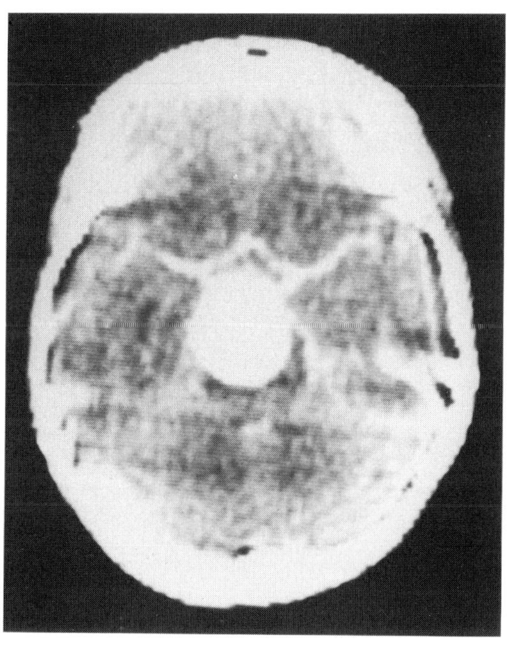

Giant Aneurysm Of The Basilar Artery.

Case 320

45-year-old man.

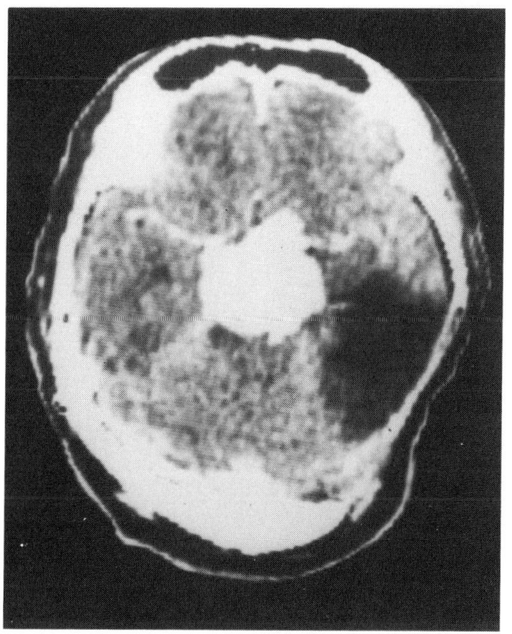

Recurrent Clivus Meningioma.

Occasionally the lumen of a giant aneurysm is entirely patent, as seen in Case 319. The uniform precontrast density of circulating blood and the intense enhancement following injection of contrast may then mimic a meningioma.

The patient in Case 319 had presented with hydrocephalus due to the mass effect of the aneurysm. When shunt surgery was performed the aneurysm expanded and bled. This case emphasizes that giant aneurysms may be dangerous both as masses and as sources of hemorrhage.

The meningioma in Case 320 was densely calcified. The left temporal craniotomy and encephalomalacia were due to previous surgery.

Case 321A

60-year-old woman.

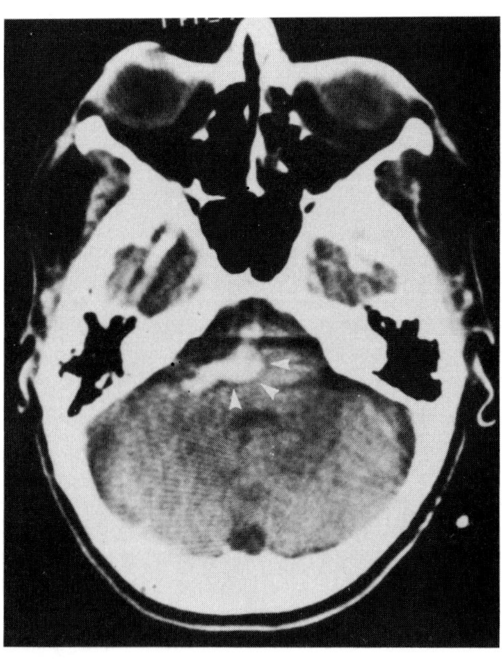

Two categories of aneurysms may involve the basilar artery. Saccular or "berry" aneurysms are usually seen as discrete vascular masses near the vertebrobasilar junction or at the basilar artery tip. Fusiform, atherosclerotic ectasia of the artery may reach aneurysmal proportions in the midbasilar region, often combined with elongation of the vessel (see "dolichoectasia," Case 322).

Some cases present a combination of these features, with focal dilatation superimposed on generalized ectasia. Here a saccular aneurysm *(arrows)* arises from an ectatic and tortuous vertebrobasilar junction.

Case 321B

Same patient.

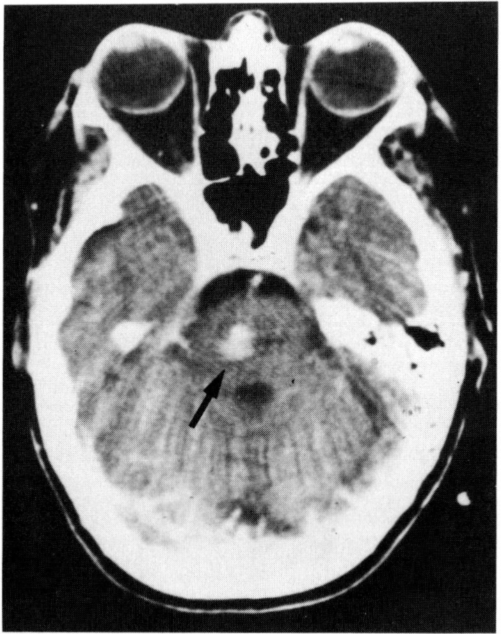

Prepontine extra-axial lesions may indent the ventral surface of the brain stem. Axial scans passing through the superoposterior portion of such embedded lesions cause them to appear intra-axial.

The dome of the aneurysm in Case 321A is partially imaged on this scan, mimicking a brain stem lesion. The course of the basilar artery should be carefully followed on adjacent scans when this appearance is encountered.

This scan incidentally demonstrates two pseudolesions: (1) partial volume of the petrous ridge appears as a calcification within the inferior temporal lobe (see Case 336A), and (2) prominent veins near the tentorium could be misinterpreted as a vascular malformation (see Case 284).

DOLICHOECTASIA

Case 322

70-year-old woman.

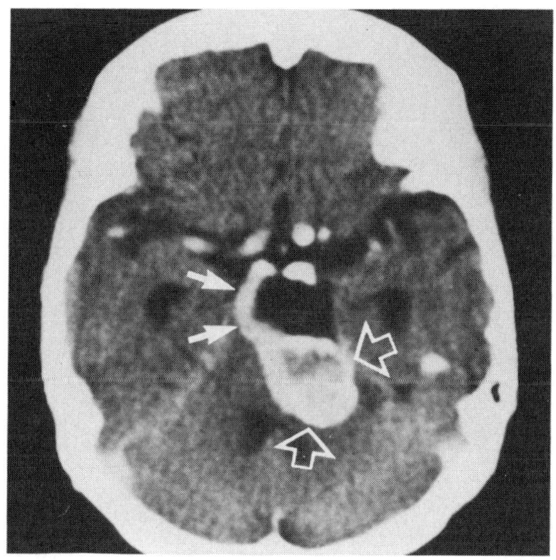

The basilar artery may undergo striking elongation and ectasia in elderly patients. This so-called "dolichoectasia" may cause the tip of the artery to rise as far superiorly as the foramen of Monro. The vessel may then appear as an enhancing mass impinging on the third ventricle and causing hydrocephalus. (Hydrocephalus may alternatively be caused by increased intraventricular "pulse pressure" due to the invaginating basilar artery tip.) The "lesion" can usually be followed inferiorly through the series of scans and identified as a tubular structure originating in the prepontine region.

An elongated basilar artery is often tortuous, and its aberrant course may distort cranial nerves. Hemorrhages are rare in true dolichoectasia; brain stem infarction is more common. (Hemorrhage does occur from more fusiform atherosclerotic aneurysms of the basilar artery.)

This case demonstrates a combination of dolichoectatic and aneurysmal features. A calcified aneurysm *(open arrows)* is superimposed on an elongated basilar artery *(solid arrows)*. This long-standing extra-axial mass has become embedded in the brain stem, deforming the fourth ventricle. Posterior displacement of the brain stem has widened the prepontine cistern.

Case 323

70-year-old man (noncontrast scan).

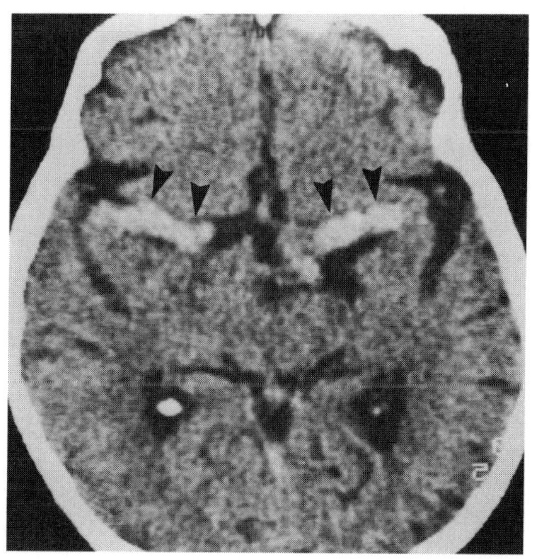

Dolichoectasia of the internal carotid or middle cerebral arteries may accompany or exceed involvement of the basilar artery. In this case, the horizontal segments of the middle cerebral arteries are grossly ectatic *(arrows)*, appearing dense because of their blood content. (Compare this scan with the noncontrast density of dilated veins in Case 281).

SPONTANEOUS INTRACEREBRAL HEMATOMAS

Case 324

63-year-old man presenting with a CVA.

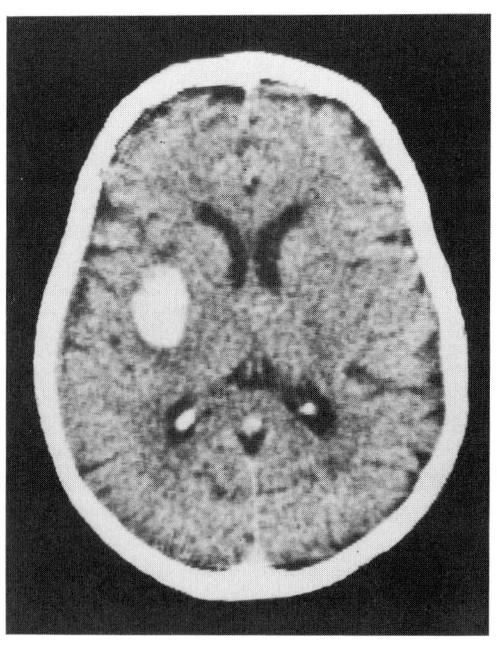

The clear demonstration of intracerebral hemorrhage was one of the earliest achievements of cerebral CT scanning. The characteristic high attenuation of hematomas is due primarily to the x-ray absorption (via Compton scatter) of the globin protein in red cells.

Spontaneous intraparenchymal hemorrhages tend to occur in a few specific locations, notably the basal ganglia, thalamus, pons, and cerebellum. Many patients experiencing "spontaneous" hemorrhages have a history of systemic hypertension. In these cases, angiopathic changes of small arteries (e.g., Charcot's aneurysm formation) may predispose to bleeding.

Here the deep hemisphere hematoma is of medium size. It has arisen in the putamen, the site of most ganglionic hemorrhages.

Small hematomas displace more tissue than they destroy. They may have a better long-term prognosis than cerebral infarctions causing equal initial deficits.

Case 325

48-year-old woman presenting with a CVA.

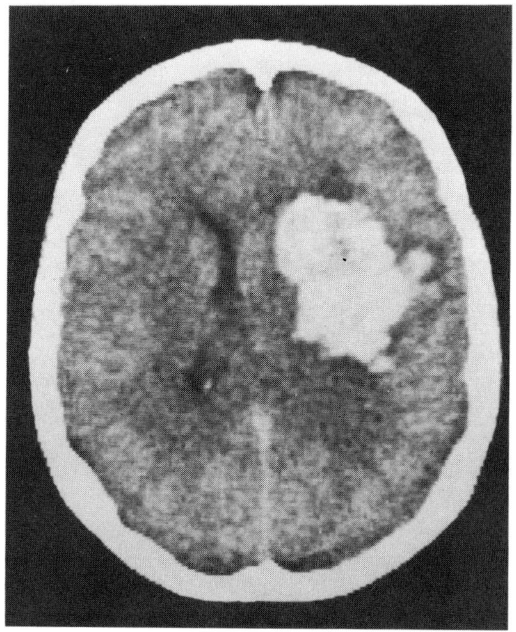

Spontaneous and/or hypertensive intracerebral hemorrhages may become very large, occupying much of the cerebral hemisphere and causing rapid uncal herniation. Ganglionic hematomas frequently rupture into the ventricular system (see Case 335).

In this case, the large hematoma remains separated from the compressed and shifted ventricles.

Case 326

80-year-old woman with acute onset of coma.

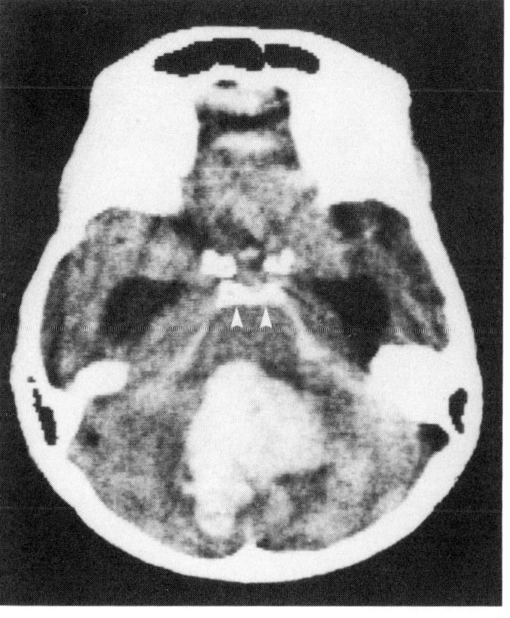

About 10% to 15% of spontaneous and/or hypertensive hematomas occur in the posterior fossa. They may involve the cerebellum or the brain stem, usually the pons. It is important to distinguish between cerebellar and brain stem hemorrhages, since the former may be evacuated, with life-saving results.

Cerebellar hematomas may be midline or hemispheric. Here a large vermian hematoma has effaced the fourth ventricle, causing obstructive hydrocephalus. The brain stem is displaced anteriorly, with its ventral margin compressed against the clivus and dorsum *(arrows)*.

The apparent AP diameter of the brain stem varies with the angle of the scan. When the head is flexed, the usual axial scan (0 degree gantry angle) passes obliquely through the brain stem from anterosuperior to posteroinferior. For example, a typical scan may demonstrate the cerebral peduncles (midbrain) ventrally while passing through the fourth ventricle (pons) dorsally. Routine axial scans performed with head extension result in a truer cross-section of the brain stem with less elongation. This apparently "small" brain stem diameter may cause confusion in localizing lesions. The cerebellar hemorrhage in this case had originally been misinterpreted as a brain stem hematoma because of its apparent anterior location (caused by head extension of the intubated patient and brain stem compression by the cerebellar mass).

Case 327

32-year-old woman with acute onset of headache and facial paresis.

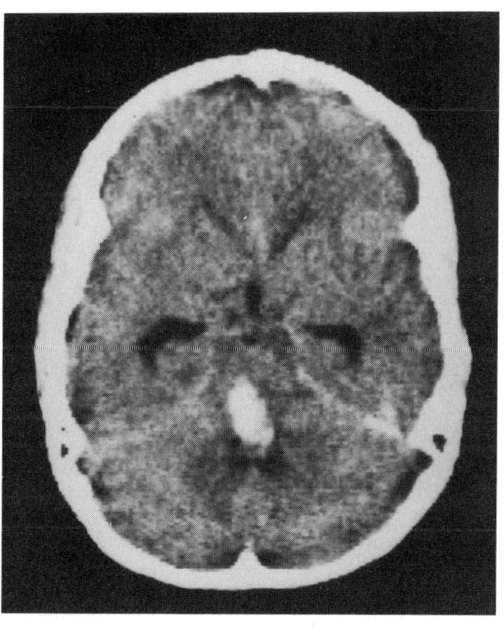

Brain stem hematomas are seen anterior to the plane of the fourth ventricle, as illustrated in this case. Compression of the fourth ventricle or aqueduct usually causes superimposed hydrocephalus, indicated here by the large temporal horns.

Although spontaneous and/or hypertensive hemorrhages are seen in the brain stem, the age of this patient suggests a possible underlying vascular malformation. (Compare the location of this hematoma with that of the AVM in Case 292).

DIFFERENTIAL DIAGNOSIS: ATYPICAL INTRACEREBRAL HEMATOMA

Case 328

20-year-old Vietnamese man presenting with seizures.

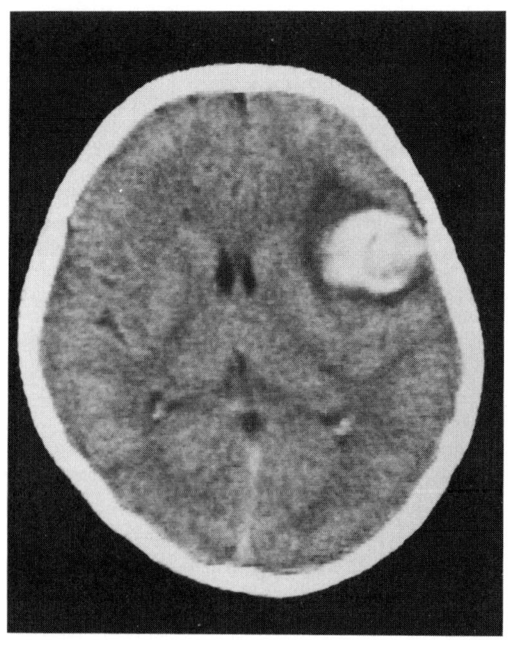

Hemorrhage From A Mycotic Aneurysm.

Case 329

30-year-old man presenting with a CVA.

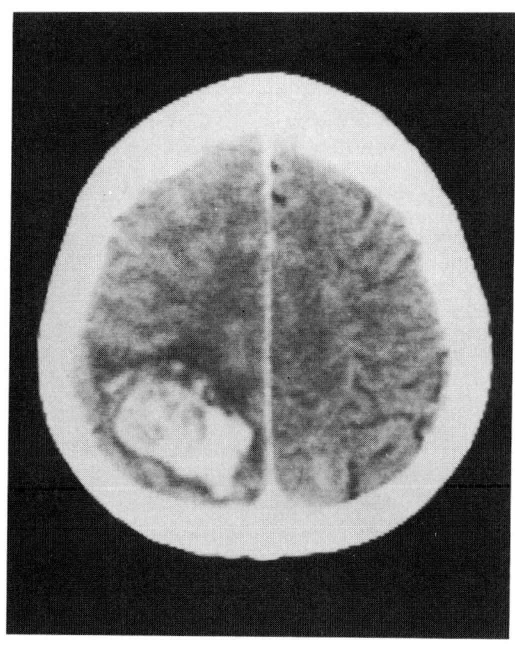

Hemorrhage Into Metastatic Melanoma.

The discovery of an intracerebral hematoma should be followed by critical assessment of its location and morphology. The diagnosis of "spontaneous hemorrhage" is reserved for hematomas occupying typical sites and demonstrating no unusual features. Superficial hematomas as seen in these cases are highly suspicious, and clues to an underlying cause should be sought.

In Case 328, the history of recent immigration and the appearance of concentric hemorrhage originating near the cortical surface suggested the correct diagnosis of mycotic aneurysm. Hemorrhage from other peripheral aneurysms (e.g., those associated with tumor emboli or meningitis) or from a small AVM could cause a similar appearance.

In Case 329, the structure of an underlying mass can be seen through the hematoma. Melanoma is one of the primary tumors known to cause vascular metastases, and intracerebral hemorrhage is a recognized presentation of this disease (compare with Cases 9 and 10).

Postcontrast scans performed days or weeks after intracerebral hemorrhage may demonstrate peripheral enhancement attributable to the organizing hematoma itself (see Cases 332 and 333). Such enhancement does not imply (or exclude) an underlying lesion.

Case 330

27-year-old woman presenting with sudden headache.

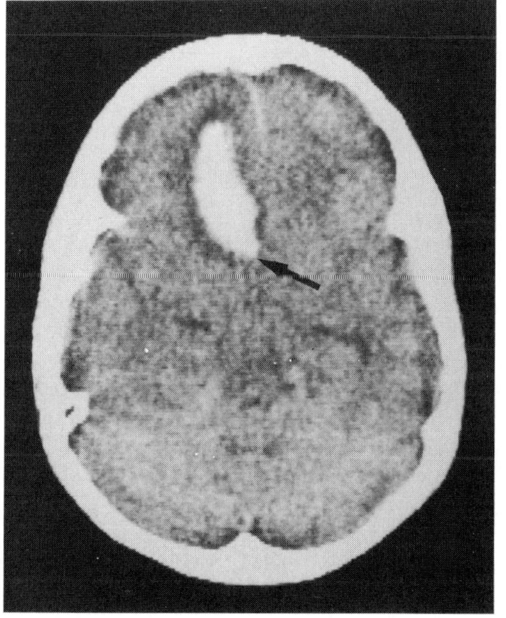

Ruptured Aneurysm Of The Anterior Communicating Artery.

Case 331

19-year-old man presenting with acute onset of headache, nausea, and stiff neck.

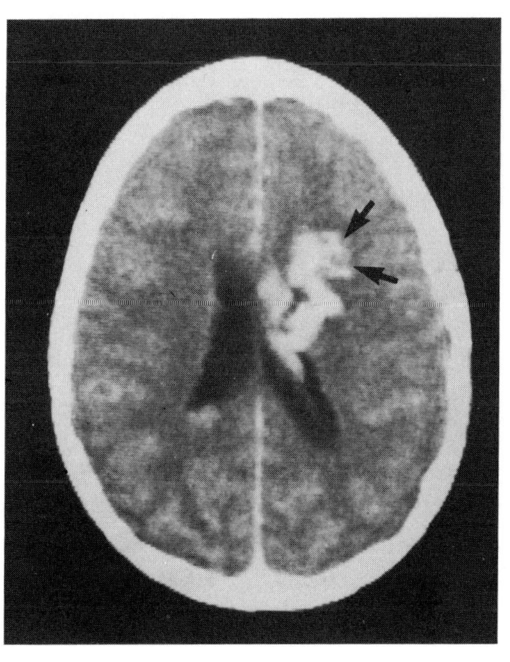

Ruptured AVM

The frontal lobe hematoma in Case 330 is unusual in location and morphology. The posteromedial margin of the hemorrhage approaches the midline near the anterior circle of Willis *(arrow)*. When a hematoma can be traced to a common aneurysm site in this manner, a clue to the origin of the hemorrhage is obtained.

Although the hematoma in Case 331 occupies a deep hemisphere location, its occurrence in a teenager argues strongly against a "spontaneous" etiology. The statistically best choice for an underlying lesion in these circumstances is an AVM.

Careful comparison of the precontrast and postcontrast scans in Case 331 established abnormal contrast enhancement in a small region at the margin of the hematoma *(arrows)*. Angiography and surgery confirmed a small AVM at this site.

When hematomas are found in an atypical location with no other clues to cause, the possibility of underlying coagulopathy or vasculitis (e.g., amyloid angiopathy; see Case 333) should be considered.

Case 332

73-year-old woman.

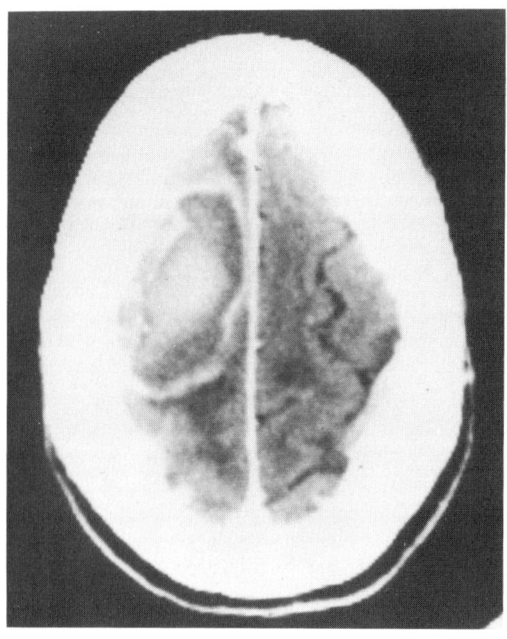

The attenuation values of an intracerebral hematoma decrease gradually over a period of weeks. Dissolution and organization of the clot simultaneously begin from the periphery. This process leads to a rim of contrast enhancement at the margins of a resolving hematoma.

A scan performed several weeks after hemorrhage may demonstrate the enhancing rim of the lesion, with little remaining high attenuation. The resolving hematoma may then resemble an abscess or neoplasm, as seen here. The lesion in this scan represented an unusual superior extension of a large, but otherwise typical, ganglionic hematoma.

Clues to the correct diagnosis in most cases are: (1) a history of a recent CVA; (2) location at a common site of spontaneous hemorrhage; (3) a smooth, uniform rim, *not* well seen on the precontrast scan; (4) faint residual high attenuation near the center of the mass; and (5) lack of adjacent edema.

Case 333

53-year-old woman, one month after intracerebral hemorrhage due to amyloid angiopathy.

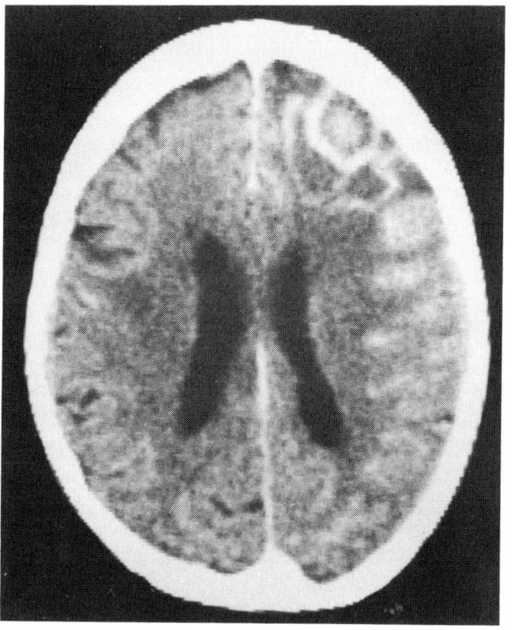

Hematomas may occur in unusual locations, have irregular contours, and cause marked edema. Such lesions create bizarre rim-enhancement patterns as they resolve, as seen in this case. Since hemorrhage may secondarily occur into preexisting lesions, enhancement patterns must be closely evaluated before being ascribed to evolution of a spontaneous hematoma.

"Benign" enhancement around an intracerebral hematoma has been seen within days of the original hemorrhage. The finding may persist for one or two months.

Case 334

80-year-old woman in coma. (Same patient as in Case 326.)

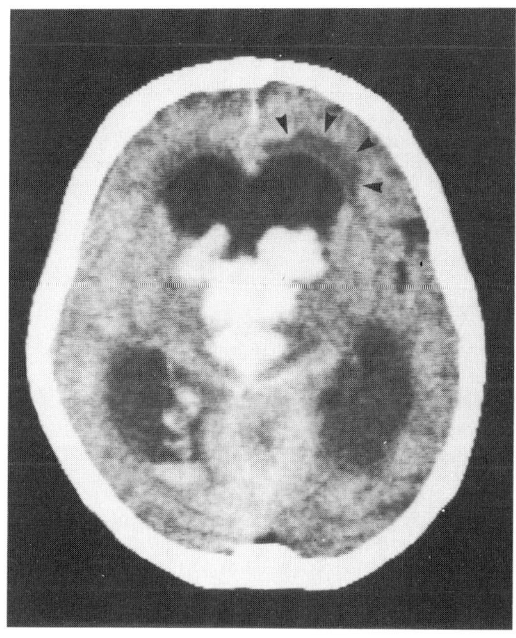

Hematomas in the posterior fossa or basal ganglia may rupture into the fourth or third ventricles. The ventricles may be grossly expanded by clot, as in this case. The intraventricular hematoma acts as a mass lesion and causes obstructive hydrocephalus.

Here the massa intermedia is faintly seen as a filling defect in the distended third ventricle. Clot extends through the foramina of Monro into the frontal horns. Transependymal cerebrospinal fluid (CSF) passage due to acute hydrocephalus is seen in the frontal lobes *(arrows)*. Ascending, transtentorial herniation has impacted the cerebellar vermis and brain stem at the tentorial hiatus.

Case 335

68-year-old man.

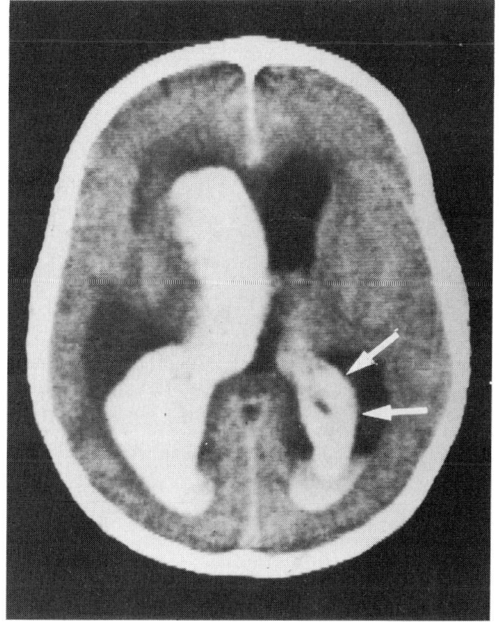

In this case, a primary hematoma within the caudate nucleus has ruptured into the ventricular system. The right lateral ventricle has filled with blood.

Such "casting" forms a clot having the shape and size of the ventricle at the time of hemorrhage. A small cast is present within the trigone of the left ventricle *(arrows),* which has evidently enlarged since the original hemorrhage. Superimposed on the cast is a sedimentation level.

Intraventricular hemorrhage is a common occurrence in premature infants. The hemorrhage usually arises from fragile vessels in the periventricular layer of germinal matrix (see Case 176). Hydrocephalus is often superimposed. Cribside ultrasound (using the open fontanelles as acoustic windows) is the procedure of choice for following the course of such cases.

REFERENCES

1. Adams H.P. Jr., Kassell N.F., Torner J.C., et al.: CT and clinical correlations in recent aneurysmal subarachnoid hemorrhage: A preliminary report of the cooperative aneurysm study. *Neurology* 33:981–988, 1983.
2. Albright L., Fellows R.: Sequential CT scanning after neonatal intracerebral hemorrhage. *A.J.N.R.* 2:133–137, 1981.
3. Becker D.H., Townsend J.J., Kramer R.A., Newton T.H.: Occult cerebrovascular malformations. *Brain* 102:249–287, 1979.
4. Byrd S.E., Bentson J.R., Winter J., et al.: Giant intracranial aneurysms simulating brain neoplasms on computed tomography. *J. Comput. Assist. Tomogr.* 2:303–307, 1978.
5. Davis J.M., Ploetz J., Davis K.R., et al.: Cranial computed tomography in subarachnoid hemorrhage: Relationship between blood detected by CT and lumbar puncture. *J. Comput. Assist. Tomogr.* 4:794–796, 1980.
6. Davis K.R., Kistler J.P., Heros R.C., et al.: Neuroradiologic approach to the patient with the diagnosis of subarachnoid hemorrhage. *Radiol. Clin. North Am.* 20:87–94, 1982.
7. Diebler C., Dulac O., Renier D., et al.: Aneurysms of the vein of Galen in infants aged 2 to 15 months: Diagnosis and natural evolution. *Neuroradiology* 21:185–197, 1981.
8. Fierstien S.B., Pribham H.W., Hieshima G.: Angiography and computed tomography in the evaluation of cerebral venous malformations. *Neuroradiology* 17:137–148, 1979.
9. Golding R., Peatfield R.C., Shawdon H.H., et al.: Computer tomographic features of giant intracranial aneurysms. *Clin. Radiol.* 31:41, 1980.
10. Goldstein S.J., Sacks J.G., Lee C., et al.: Computed tomographic findings in cerebral arterial ectasia. *A.J.N.R.* 4:501–504, 1983.
11. Graeb D.A., Robertson W.D., Lapointe J.S., et al.: Computed tomographic diagnosis of intraventricular hemorrhage: Etiology and prognosis. *Radiology* 143:91–96, 1982.
12. Inoue Y., Saiwai S., Miyamoto T., et al.: Post-contrast computed tomography in subarachnoid hemorrhage from ruptured aneurysms. *J. Comput. Assist. Tomogr.* 5:341–344, 1981.
13. Kistler J.P., Crowell R.M., Davis K.R., et al.: The relation of cerebral vasospasm to the extent and location of subarachnoid blood visualized by CT scan: A prospective study. *Neurology* 33:424–436, 1983.
14. Laster D.W., Moody D.M., Ball M.R.: Resolving intracerebral hematoma: alteration of the ring sign with steroids. *A.J.R.* 130:935–939, 1978.
15. Lazzara A., Ahmann P., Dykes F., et al.: Clinical predictability of intraventricular hemorrhage in preterm infants. *Pediatrics* 65:30–34, 1980.
16. Leblanc R., Ethier R., Little J.R.: Computerized tomography findings in arteriovenous malformations of the brain. *J. Neurosurg.* 51:765–772, 1979.
17. Liliequist B., Lindqvist M.: Computer tomography in the evaluation of subarachnoid hemorrhage. *Acta Radiol. (Diag).* 21:327, 1980.
18. Little J.R., Tubman D.E., Ethier R.: Cerebellar hemorrhage in adults. *J. Neurosurg.* 48:575–579, 1978.
19. Martell A., Scotti G., Harwood-Nash D.C.: Aneurysms of the vein of Galen in children: CT and angiographic correlations. *Neuroradiology* 20:123–133, 1980.
20. Messina A.V., Chernik N.L.: Computed tomography: The 'resolving' intracerebral hemorrhage. *Radiology* 118:609–613, 1976.
21. Mitnick J.S., Pinto R.S., Lin J.P., et al.: CT of thrombosed arteriovenous malformations in children. *Radiology* 150:385–389, 1984.
22. Modic M.T., Weinstein M.A.: Cerebrovascular disease of the brain, in Haaga J.R., Alfidi R.J., (eds.): *Computed Tomography of the Whole Body.* St. Louis, C.V. Mosby Co., 1983, pp. 136–169.
23. Mosely I.F., Holland I.M.: Ectasia of the basilar artery: The breadth of the clinical spectrum and the diagnostic value of computed tomography. *Neuroradiology* 18:83–91, 1979.
24. Norman D., Price D., Boyd D., et al.: Quantitative aspects of computed tomography of the blood and cerebrospinal fluid. *Radiology* 123:335–338, 1977.
25. Olson E., Gilmor R.L., Richmond B.: Cerebral venous angiomas. *Radiology* 151:97–104, 1984.
26. Patel, D.V., Hier D.B., Thomas C.M., et al.: Intracerebral hemorrhage secondary to cerebral amyloid angiopathy. *Radiology* 151:397–400, 1984.
27. Pinto R.S., Cohen W.A., Kricheff I.I., et al.: Giant intracranial aneurysms: Rapid sequential computed tomography. *A.J.N.R.* 3:495–499, 1982.
28. Pinto R.S., Kricheff I.I., Butler A.R.: Correlation of computed tomographic, angiographic, and neuropathological changes in giant intracranial aneurysms. *Radiology* 132:85–92, 1979.
29. Rothfus W.E., Albright A.L., Casey K.F., et al.: Cerebellar venous angioma: 'Benign' entity? *A.J.N.R.* 5:61–66, 1984.
30. Schubiger O., Valavanis A., Hayek J.: Computed tomography in cerebral aneurysms with special emphasis on giant intracranial aneurysms. *J. Comput. Assist. Tomogr.* 4:24–32, 1980.
31. Shirkhoda A., Whaley R.A., Boone S.C., et al.: Varied CT appearance of aneurysm of the vein of Galen in infancy. *Neuroradiology* 21:265–270, 1981.
32. Silver A.J., Pederson M.E., Ganti S.M., et al.: CT of subarachnoid hemorrhage due to ruptured aneurysm. *A.J.N.R.* 2:13–22, 1981.
33. Sobel D., Li F.C., Norman D., et al.: Cisternal enhancement after subarachnoid hemorrhage. *A.J.N.R.* 2:549–552, 1981.
34. Terao H., Hori T., Matsutani M., et al.: Detection of cryptic vascular malformations by computerized tomography. *J. Neurosurg.* 51:546–551, 1979.
35. Valavanis A., Wellauer J., Yasargil M.G.: The radiological diagnosis of cerebral venous angioma: Cerebral angiography and computed tomography. *Neuroradiology* 24:193–199, 1983.
36. Volpe J.J.: Neonatal intraventricular hemorrhage. *N. Engl. J. Med.* 304:886–890, 1981.
37. Wagle W.A., Smith T.W., Weiner M.: Intracerebral hemorrhage caused by cerebral amyloid angiopathy: Radiographic-pathologic correlation. *A.J.N.R.* 5:171–176, 1984.
38. Wharen R.E., Scheithauer B.W., Laws E.R.: Thrombosed arteriovenous malformations of the brain. *J. Neurosurg.* 57:520–526, 1982.
39. Yeates A., Enzmann D.: Cryptic vascular malformations involving the brain-stem. *Radiology* 146:71–75, 1983.
40. Yock D.H. Jr., Larson D.A.: Computed tomography of hemorrhage from anterior communicating artery aneurysms with angiographic correlation. *Radiology* 134:399–407, 1980.
41. Zimmerman R.D., Leeds N.E., Naidich T.P.: Ring blush associated with intracerebral hematoma. *Radiology* 122:707–711, 1977.

CHAPTER 11

HYDROCEPHALUS, CYSTS, AND DEVELOPMENTAL ABNORMALITIES

COMMUNICATING HYDROCEPHALUS: INFANTS

Case 336A

19-month-old girl.

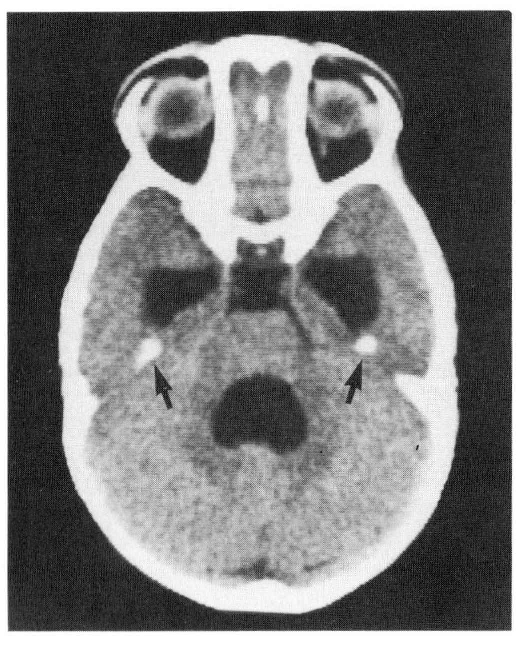

Case 336B

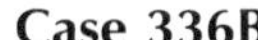

Same patient.

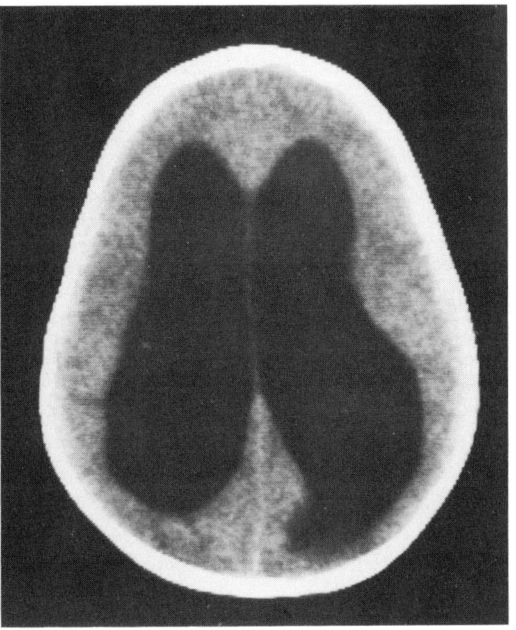

Hydrocephalus ranks among the pathologic conditions most clearly demonstrated on CT scans. Expanded components of the ventricular system are easily defined because of the contrast provided by spinal fluid.

In this case, the fourth ventricle is enlarged along with the temporal horns. The dilated anterior recesses of the third ventricle occupy the suprasellar cistern (compare with Case 347).

Hydrocephalic expansion of all four ventricles suggests impairment of cerebrospinal fluid (CSF) flow or absorption along the surface pathways from the foramen magnum through the tentorial incisura to the parasagittal arachnoid granulations. This "communicating" pathophysiology contrasts with intraventricular obstruction and is one of the common causes of infantile hydrocephalus. It is usually idiopathic, but may follow perinatal meningitis or intracranial hemorrhage.

Small densities in the posterior temporal region are seen where the scan passes along the superior surface of the petrous bones *(arrows)*. The "arcuate eminence" roofing the superior semicircular canal is partially imaged on such sections.

Hydrocephalic lateral ventricles may become hugely dilated, occupying most of the supratentorial compartment. Except in extreme cases, the thinness of the residual cortical mantle is an unreliable predictor of postshunt recovery.

In severe hydrocephalus the septum pellucidum may become markedly thinned or frankly dehiscent. The resulting communication between the lateral ventricles may resemble lobar holoprosencephaly (see Case 337).

The posterior bodies, atria, and occipital horns of hydrocephalic ventricles are often larger than the frontal horns. This disparity may increase after shunting, with the greatest reduction in ventricular size occurring anteriorly.

DIFFERENTIAL DIAGNOSIS: DEVELOPMENTAL ABNORMALITY WITH LARGE SUPRATENTORIAL FLUID SPACES

Case 337

3-week-old boy.

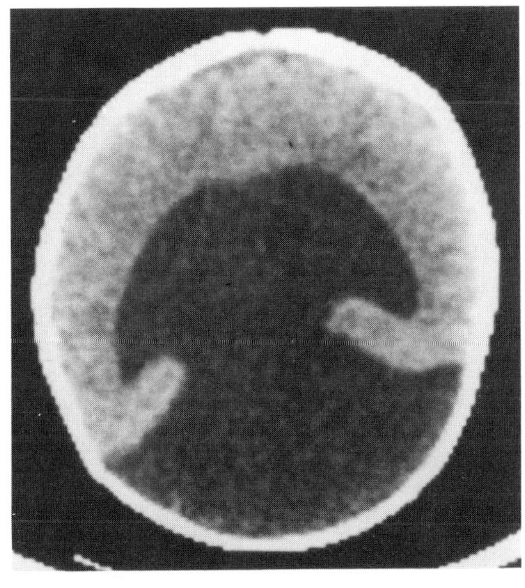

Holoprosencephaly.

Case 338

Newborn boy.

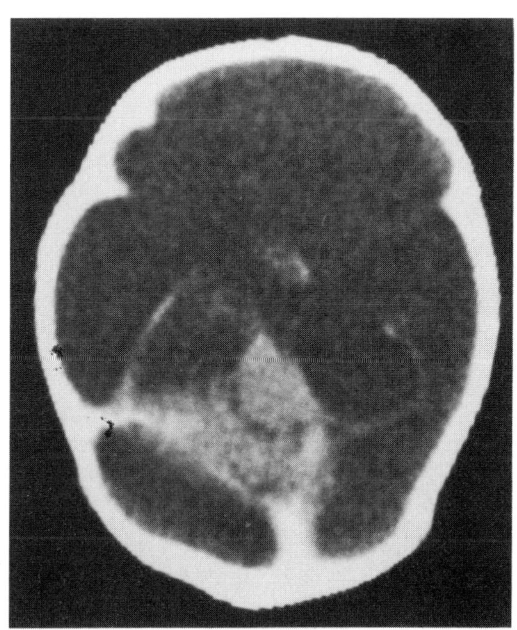

Hydranencephaly.

Several congenital abnormalities are associated with large supratentorial CSF spaces that may resemble hydrocephalic ventricles.

Holoprosencephaly is a developmental malformation (absent or incomplete cerebral hemispherization) in which a horseshoe-shaped forebrain surrounds a central monoventrical. The characteristic "bat-wing" morphology of the single-chambered ventricle is seen anteriorly in Case 337. A midline "dorsal cyst" may be found above the brain in association with holoprosencephaly, as seen posteriorly in this case. (The posterior fossa was normal; the diencephalon was mildly malformed.)

Hydranencephaly represents a loss of normal cerebral tissue due to an embryologic insult. The cerebral hemispheres are nearly or completely absent, and the supratentorial region is filled with fluid. The posterior fossa and diencephalon are characteristically preserved. This finding suggests that the hemisphere deficiency is due to agenesis, hypoplasia, and/or occlusion of the supraclinoid internal carotid arteries.

Hydranencephaly may be mistaken for severe hydrocephalus. However, the scattered remnants of cortex in hydranencephaly do not form a rim around the hemisphere, as does the compressed cortical mantle of hydrocephalus.

A diffuse anoxic or ischemic insult may also resemble hydranencephaly due to widespread low attenuation with relative sparing of the posterior fossa and diencephalon. However, a "ghost" of once-normal structure is usually visible in the former circumstances (see Case 153).

DIFFERENTIAL DIAGNOSIS: LARGE LATERAL VENTRICLES IN A CHILD

Case 339

2-year-old boy examined for large head size.

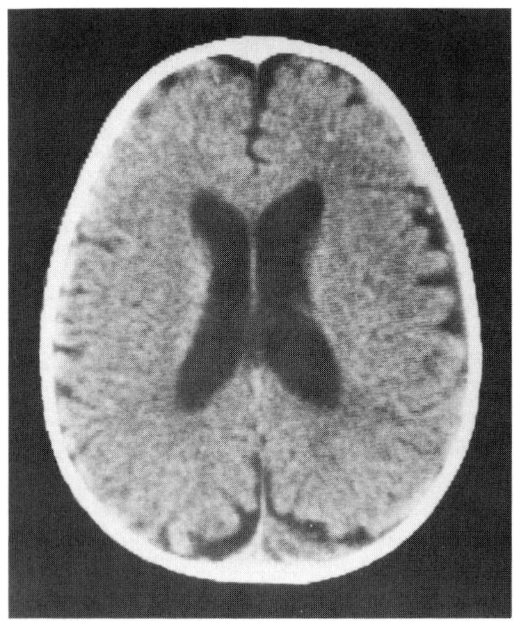

Megalencephaly.

Case 340

7-year-old boy retarded since birth.

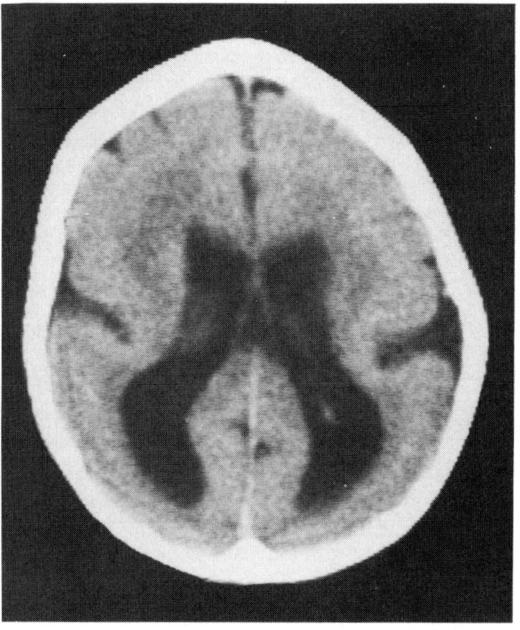

Developmental Abnormality (Pachygyria; Dysgenesis Of The Corpus Callosum).

Some children have large heads as a consequence of having large brains. Several pathological syndromes (e.g., mucopolysaccharidoses, gangliosidoses) are associated with "megalencephaly," but many children with large brains are functionally normal. Clinical clues to "benign megalencephaly" include normal head shape, head growth curves parallel to standards, the absence of increased intracranial pressure, normal neurologic development, and large head size of a parent. The child in Case 339 is a functionally normal boy whose father wears a cap over an unusually large head.

Children with benign megalencephaly often have large ventricles. They may also demonstrate prominent subarachnoid spaces. The latter finding provides a clue to the diagnosis, since hydrocephalic expansion of ventricles usually effaces sulcal markings. Occasionally "benign" communicating hydrocephalus causes large ventricles and sulci in a child, with a stable appearance or improvement on follow-up scans.

Poor brain growth in childhood may also result in ventricular enlargement. Distinction from hydrocephalus is usually aided by small head size and a history of developmental delay. In Case 340 the abnormal morphological character of the sylvian fissures ("fetal" lack of opercularization) and the paucity of normal sulcal markings also suggest a developmental problem. The terms "lissencephaly" and "pachygyria" are used to describe the surface of brains with no or few cortical gyri.

DIFFERENTIAL DIAGNOSIS: LARGE VENTRICLES WITH PERIPHERAL ZONES OF LOW ATTENUATION IN AN INFANT

Case 341

1-month-old boy.

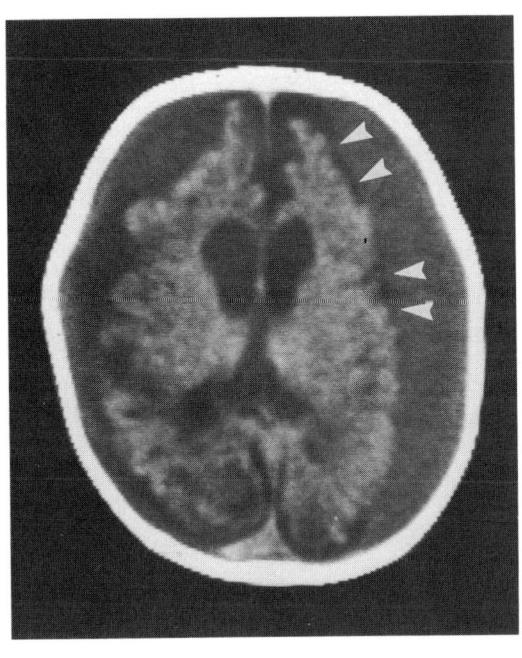

Viral Meningoencephalitis; Subdural Fluid Collections.

Case 342

8-month-old girl, three months after smoke inhalation.

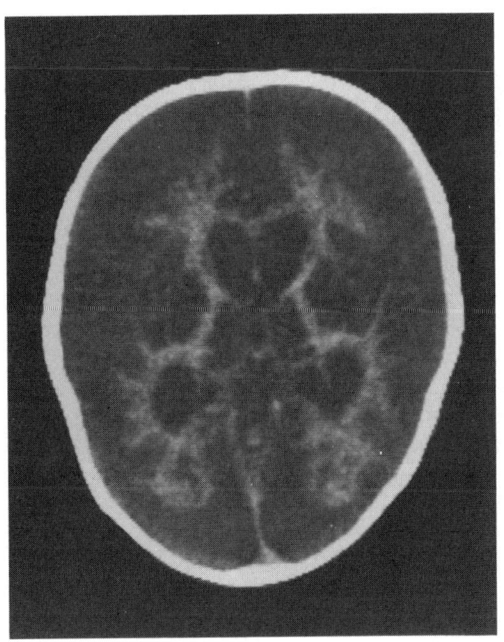

Cerebral Anoxia.

Perinatal viral meningitis and/or encephalitis often causes rapid and extensive damage to the immature brain. The result is a diffuse loss of parenchymal volume, which presents the appearance of atrophy.

In Case 341 the cerebral cortex has collapsed away from the inner table. Large subdural fluid collections have developed. The subdural fluid is higher in attenuation than the thin ribbon of CSF surrounding the collapsed hemispheres *(arrows)*. Despite the severe infectious parenchymal damage, the morphology of cortical gray matter is relatively preserved, in contrast to that of Case 342.

Primary subdural hematomas may cause communicating hydrocephalus with secondary ventricular enlargement. The atrophic cortical surface and large sulci in Case 341 argue against this interpretation.

Acute anoxia causes swelling (see Cases 271 and 274), which is rapidly replaced by parenchymal loss. In Case 342 the enlarged ventricles are surrounded by a halo of relatively preserved white matter. Cortical regions are seen as a featureless zone of low attenuation. (Compare Case 342 with the acute changes in Case 274.)

CONGENITAL ETIOLOGIES OF HYDROCEPHALUS: CHIARI II ("ARNOLD-CHIARI") MALFORMATION

Case 343

5-month-old girl.

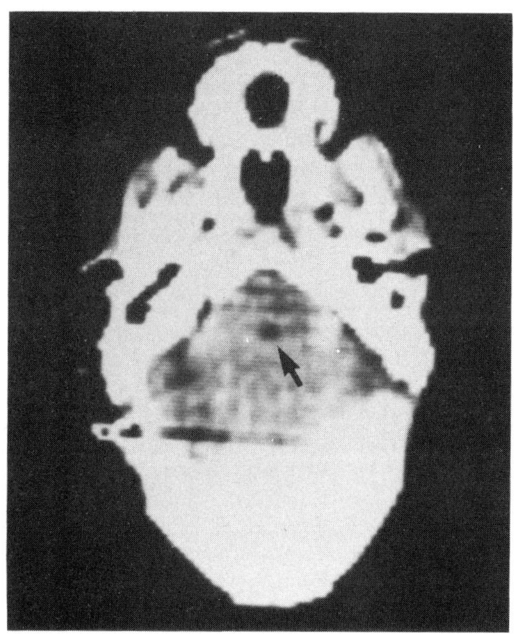

The Chiari II malformation ranks with communicating hydrocephalus and aqueductal stenosis as a major cause of infantile hydrocephalus. The malformation is a complex developmental abnormality including caudal herniation of the hindbrain through the foramen magnum into the cervical spinal canal.

In combination with associated hydrocephalus, this deformity causes a large supratentorial compartment and a small posterior fossa. Findings on CT may reflect infratentorial crowding with scalloped erosion of the petrous ridges and enlargement of the foramen magnum. An additional clue to the diagnosis is the associated skull dysplasia called "craniolacunae" or "lückenschädel skull."

In this case the posterior fossa is tiny, and the fourth ventricle *(arrow)* is caudally located at the level of a large foramen magnum.

Case 344

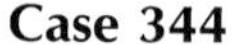

1-year-old girl (after shunting for hydrocephalus).

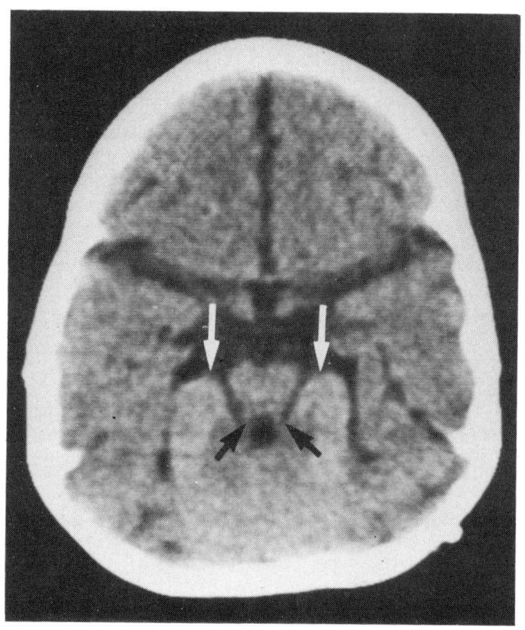

In addition to the calvarial abnormalities discussed in Case 343, several parenchymal deformities are characteristic of the Chiari II malformation. The dorsal midbrain is typically "beaked," with the colliculi fused into a single peak *(black arrows)*. The crowded cerebellum wraps around the brain stem bilaterally *(white arrows)*. After shunting, the cerebellum towers superiorly near the midline as a pseudomass. Hypoplasia or fenestration of the falx and tentorium may also be noted.

The CT features described in Cases 343 and 344 are characteristic of the Chiari II malformation. The almost invariable association with myelomeningocele further supports the diagnosis.

Case 345

24-year-old man presenting with increased intracranial pressure. Aqueductal stenosis.

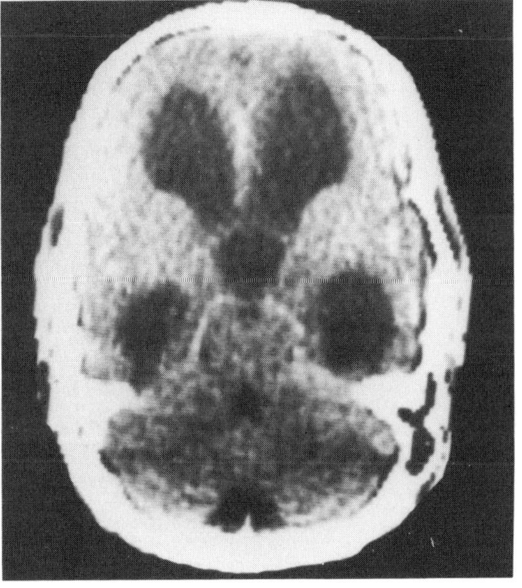

Aqueductal stenosis, a major cause of infantile hydrocephalus, may also present in adulthood. The CT diagnosis is suggested by (1) enlargement of lateral and third ventricles without fourth ventricular expansion and (2) the absence of other lesions mimicking obstruction at the aqueductal level (see Cases 348 through 350).

In this case, the small fourth ventricle contrasts with the dilated third and lateral ventricles. The posterior fossa is relatively small, since the long-standing distension of the lateral ventricles has led to expansion of the supratentorial compartment.

Most cases of benign aqueductal stenosis are due to a congenital abnormality (usually "forking" or "gliosis"). Acquired stenosis may also follow ependymitis from infection or intraventricular hemorrhage. Cases of congenital origin may present in adulthood when the borderline capacity of a narrowed lumen is further compromised or exceeded by some superimposed event.

Case 346

1-year-old boy. Dandy-Walker malformation.

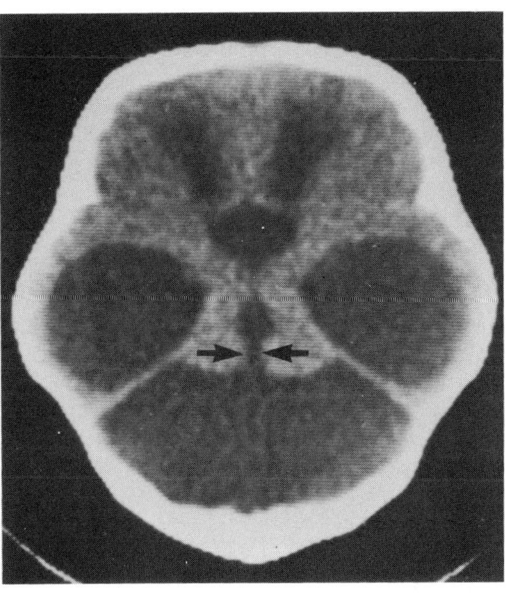

The Dandy-Walker malformation is a less common cause of congenital hydrocephalus. Aplasia or hypoplasia of the cerebellar vermis is associated with a "roofless" fourth ventricle opening dorsally *(arrows)* into a large posterior fossa cyst. The cyst typically surrounds hypoplastic cerebellar hemispheres. Expansion of the posterior fossa associated with the Dandy-Walker malformation contrasts with the small posterior fossas seen in aqueductal stenosis and the Chiari II malformation.

This scan demonstrates a large infratentorial compartment at a level above the petrous ridges. The vermis defect is outlined by arrows. Chronic enlargement of the temporal horns has caused molding of the adjacent calvarium and outlines the tentorium.

Posterior fossa arachnoid cysts (see Case 364) and large cisterna magnas may mimic the Dandy-Walker malformation. However, these structures are often less symmetric than the Dandy-Walker cyst. The integrity of the cerebellar vermis provides the key to differential diagnosis.

DIFFERENTIAL DIAGNOSIS: SUPRASELLAR CYST ASSOCIATED WITH HYDROCEPHALUS

Case 347

20-year-old man.

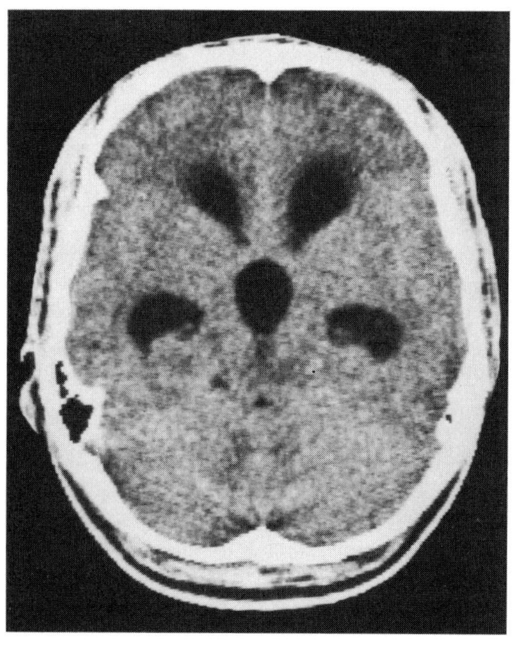

Hydrocephalic Third Ventricle (Aqueductal Obstruction Due To A Midbrain Mass).

Case 348

8-year-old boy.

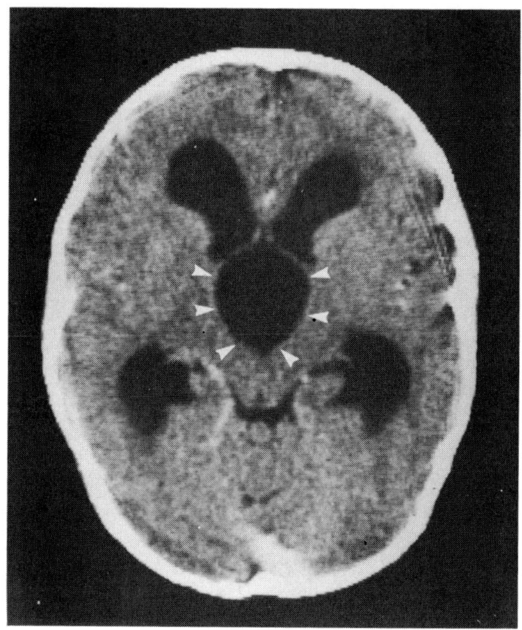

Suprasellar Arachnoid Cyst Obstructing The Third Ventricle.

The diagnosis of "benign" aqueductal stenosis requires careful exclusion of other lesions with similar CT appearances. Small midbrain masses can obstruct the aqueduct while causing minimal abnormalities of density or contour. Alternatively, low-attenuation lesions may be overlooked as they occupy or compress the third ventricle. Such lesions can be hidden within CSF density (see Cases 349 and 350) or mistakenly interpreted as a dilated ventricle.

A hydrocephalic third ventricle is seen in Case 347. This structure may act as a suprasellar mass, causing erosion of the dorsum sella and expansion of the sella itself.

The suprasellar arachnoid cyst in Case 348 *(arrows)* mimics an enlarged third ventricle. The diagnosis of aqueductal stenosis could be assumed, although the very round margins of the cyst are unusual for third ventricular dilatation. Subsequent evaluation demonstrated a suprasellar cyst compressing the third ventricle and causing obstructive hydrocephalus. An ependymal cyst arising *within* the third ventricle could present an identical image.

Other midline lesions that may mimic third ventricular distention include low-density hypothalamic gliomas and low-attenuation craniopharyngiomas.

DIFFERENTIAL DIAGNOSIS: LOW-ATTENUATION LESION WITHIN THE THIRD VENTRICLE

Case 349

9-year-old girl with neurofibromatosis.

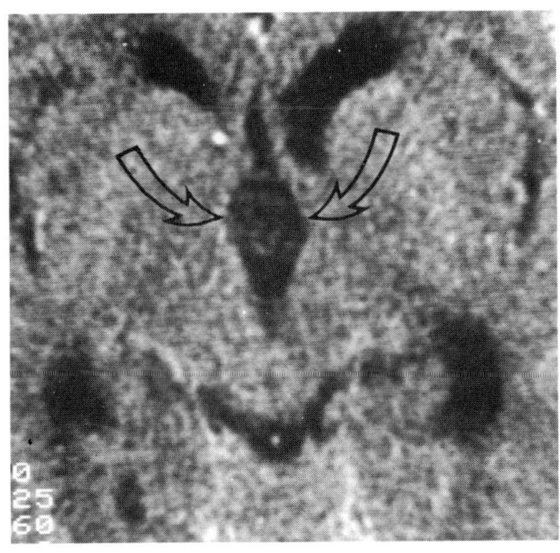

Pilocytic Astrocytoma.

Case 350

17-year-old girl.

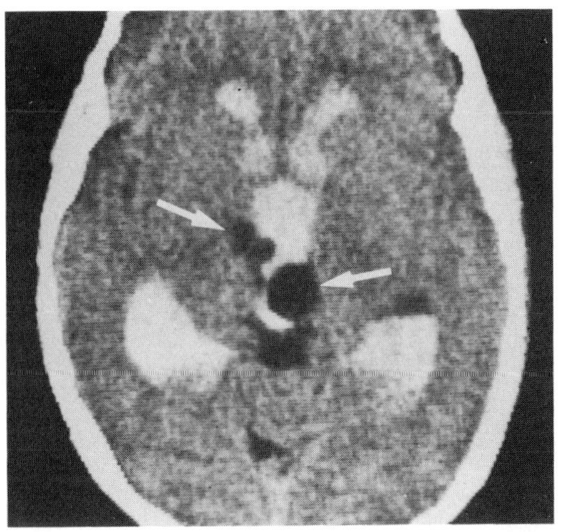

Intraventricular Cysts (Possible Cysticercosis).

Cysts or tumors of low attenuation (e.g., ependymal cyst, parasitic cyst, glioma, epidermoid tumor) may obstruct the third ventricle while blending with the surrounding spinal fluid. These masses can be easily overlooked, leading to the incorrect diagnosis of aqueductal stenosis.

The density of such lesions may differ slightly from CSF, allowing detection by close examination of standard scans (as in Case 349).

Other lesions may be completely hidden, requiring intraventricular contrast for diagnosis (as in Case 350).

DIFFERENTIAL DIAGNOSIS: LARGE LATERAL VENTRICLES IN AN ELDERLY PATIENT

Case 351

75-year-old man.

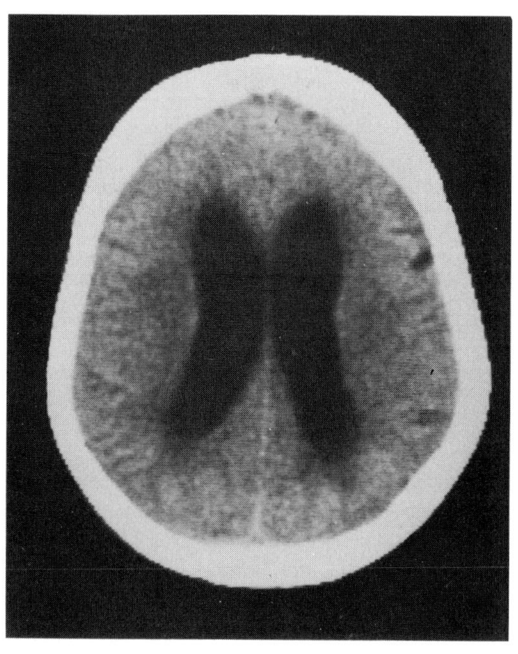

Hydrocephalus (Acoustic Schwannoma).

Case 352

63-year-old man.

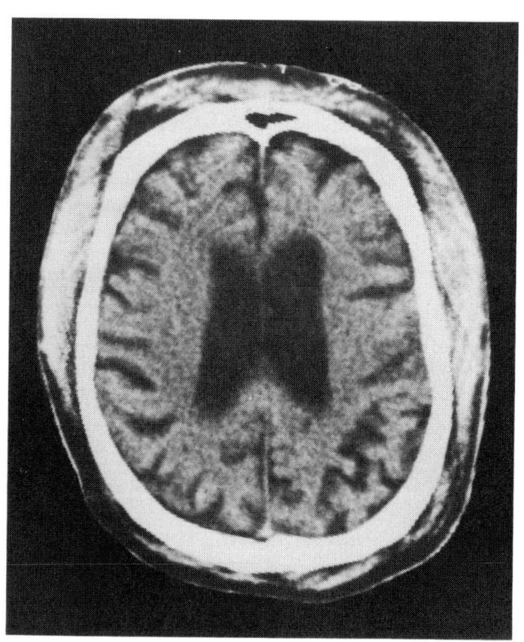

Atrophy.

Hydrocephalus can usually be distinguished from atrophic ventricular enlargement in most cases, as illustrated here. In some patients the diagnosis of hydrocephalus may be obscured by a background of atrophy. (See Case 354, which demonstrates features intermediate between Cases 351 and 352).

Several CT clues may be helpful in this situation: (1) The margins of hydrocephalic ventricles appear tight and stretched, while the margins of atrophic ventricles are more slack and undulating. (2) A halo or fringe of periventricular edema may cause the borders of hydrocephalic ventricles to become indistinct (see Cases 355 and 356), while atrophic ventricles are sharply defined. (3) Hydrocephalic expansion of the lateral ventricles includes prominent temporal horn enlargement, while the temporal horns are less dilated in the usual case of cerebral atrophy (except in Pick's disease; see Case 183). (4) Third-ventricular enlargement is definite in hydrocephalus but less impressive in patients with atrophy.

Fourth-ventricular enlargement favors hydrocephalus when present, but many cases of communicating hydrocephalus do not show significant expansion of the fourth ventricle. Large sulci favor atrophy, but patients with atrophy may develop superimposed hydrocephalus.

Case 351 shows tight ventricular margins, mild periventricular edema, and small sulcal size relative to ventricular enlargement.

Case 352 shows slack, sharply defined ventricular margins, and proportionate enlargement of sulci. Massive scalp hematomas are present due to a severe beating that led to admission.

Case 353

57-year-old woman, ten days after subarachnoid hemorrhage.

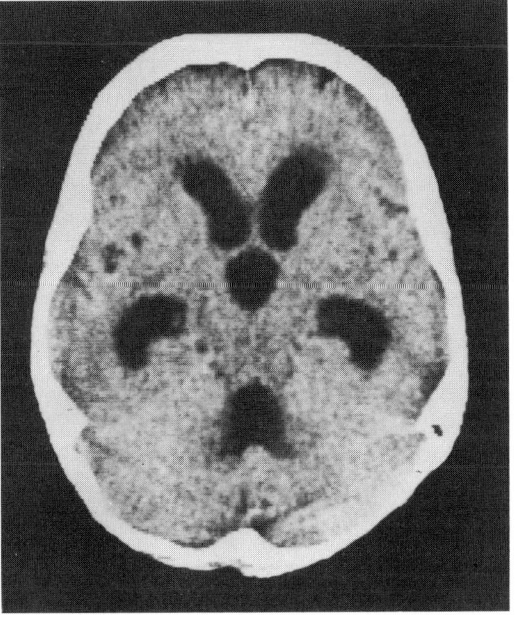

The enlargement of lateral, third, and fourth ventricles in this case places the impairment to CSF flow outside the ventricular system. Communicating hydrocephalus in adults often follows an inflammatory meningeal process, either infectious (meningitis) or hemorrhagic (trauma or aneurysm rupture). Such patients are usually good candidates for shunt procedures.

Case 354

71-year-old woman. "Normal pressure hydrocephalus."

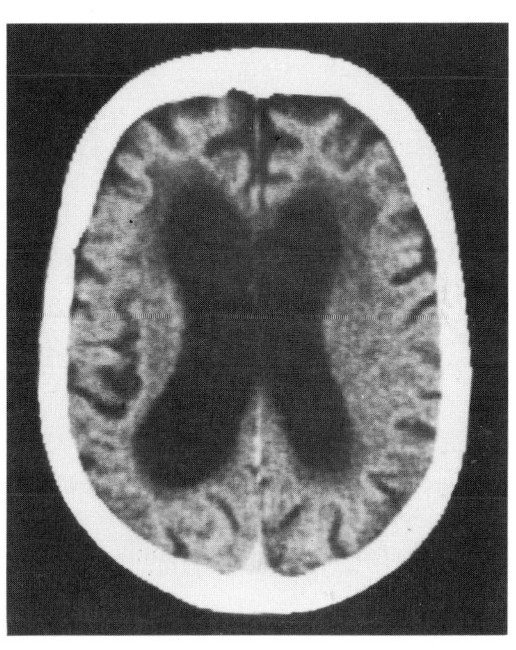

Some adults develop low-grade, communicating hydrocephalus with no history of meningitis or subarachnoid hemorrhage. This "normal pressure hydrocephalus" is often superimposed on a background of atrophy in an elderly patient. Associated periventricular edema may mimic the low attenuation "normally" seen in "old" white matter. For these reasons, the distinction between atrophic ventricular expansion and true hydrocephalus can sometimes be difficult (see discussion of Cases 351 and 352).

Tests of CSF dynamics using subarachnoid contrast materials may be useful. However, the best predictor of shunt response appears to be the clinical triad of gait abnormality, urinary incontinence, and dementia. A short history and a prominent degree of hydrocephalus also favor a good result.

Patients with aqueductal stenosis or communicating hydrocephalus may do well for years with a "compensated" or "arrested" state of ventricular enlargement (see Case 345). Symptoms of progressive hydrocephalus may subsequently develop due to an undetermined alteration of equilibrium.

SECONDARY FINDINGS IN HYDROCEPHALUS: PERIVENTRICULAR EDEMA (TRANSEPENDYMAL CSF ABSORPTION)

Case 355

57-year-old woman. Hydrocephalus due to a colloid cyst of the third ventricle.

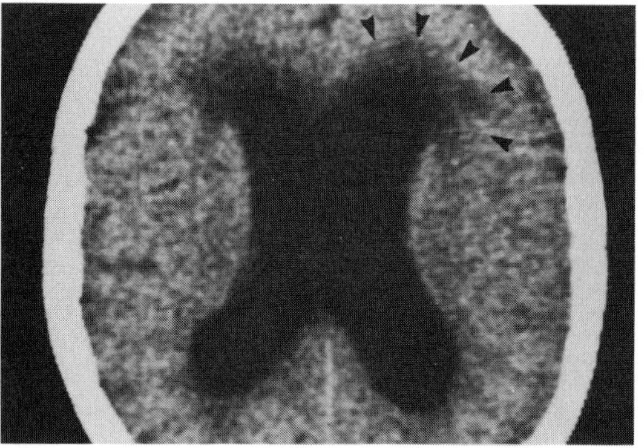

As the lateral ventricles enlarge in hydrocephalus, the tight junctions between ependymal cells are eventually disrupted. This discontinuity may allow spinal fluid under pressure to "leak" into the periventricular white matter.

The apparent transependymal movement of CSF causes a localized or diffuse "fringe" of low attenuation around the ventricles. The low density may be appreciated as a definite zone, as in this case *(arrows)*, or as indistinctness of the normally sharp ventricular margins (see Case 351).

When diffuse transependymal edema occurs in an elderly patient, the appearance can mimic the aging white matter pattern illustrated in Case 174.

Case 356

15-month-old boy. Hydrocephalus due to an optic glioma (narrow window width).

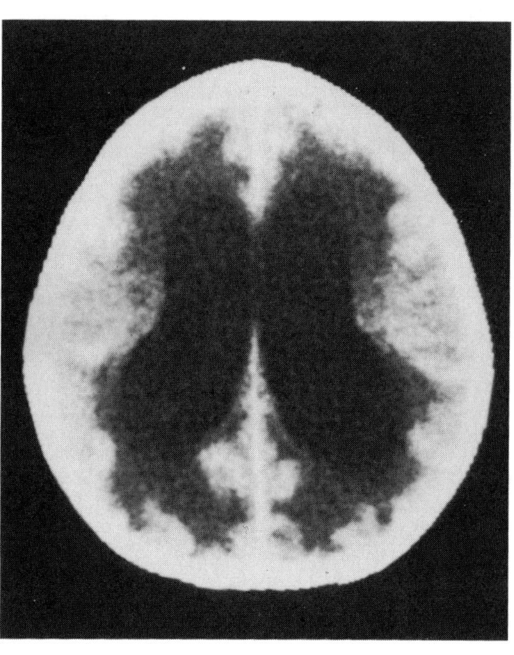

The zone of periventricular edema may be strikingly demonstrated in some cases of acute, severe hydrocephalus. Here the low-attenuation "halo" surrounding the ventricles has been accentuated by photographing at a narrow window width. Hydrocephalus could be considered a type of white matter disease, since distortion and edema of white matter are prominent features of the condition.

Case 45, 163, and 334 illustrate other examples of periventricular edema in hydrocephalus. This finding is also well demonstrated by magnetic resonance imaging.

Case 357

15-month-old boy. Diverticulum of the third ventricle.

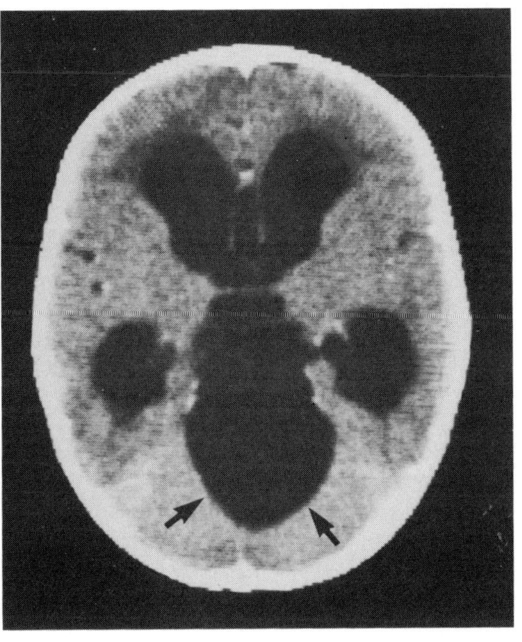

Hydrocephalic ventricles may bulge into areas of relatively low resistance. For example, the posterior third ventricle may bulge into the quadrigeminal cistern. Continued enlargement of this diverticulum may extend inferiorly through the tentorial hiatus.

The diverticulum is then seen as a midline mass in the posterior fossa, as in this case. Such diverticula may be confused with primary cysts or masses and erroneously implicated as the cause of hydrocephalus.

The thinned walls of distended ventricles may also perforate, immediately relieving symptoms ("spontaneous ventriculostomy").

Case 358

1-year-old boy. Diverticulum of the lateral ventricular trigone.

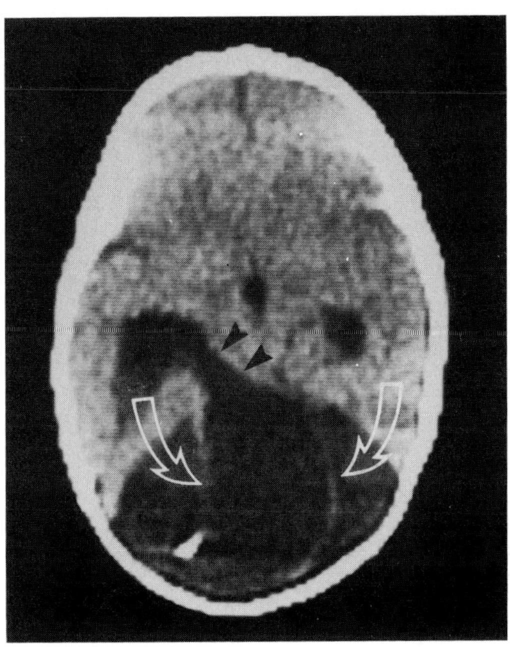

Another common location for the formation of ventricular diverticula is the medial wall of the trigone (lateral ventricle). A diverticulum from this site *(arrowheads)* often extends into the posterior fossa.

Here, shunting of a Dandy-Walker cyst has allowed infratentorial expansion of the ventricular diverticulum *(arrows)*.

Case 359

8-year-old boy. Subdural hematomas.

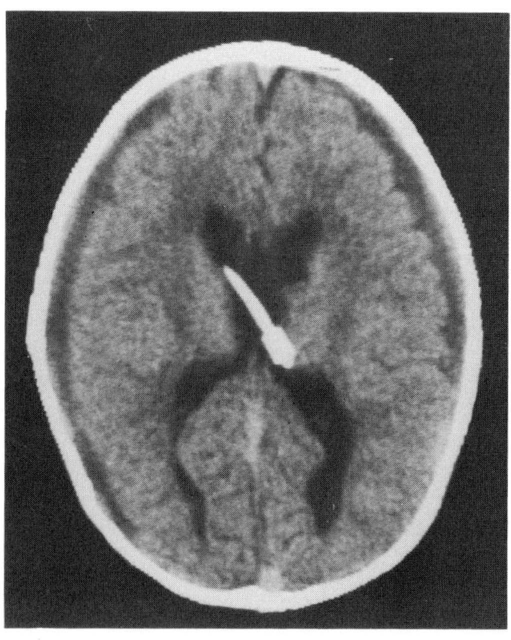

Decompression of dilated ventricles may lead to collapse of the cerebral cortex, favoring the development of secondary subdural hematomas. Large subdural collections may present acutely, while smaller lesions follow a more chronic course (as in this case). Subdural hematomas should be a primary consideration (along with shunt malfunction) when symptoms recur or head size increases in a patient who has undergone shunting.

Case 360

5-month-old girl. "Slit-like" (collapsed) ventricles.

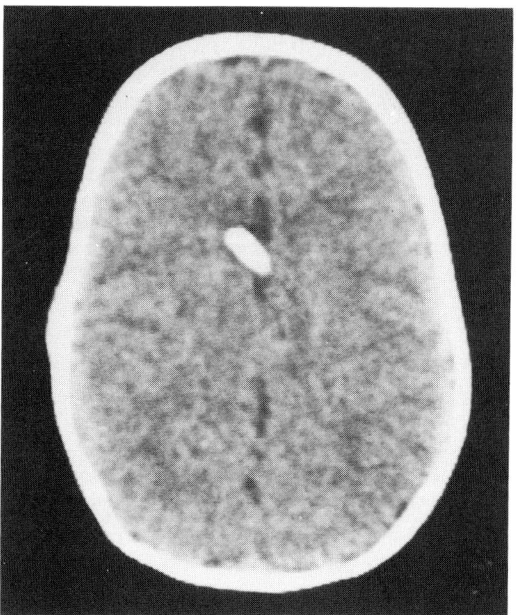

Shunted ventricles sometimes collapse to tiny residual slits. In this case, the lateral ventricles are essentially invisible.

Chronic ventricle collapse may be associated with low compliance. Subsequent shunt malfunction can cause a rapid increase in pressure with little expansion of ventricular volume. Small ventricular size does not exclude shunt obstruction in such cases.

Infection is another complication of ventricular shunts, occurring in about 1% to 10% of cases. Shunt-related infection often involves the subependymal tissue. Periventricular cysts or loculations may form. These can enlarge and bulge into the ventricle, mimicking intraventricular septations.

Case 361

30-year-old woman injured in an automobile accident.

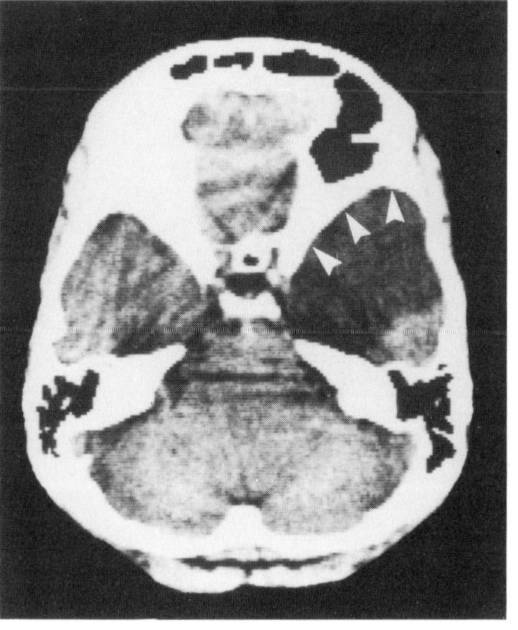

Arachnoid cysts account for about 1% of intracranial lesions. They are often discovered incidentally, presenting as low-attenuation masses in a number of characteristic locations. The middle cranial fossa is a common site, as illustrated here.

Long-term exertion of pressure from arachnoid cysts often causes expansion or erosion of bone. In this case, the sphenoid wing has been anteriorly displaced *(arrows)*, expanding the middle cranial fossa. The anterior temporal lobe is compressed posteriorly.

A similar appearance is occasionally seen in children with chronic "juvenile" subdural hematomas of the middle cranial fossa. In adults, the major differential diagnosis is a middle fossa epidermoid cyst.

Case 362

42-year-old woman examined because of a "lytic lesion" on skull roentgenograms.

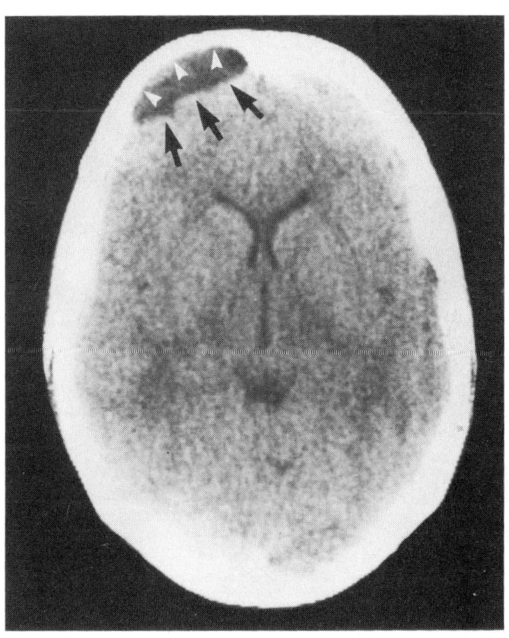

Arachnoid cysts are most common near the skull base but may occur over cerebral convexities. Erosion of the adjacent inner table is commonly associated with such lesions *(white arrows)*. The medial margin or cerebral interface of the cysts is often characteristically straight and angular *(black arrows;* see also Case 366).

Case 363

9-year-old girl.

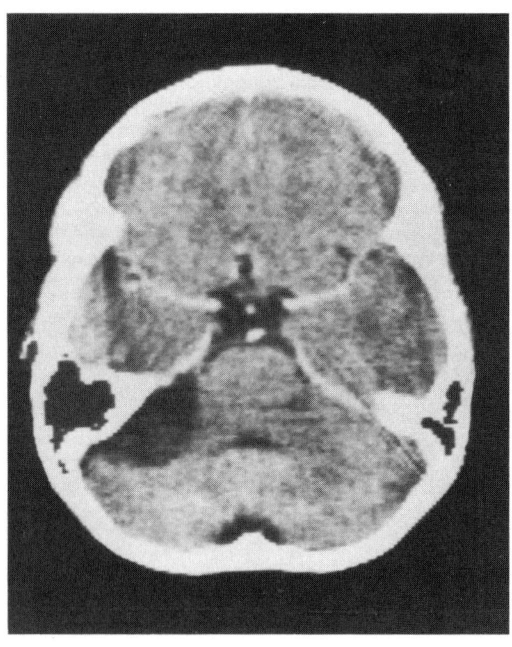

The cerebellopontine angle is another common location for arachnoid cysts. They should be included in the differential diagnosis of low-attentuation, extra-axial lesions at this site, along with epidermoid cysts and occasional acoustic schwannomas (compare this case to Cases 131 and 132).

The distinction between epidermoid cysts and arachnoid cysts can be made with subarachnoid contrast agents (see Case 130). Epidermoid cysts characteristically have a papillary surface, which contrasts with the smooth margins of an arachnoid cyst. Arachnoid cysts may fill with subarachnoid contrast material, particularly on delayed scans.

Case 364

77-year-old woman.

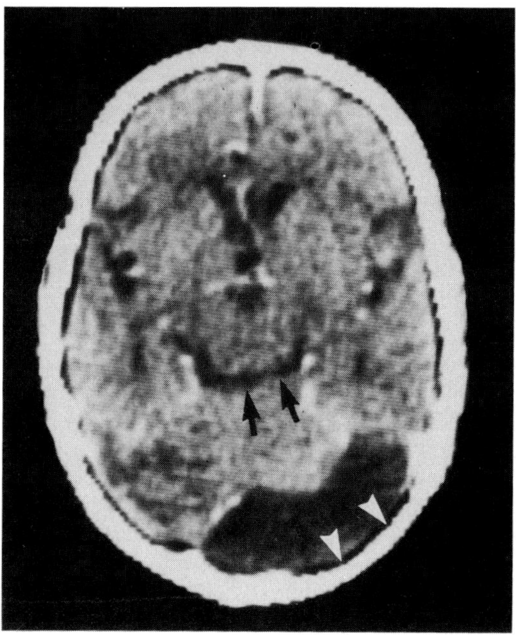

Arachnoid cysts near the occipital bone may be confused with a large and/or asymmetric cisterna magna. Evidence of mass effect favors the diagnosis of a true cyst.

In this case, the quadrigeminal cistern is flattened *(black arrows)* and cerebellar sulci are effaced on the side of the cyst. The cyst has also caused erosion of the inner table *(white arrows),* a finding sometimes also seen with a large cisterna magna. Some lesions have features intermediate between those of an obvious cyst and an asymmetric cisterna magna.

Posterior fossa arachnoid cysts should not be confused with the Dandy-Walker malformation (see Case 346), since they are usually asymmetric and are not associated with defects of the vermis.

DIFFERENTIAL DIAGNOSIS: LOW-ATTENUATION LESION EXTENDING OVER THE CEREBRAL CONVEXITY

Case 365

54-year-old woman.

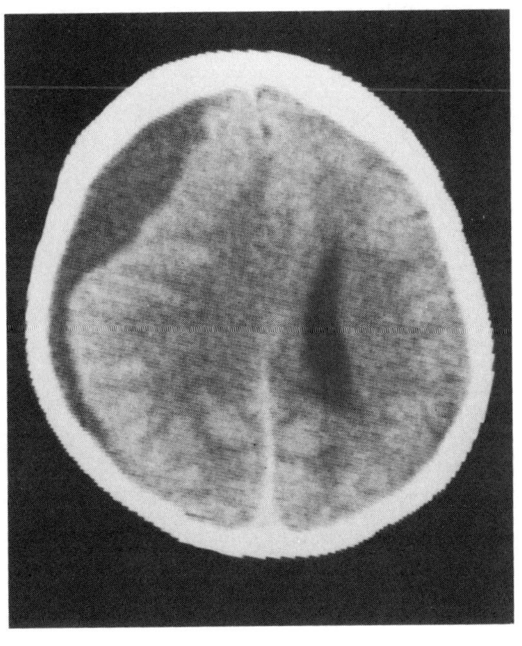

Chronic Subdural Hematoma.

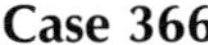

Case 366

48-year-old man.

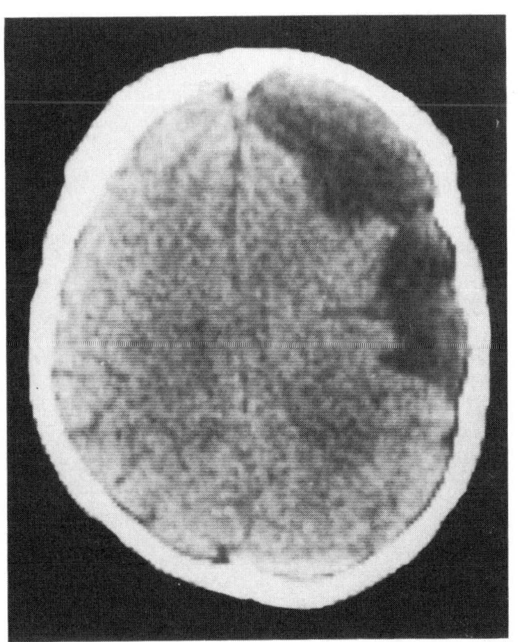

Arachnoid Cyst.

Arachnoid cysts may extend over large portions of the cerebral convexity. The appearance of such lesions can resemble a chronic subdural hematoma.

A useful diagnostic feature of arachnoid cysts is the frequently linear or angular contour of their medial margin, as demonstrated in Case 366. This jagged boundary contrasts with the smoothly compressed cerebral cortex underlying a subdural hematoma, as in Case 365.

DIFFERENTIAL DIAGNOSIS: LOW-ATTENUATION MASS OCCUPYING THE QUADRIGEMINAL CISTERN

Case 367

14-year old girl.

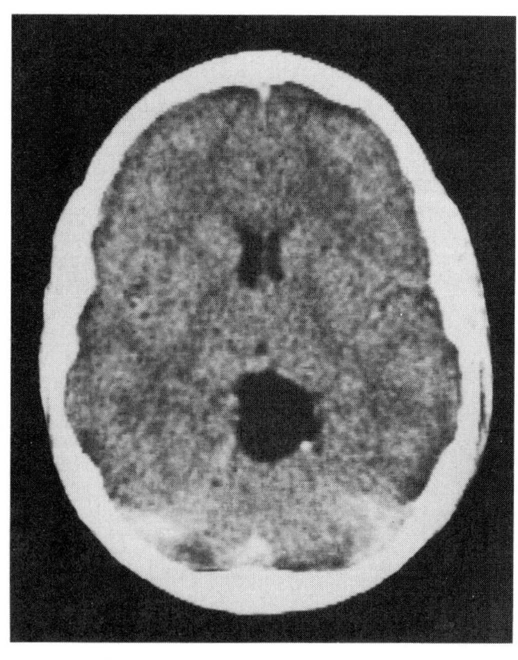

Epidermoid Cyst.

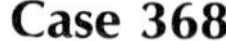

Case 368

40-year-old man.

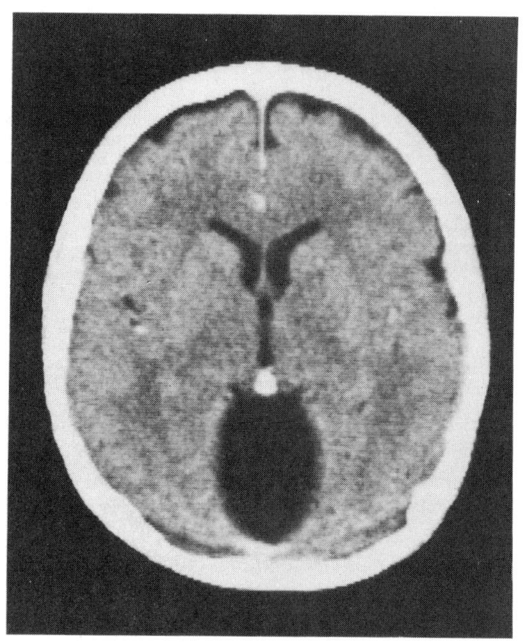

Arachnoid Cyst.

The quadrigeminal cistern is a common location for both epidermoid cysts and arachnoid cysts.

The epidermoid cyst in Case 367 has expanded in the plane between the brain stem and superior vermis. The brain stem is compressed anteriorly, while the vermis is displaced posteriorly.

The arachnoid cyst in Case 368 has displaced the vermis inferiorly to occupy the apex of the posterior fossa, defined by the tentorial margins.

Small lipomas are also commonly found in the quadrigeminal cistern, but their very low attenuation values prevent confusion with the lesions illustrated here.

DIFFERENTIAL DIAGNOSIS: LOW-ATTENUATION SUPRASELLAR MASS

Case 369

52-year-old man (same patient as Case 130).

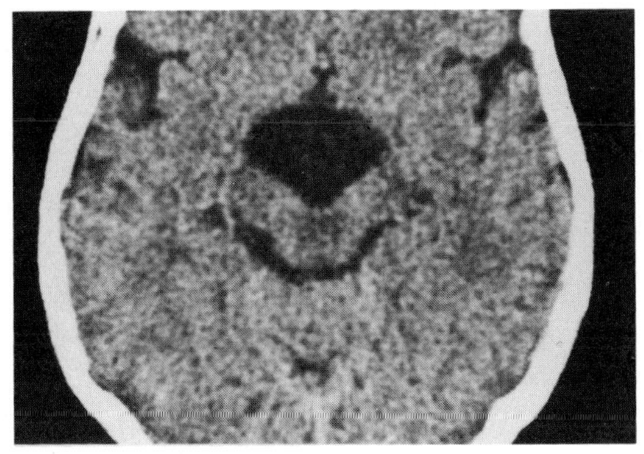

Epidermoid Cyst.

Case 370

8-year-old boy.

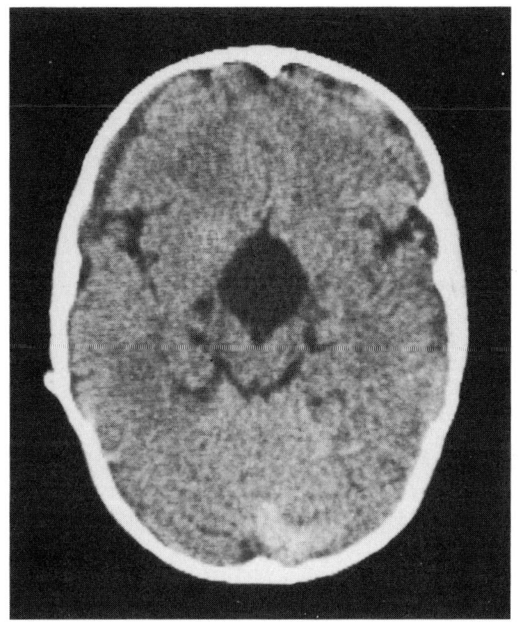

Arachnoid Cyst.

Both arachnoid cysts and epidermoid cysts may occur in the suprasellar region. Cysts or low-density tumors in this location may mimic an enlarged third ventricle (see Cases 347 and 348). The suprasellar masses in Cases 369 and 370 have extended posteriorly into the interpeduncular cistern, splaying the cerebral peduncles.

Attenuation values within an arachnoid cyst are often lower and usually more homogeneous than those of an epidermoid. The distinction may also be made with subarachnoid contrast material (see Case 130) or by magnetic resonance imaging.

PORENCEPHALIC CYSTS

Case 371

51-year-old woman with history of a childhood "stroke," now presenting with seizures.

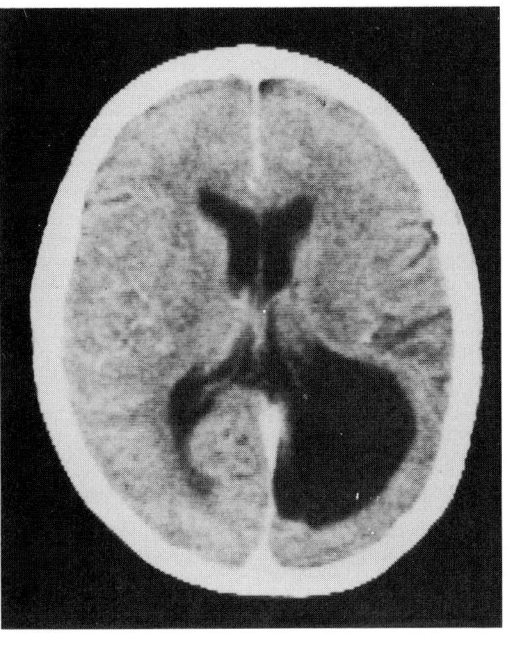

The term "porencephalic cyst" is variously applied to cystic lesions that form in a region of cerebral encephalomalacia. The strict application of the term refers to a localized expansion of the ventricular system into an area of parenchymal damage.

In this case the porencephalic expansion of the ventricular trigone probably indicates the site of the childhood cerebrovascular accident. Compare this scan to Case 232.

Case 372

72-year-old woman with a history of an old stroke.

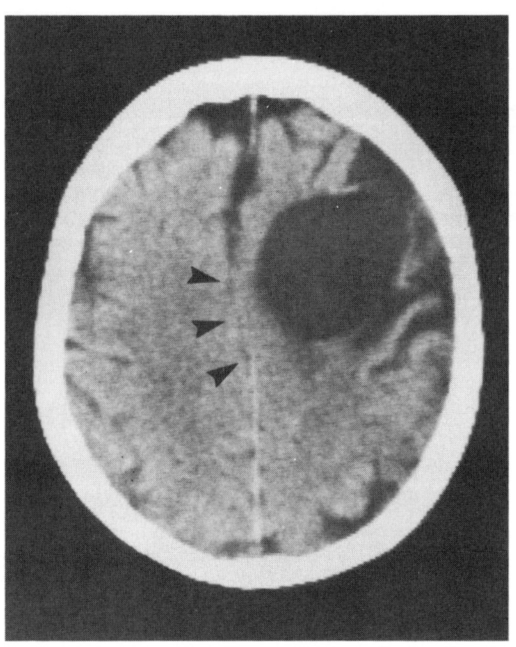

Porencephalic cysts may grow and exert pressure, probably due to incomplete communication with the parent ventricle or subarachnoid pathways. Such lesions present a paradoxical appearance of mass effect in the midst of atrophy.

The cyst in this case is surrounded by large sulci, reflecting an old parenchymal insult. The cyst itself appears "tight," with mass effect evidenced by mild subfalcial herniation *(arrows).*

AGENESIS OF THE CORPUS CALLOSUM

Case 373A

32-year-old woman presenting with seizures .

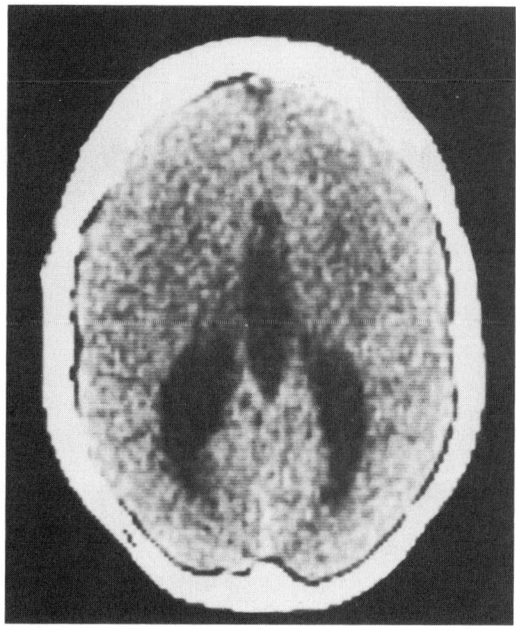

Case 373B

Same patient.

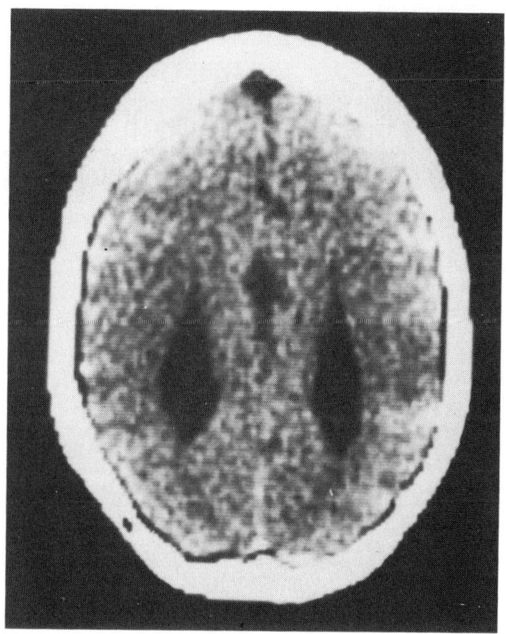

Agenesis of the corpus callosum may present a variety of appearances on CT scans. The most characteristic pattern is seen when the absence of the corpus callosum allows the third ventricle to rise high in the midline as an interhemispheric cyst.

This "high-riding" third ventricle is best appreciated on coronal scans, which may also demonstrate deep extension of the falx and comma-shaped frontal horns. Dilatation of the posterior portions of the lateral ventricles is a common associated finding.

The bodies of the lateral ventricles are separated, with an abnormally parallel or parasagittal orientation. This "classic" ventricular configuration is not seen in all cases, and other CT features are more reliable (see Case 375).

Agenesis of the corpus callosum may be incomplete, with absence of only the posterior portion. In such cases, the CT findings may be correspondingly less characteristic.

DIFFERENTIAL DIAGNOSIS: MIDLINE CYST BETWEEN THE LATERAL VENTRICLES

Case 374

40-year-old woman.

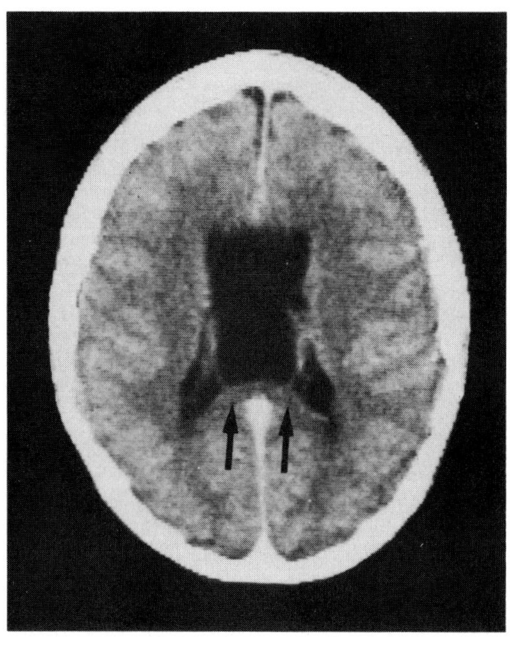

Cavum Septi Pellucidi And Cavum Vergae.

Case 375

1-year-old boy.

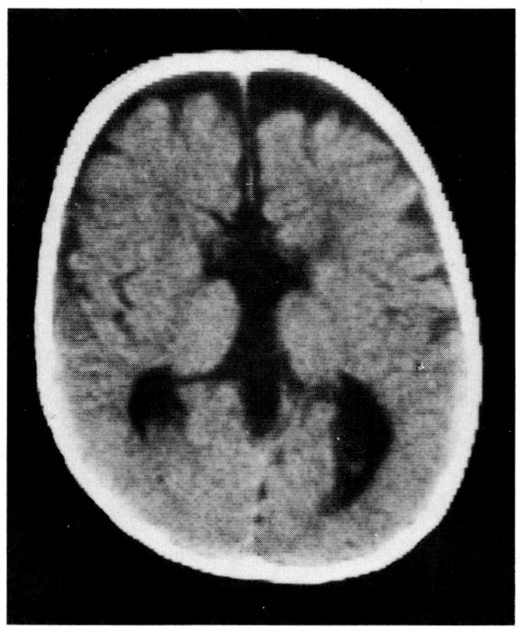

Agenesis Of The Corpus Callosum.

Cysts within the septum pellucidum are a normal feature of developing brains. They are usually obliterated soon after birth. Persistent cysts are often found at the level of the frontal horns and are termed "cavum septi pellucidi."

Larger cysts occupying most of the septum pellucidum and extending posterior to the fornix ("cavum vergae"), as in Case 374, are unusual. Case 374 has no other features to suggest agenesis of the corpus callosum; the splenium is clearly seen posteriorly *(arrows)*.

In Case 375, the midline "cyst" represents the third ventricle and adjacent interhemispheric fissure. The absence of the normal callosal tissue allows the anterior interhemispheric fissure to adjoin the elevated third ventricle. This continuity of interhemispheric fissure and superior third ventricle is a reliable sign of callosal agenesis.

Postcontrast scans in cases of agenesis of the corpus callosum may show the pericallosal arteries following an abnormally straight and posterior course as they ascend close to the anterior wall of the third ventricle. The high position of the third ventricle may separate the internal cerebral veins (see Case 376).

DIFFERENTIAL DIAGNOSIS: MIDLINE LOW-ATTENUATION LESION AT THE LEVEL OF THE CORPUS CALLOSUM

Case 376

32-year-old woman with seizures.

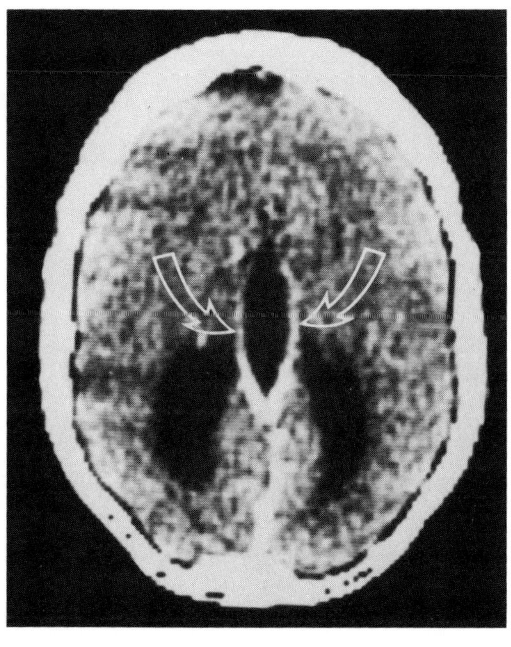

Agenesis Of The Corpus Callosum (Postcontrast Scan).

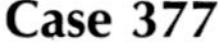

Case 377

10-month-old girl with seizures.

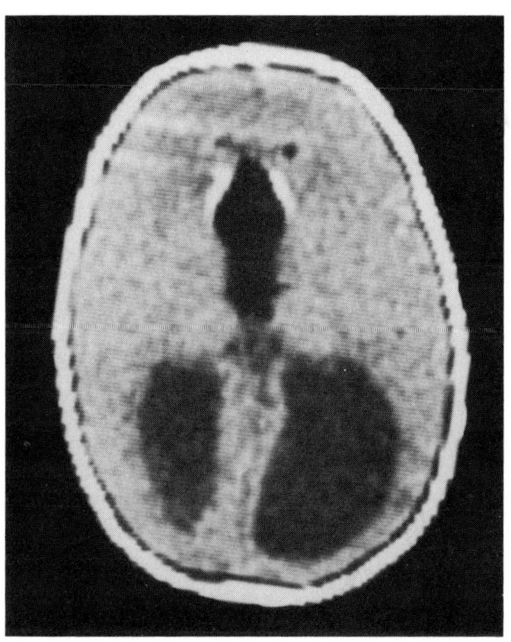

Lipoma Of The Corpus Callosum (Noncontrast Scan).

The high-riding third ventricle seen with agenesis of the corpus callosum often separates the internal cerebral veins, as seen in Case 376 (*arrows;* see Case 170 for an example of normal internal cerebral veins above the third ventricle). This appearance may superficially resemble the typical arcs of calcification surrounding a lipoma of the corpus callosum, demonstrated in Case 377.

Both lesions are often associated with dilatation and deformity of the posterior portions of the lateral ventricles. The attenuation values within a lipoma are much lower than those of spinal fluid, distinguishing these two congenital abnormalities.

REFERENCES

1. Altman N.R., Altman D.H., Sheldon J.J., et al.: Holoprosencephaly classified by computed tomography. *A.J.N.R.* 5:433–437, 1984.
2. Archer C.R., Darwish H., Smith K.: Enlarged cisternae magnae and posterior fossa cysts simulating Dandy-Walker syndrome on computed tomography. *Radiology* 127:681-686, 1978.
3. Armstrong E.A., Harwood-Nash D.C., Hoffman H., et al.: Benign suprasellar cysts: The CT approach. *A.J.N.R.* 4:163–166, 1983.
4. Byrd S.E., Harwood-Nash D.C., Fitz C.R.: Absence of the corpus callosum: Computed tomographic evaluation in infants and children. *J. Assoc. Can. Radiol.* 29:108–112, 1978.
5. Day R.E., Schutt W.H.: Normal children with large heads: Benign familial megalencephaly. *Arch. Dis. Child.* 54:512–517, 1979.
6. Drayer B.P., Rosenbaum A.E.: Studies of the third circulation: Amipaque CT cisternography and ventriculography. *J. Neurosurg.* 48:946–956, 1978.
7. Dublin A.B., French B.N.: Diagnostic image evaluation of hydranencephaly and pictorially similar entities, with emphasis on computed tomography. *Radiology* 137:81–91, 1980.
8. Fitz C.R.: Midline anomalies of the brain and spine. *Radiol. Clin. North Am.* 20:95–104, 1982.
9. Fitz C.R.: Holoprosencephaly and related entities. *Neuroradiology* 25:225–238, 1983.
10. Fitz C.R., Harwood-Nash D.C., Chuang S., et al.: Metrizamide ventriculography and computed tomography in infants and children. *Neuroradiology* 16:6–9, 1978.
11. Hayashi T., Yoshida M., Kuramoto S., et al.: Radiological features of holoprosencephaly. *Surg. Neurol.* 12:261–265, 1979.
12. Heinz E.R., Ward A., Drayer B.P., et al.: Distinction between obstructive and atrophic dilatation of ventricles in children. *J. Comput. Assist. Tomogr.* 4:320–325, 1980.
13. Hiratsuka H., Fujiwara K., Okada K., et al.: Modification of periventricular hypodensity in hydrocephalus with ventricular reflux in metrizamide CT cisternography. *J. Comput. Assist. Tomogr.* 3:204–208, 1979.
14. Hoffman H.J., Hendrick R.B., Humphreys R.P., et al.: Investigation and management of suprasellar arachnoid cysts. *J. Neurosurg.* 57:597–602, 1982.
15. Huckman M.S.: Normal pressure hydrocephalus: evaluation of diagnostic and prognostic tests. *A.J.N.R.* 2:385–395, 1981.
16. Kapila A., Naidich T.P.: Spontaneous lateral ventriculocisternostomy documented by metrizamide CT ventriculography. *J. Neurosurg.* 54:101–104, 1981.
17. Kendall B.E.: Dysgenesis of the corpus callosum. *Neuroradiology* 25:239–256, 1983.
18. Kendall B., Holland I.: Benign communicating hydrocephalus in children. *Neuroradiology* 21:93–96, 1981.
19. Leo J.S., Pinto R.S., Hulvat G.F., et al.: Computed tomography of arachnoid cysts. *Radiology* 130:675–680, 1979.
20. Masdeu J.C., Dobben G.D., Akar-Kia B.: Dandy-Walker syndrome studied by computed tomography and pneumoencephalography. *Radiology* 147:109–114, 1983.
21. Ment L.R., Duncan C.C., Geehr R.: Benign enlargement of the subarachnoid spaces in the infant. *J. Neurosurg.* 54:504–508, 1981.
22. Modic M.T., Kaufman B., Bonstelle C., et al.: Megalocephaly and hypodense extracerebral fluid collections. *Radiology* 141:93–100, 1981.
23. Mori K., Handa H., Murata T., et al.: Periventricular lucency in computed tomography of hydrocephalus and cerebral atrophy. *J. Comput. Assist. Tomogr.* 4:204–209, 1980.
24. Nabawi P., Dobben G.D., Mafee M., et al.: Diagnosis of lipoma of the corpus callosum by CT in five cases. *Neuroradiology* 21:159–162, 1981.
25. Naidich T.P., McLone D.G., Hahn Y.S., et al.: Atrial diverticula in severe hydrocephalus. *A.J.N.R.* 3:257–266, 1982.
26. Naidich T.P., Schott L.H., Baron R.L.: Computed tomography in evaluation of hydrocephalus. *Radiol. Clin. North Am.* 20:143–167, 1982.
27. Naidich T.P., Pudlowski R.M., Naidich J.B., et al.: Computed tomographic signs of the Chiari II malformation: I. Skull and dural partitions. *Radiology* 134:65–71, 1980.
28. Naidich T.P., Pudlowski R.M., Naidich J.B.: Computed tomographic signs of Chiari II malformation: II. Midbrain and cerebellum. *Radiology* 134:391–398, 1980.
29. Naidich T.P., Pudlowski R.M., Naidich J.B.: Computed tomographic signs of the Chiari II malformation: III. Ventricles and cisterns. *Radiology* 134:657–663, 1980.
30. Naidich T.P., McLone D.G., Fulling K.H.: The Chiari II malformation: IV. The hindbrain deformity. *Neuroradiology* 25:179–197, 1983.
31. New P.F., Davis K.R.: Intraventricular noncolloid neuroepithelial cysts. *A.J.N.R.* 2:569–575, 1981.
32. Ohno K., Enomoto T., Imamoto J., et al.: Lissencephaly (agyria) on computed tomography. *J. Comput. Assist. Tomogr.* 3:92–95, 1979.
33. Ramsey R.G., Huckman M.S.: Computed tomography of porencephaly and other cerebrospinal fluid-containing lesions. *Radiology* 123:73–77, 1977.
34. Rao K.C., Harwood-Nash D.C.: Craniocerebral anomalies, in Lee S.H., Rao K.C. (eds.): *Cranial Computed Tomography*, New York, McGraw Hill Inc., 1983, pp. 115–169.
35. Raybaud C.: Destructive lesions of the brain. *Neuroradiology* 25:265–291, 1983.
36. Sawar, M., Virapongse C., Bhimani S., et al.: Interhemispheric Fissure sign of dysgenesis of the corpus callosum. *J. Comput. Assist. Tomogr.* 8:637–644, 1984.
37. Servo A., Porras M., Jaaskinen J.: Diagnosis of ependymal intraventricular cysts of the third ventricle by computed tomography. *Neuroradiology* 24:155–157, 1983.
38. Watts R.W., Spellacy E., Kendall B.E., et al.: Computed tomography studies on patients with mucopolysaccharidoses. *Neuroradiology* 21:9–23, 1981.
39. Wolpert S.M., Scott R.M.: The value of metrizamide CT cisternography in the management of cerebral arachnoid cysts. *A.J.N.R.* 2:29–35, 1981.
40. Yeates A., Enzmann D.: Case report: An intraventricular arachnoid cyst. *J. Comput. Assist. Tomogr.* 3:697–700, 1979.

CHAPTER 12

ORBITAL LESIONS

VASCULAR MASSES

Case 378

Newborn boy with proptosis. Hemangioma.

CT provides a sensitive view of orbital pathology. The normal low attenuation of retrobulbar fat contrasts with lesions of soft-tissue density. In addition, the axial display of orbital anatomy allows localization of lesions with respect to the globe and muscle cone. CT also demonstrates pathologic conditions along the skull base, which may be manifested by ocular symptoms (see Case 28).

Vascular lesions are among the most common orbital masses. Although benign, these tumors may have extensive intraconal and extraconal components.

Orbital hemangiomas usually present as well-defined lesions with smooth or mildly lobulated margins. They are often located superior and lateral to the globe, sparing the orbital apex. Occasional cavernous hemangiomas contain characteristic calcified phleboliths.

Hemangiomas appear dense on precontrast scans. They typically demonstrate uniform, intense contrast enhancement. Proptosis is commonly associated, as seen here. In this case, the congenital mass is associated with a small globe.

Case 379

25-year-old man with a history of proptosis when bending over. Orbital varix.

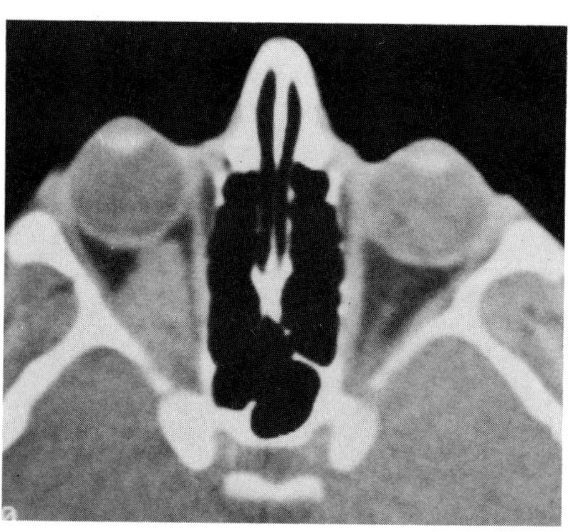

The subcategories of vascular masses within the orbit may be indistinguishable on CT scans. This varix demonstrates well-defined margins, slightly lobular contour, homogeneous density, and uniform contrast enhancement, comparable with a hemangioma or a lymphangioma.

Although the clinical history is characteristic in this case, the diagnosis was confirmed by orbital venography. Jugular vein compression or a Valsalva maneuver during CT scans may demonstrate impressive enlargement of orbital varices.

Case 380

27-year-old man. Lymphangioma.

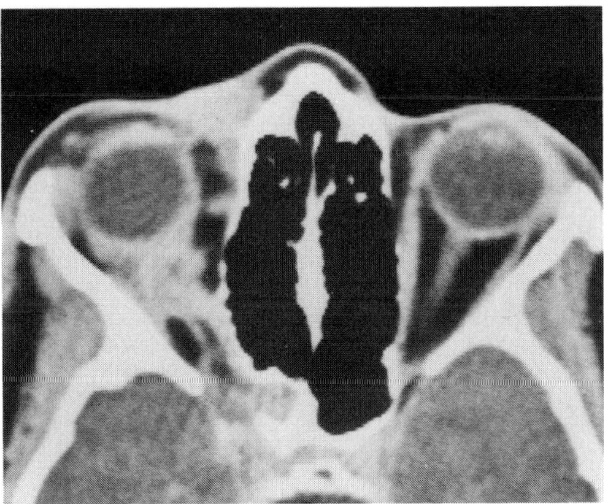

The sensitivity of orbital CT scanning exceeds the specificity of the images. The enhancing intraconal process applied to the optic nerve and globe in this case proved to be a lymphangioma. Other lymphangiomas present a more mass-like contour, identical to that of hemangiomas, while the appearance seen here resembles an inflammatory process such as orbital pseudotumor (see Case 385).

Case 381

26-year-old man injured in an automobile accident. Carotid-cavernous fistula.

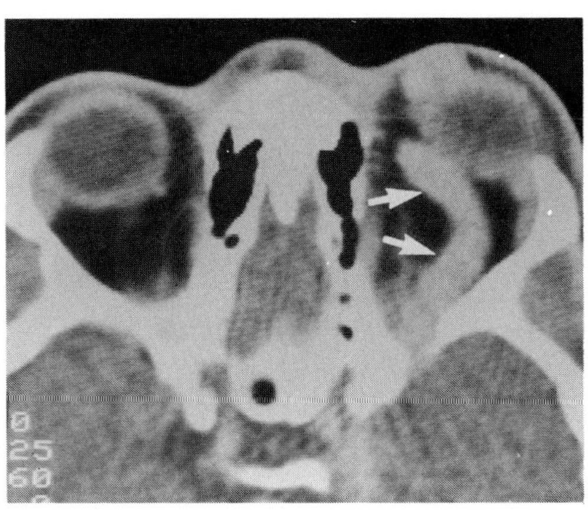

The superior ophthalmic vein is regularly seen on orbital scans as it crosses above the optic nerve on its way to the cavernous sinus. Enlargement of the vein *(arrows)* implies increased orbital blood flow, either congenital (e.g., arteriovenous malformation) or acquired (e.g., inflammatory processes such as pseudotumor or Graves' disease, carotid artery-cavernous sinus fistula).

Carotid-cavernous fistulae may be caused by a tear of the internal carotid artery as it passes through the venous compartment of the cavernous sinus. The resulting shunt of arterial blood floods the sinus and its tributaries, including the superior ophthalmic vein.

Reversal of flow in this vessel is associated with evidence of orbital vascular congestion (e.g., proptosis, conjunctival injection) and is often accompanied by a bruit transmitted from the fistula. A corroborating CT finding is distention of the ipsilateral cavernous sinus, partially visualized in this case.

Case 382

53-year-old woman. Metastatic breast carcinoma.

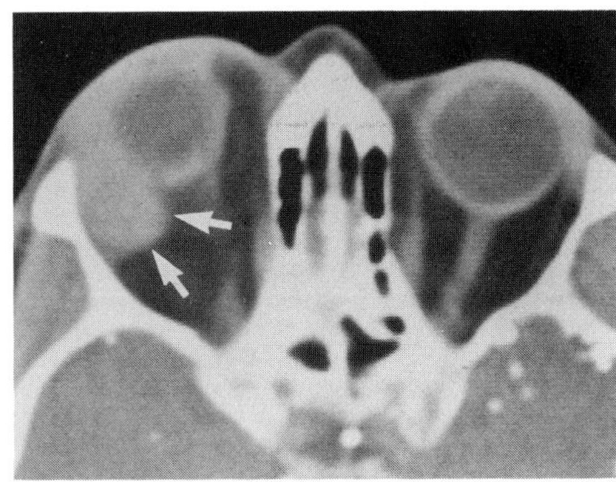

Solid tumors may arise within the globe and orbit as a primary lesion or as metastases from systemic neoplasms. In children, the most common orbital malignancies include lymphoma, leukemia, neuroblastoma, rhabdomyosarcoma, and retinoblastoma. In adults metastases from systemic carcinomas (e.g., breast, lung, kidney, colon) are more common.

The differential diagnosis of a mass in the superolateral quadrant of the orbit (as seen here) also includes tumors of the lacrimal gland (benign mixed tumors or adenocarcinomas), lymphomas, orbital dermoid cysts, sarcoidosis, and Wegener's granulomatosis. Soft-tissue prominence at this site may also be seen in thyroid ophthalmopathy and in orbital pseudotumors.

Case 383

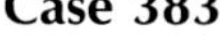

24-year-old man. Dermoid cyst.

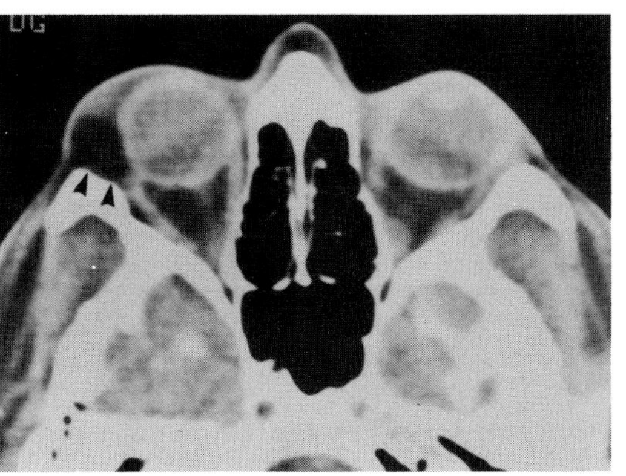

Dermoid cysts typically arise in the superolateral quadrant of the orbit, displacing the globe medially and inferiorly. Inferior displacement of one globe may be demonstrated on an axial scan by asymmetric visualization of the two lenses, as seen in this case.

The low attenuation of the lesion matches the density of retrobulbar fat and is characteristic of dermoid cysts (see Cases 98, 125, 127). Chronicity of the mass is indicated by smooth erosion of the lateral orbital rim *(arrows)*.

ORBITAL INFLAMMATION

Case 384

13-year-old girl. Orbital cellulitis.

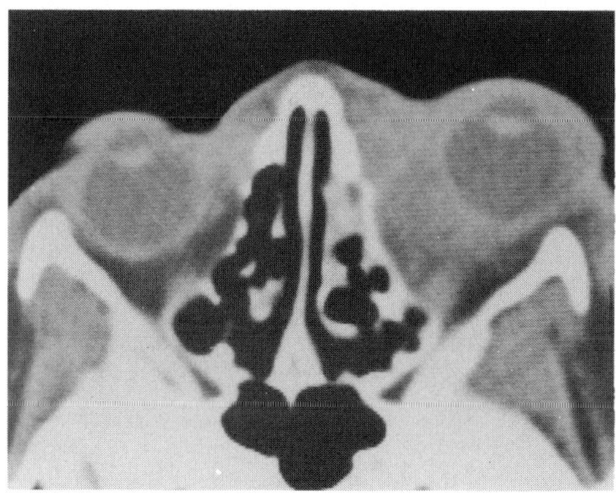

Inflammatory processes may cause edema and cellular infiltration of retrobulbar fat and/or extraocular muscles. The resulting density and swelling may mimic an orbital mass, but the clinical presentation usually clarifies the diagnosis.

In this case, the orbital inflammation is associated with midethmoid sinusitis and edema of preseptal tissue, favoring a diffuse cellulitis.

Case 385

40-year-old woman. Orbital pseudotumor.

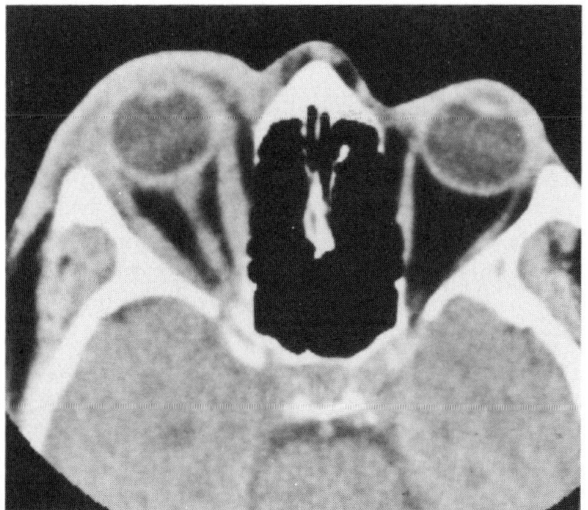

The diagnosis of "orbital pseudotumor" includes a diverse group of nonspecific lymphocytic and granulomatous inflammations. Pseudotumors may be unilateral or bilateral and may appear in many forms.

Diffuse retrobulbar infiltration may produce an appearance similar to that in Case 384, often associated with scleral enhancement. Discrete nodules of inflammatory tissue may mimic orbital tumors, although bilaterality or associated muscle changes often narrow the diagnosis. Infiltration of extraocular muscles may cause thickening that resembles Graves' disease.

This case illustrates the "myositic" form of orbital pseudotumor, with prominent swelling of the right medial and lateral rectus muscles. The appearance superficially mimics a thyroid ophthalmopathy (see Case 386). However, the associated preseptal inflammation and the shaggy prominence of the optic nerve suggest a diffuse inflammatory process. The diagnosis of orbital pseudotumor was confirmed at surgery.

Clinical features (rapid onset, pain, limitation of movement, response to steroids) also help to distinguish most pseudotumors from the tumors or endocrinopathies that they may otherwise resemble.

THYROID OPHTHALMOPATHY

Case 386A

58-year-old man with proptosis and diplopia.

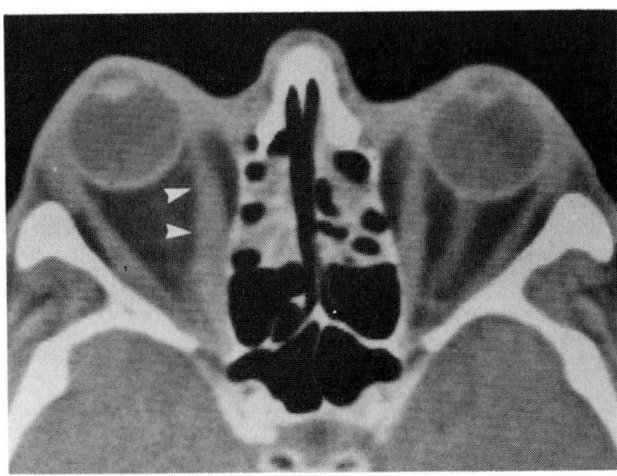

The hallmark of thyroid ophthalmopathy or "Graves' disease" is infiltration of the rectus muscles, easily detected on CT scans. The two eyes may be involved symmetrically (as in Case 388) or asymmetrically, as seen here. The medial and inferior rectus muscles are usually affected before, and to a greater extent than, the lateral rectus or superior muscle group.

This scan demonstrates right-sided proptosis with marked thickening of the medial rectus muscle *(arrows)*. Incidental ethmoid sinusitis is present.

Case 386B

Same patient. Coronal scan.

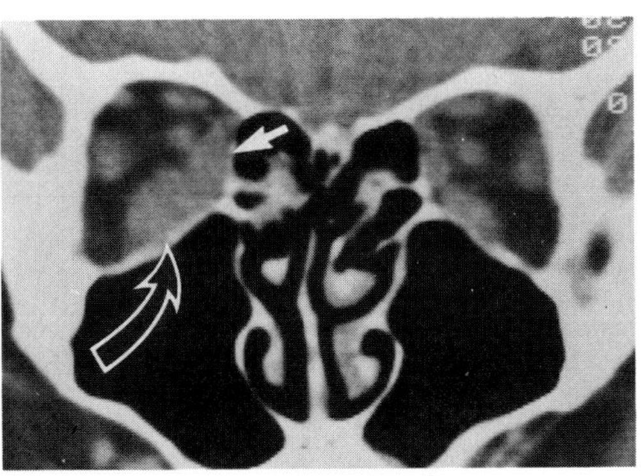

Coronal views provide a cross section of the muscle cone surrounding the optic nerve. This projection is often useful for assessing the relative intraconal and extraconal extent of a lesion. The coronal plane allows better visualization of the inferior rectus muscle and the superior muscle bundle than is possible on axial sections.

In this case, the right inferior rectus muscle *(open arrow)* is grossly enlarged, merging with the thickened medial rectus muscle *(small arrow)*.

DIFFERENTIAL DIAGNOSIS: THICKENED RECTUS MUSCLES

Case 387

44-year-old man with proptosis.

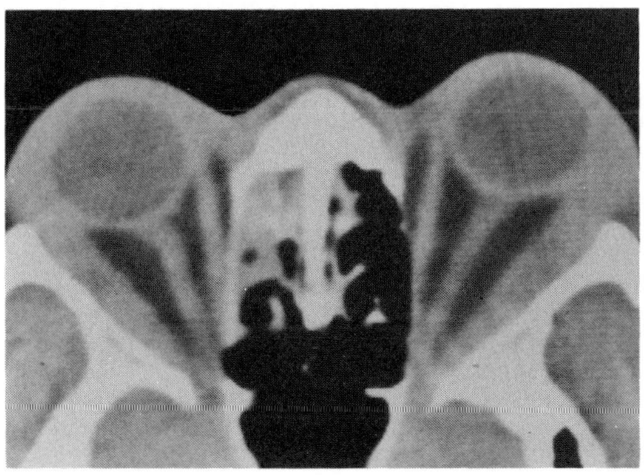

Orbital Lymphoma.

Case 388

60-year-old man with proptosis.

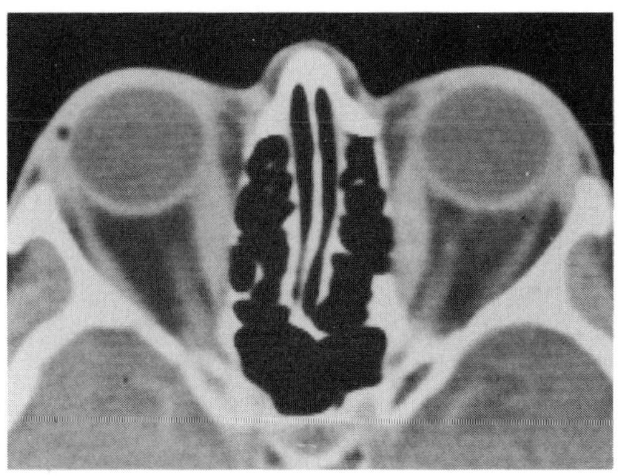

Thyroid Ophthalmopathy.

Thickening of rectus muscles may be caused by processes other than thyroid ophthalmopathy. Infiltration by neoplasms such as lymphoma, leukemia, and neuroblastoma may be observed, either unilaterally or symmetrically (as in Case 387). (Metastatic tumor is often located *adjacent* to the lateral rectus muscles in the lateral portions of the orbit.) Occasional orbital neurofibromas may also be seen as masses thickening the contour of a rectus muscle.

Inflammation localized to one or more muscles (''orbital myositis'') occurs within the spectrum of pseudotumors and is another lesion in the differential diagnosis (see Case 385). Carotid-cavernous fistulae may also be associated with swollen rectus muscles.

Masses limited to the lateral rectus muscles, as in Case 387, would be very unusual in Graves' disease. On the other hand, bilateral thickening of the medial rectus muscles, as in Case 388, is a characteristic appearance for thyroid ophthalmopathy.

DIFFERENTIAL DIAGNOSIS: THICKENING OF THE OPTIC NERVE

Case 389

7-year-old boy with neurofibromatosis.

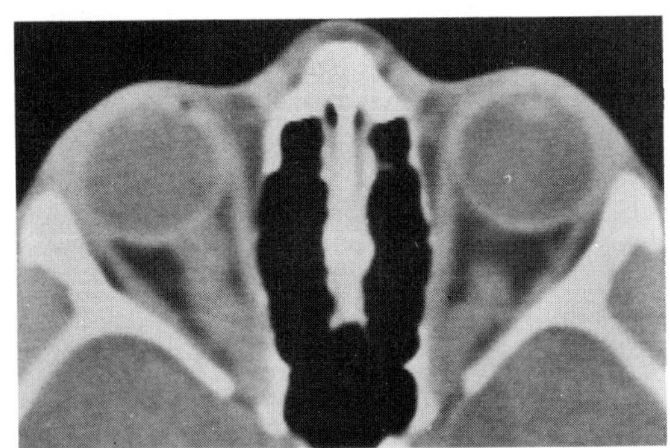

Optic Nerve Gliomas.

Case 390

24-year-old woman with neurofibromatosis.

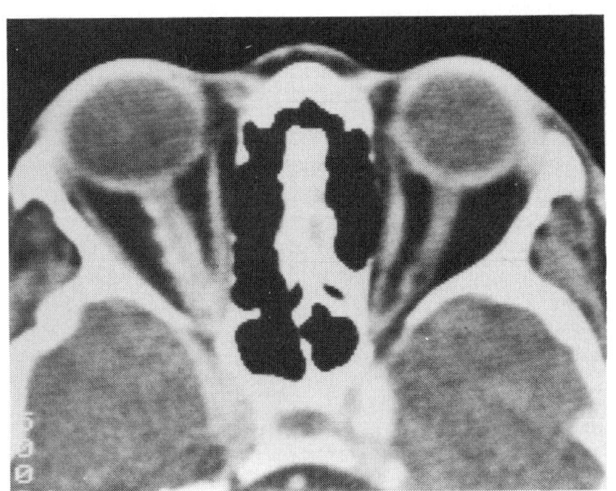

Optic Nerve Sheath Meningioma.

A wide variety of lesions may cause thickening of the optic nerve. Nonneoplastic processes such as papilledema, optic neuritis (e.g., multiple sclerosis, sarcoidosis), orbital pseudotumor, Graves' disease, and vascular malformations are included in the differential diagnosis.

Among tumors, the most important possibilities are gliomas of the nerve and meningiomas of the nerve sheath. A clinical clue to the presence of an optic nerve tumor is loss of visual acuity, which is rarely seen with other orbital masses.

As discussed in Case 105, optic nerve tumors in patients with neurofibromatosis are more often lower-grade lesions than spontaneous optic gliomas. Optic gliomas typically cause uniform thickening of the nerve, with mild undulation or lobulation.

Meningiomas of the optic nerve sheath often present as more fusiform or elliptical masses surrounding the axis of the nerve (see the calcified tumor in Case 396). Even relatively flat meningiomas are distinguished by the "tram-track" appearance of uninvolved nerve surrounded by an enhancing collar of meningioma, as seen in Case 390. (Occasionally, optic nerve involvement by orbital pseudotumor or sarcoidosis may also cause "tram-track" enhancement.) The enhancement of optic nerve sheath meningiomas is usually more intense than that of optic nerve gliomas.

When an optic nerve tumor is discovered in the orbit, the optic chiasm should be closely examined to assess intracranial extension (see Case 105). Similarly, the finding of a suprasellar mass should prompt careful evaluation of the intraorbital portions of the optic nerves.

ORBITAL EFFECTS OF SINUS DISEASE

Case 391

16-year-old boy with proptosis. Aspergillosis of ethmoid and sphenoid sinuses (noncontrast scan).

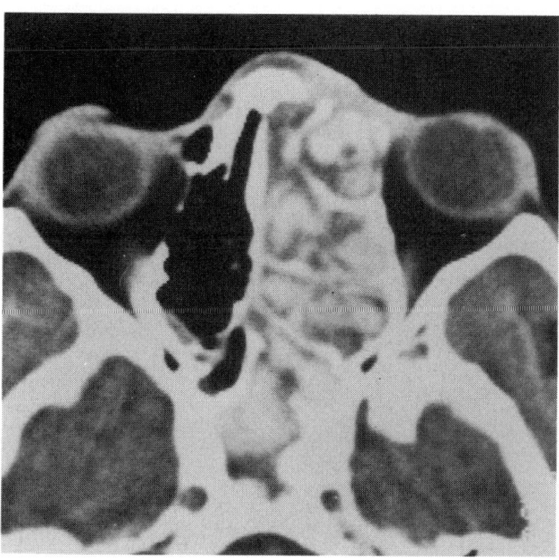

Sinus lesions are often manifested by orbital symptoms. Sinusitis may involve the orbit by direct extension as orbital cellulitis (see Case 384) or by secondary proptosis due to expansion of the sinus (mucocele or mucopyocele).

In this case, chronic infection has caused unusual enlargement of the entire ethmoid sinus system on the left side. The high attenuation within the sinus proved to be proteinacious material without hemorrhage or calcification.

Case 392

38-year-old woman with proptosis. Fibrosarcoma arising within the ethmoid sinus (coronal scan).

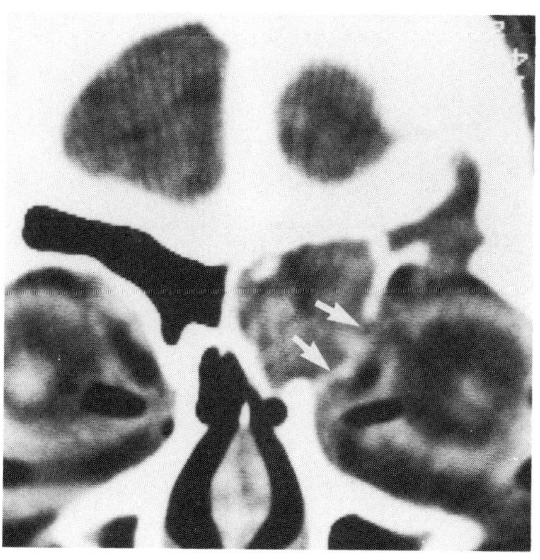

Tumors involving the paraorbital sinuses often extend into the orbit and cause secondary proptosis. Among the lesions that may present in this manner are juvenile angiofibromas, esthesioneuroblastomas, and squamous cell carcinomas.

The expansion of a sinus at the frontoethmoid junction is most commonly due to a mucocele. The irregular destruction of bone in this case *(arrows)* suggests a more aggressive lesion, as was confirmed at biopsy.

ORBITAL CALCIFICATIONS: BENIGN

Case 393

14-year-old boy noted to have swollen optic discs. Drusen.

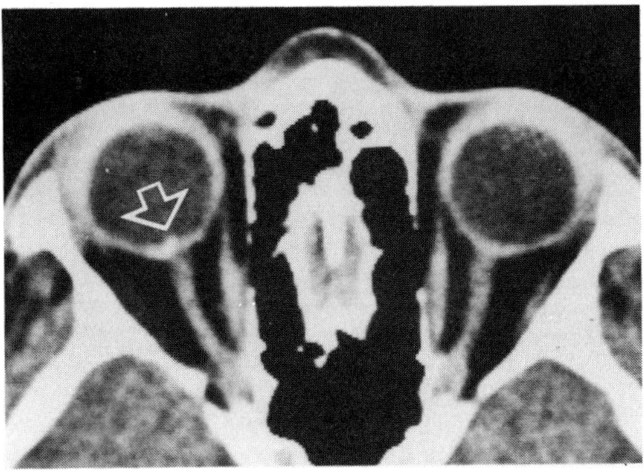

Many orbital lesions are associated with calcification. Some calcifications are diagnostically important, such as the densities marking small retinoblastomas (see Case 395). Other calcifications are merely incidental (e.g., phleboliths in hemangiomas, or calcification of a dystrophic globe in "phthisis bulbi").

The tiny calcification near the right optic disc in this case *(arrow)* is typical of optic disc drusen. These hyaline bodies are often buried in the optic discs of children, elevating the disc and mimicking papilledema. The CT demonstration of calcification establishes the specific diagnosis, while the cerebral scan excludes increased intracranial pressure.

The differential diagnosis of globe calcification would include retinal hamartoma in tuberous sclerosis, neurofibromatosis, choroidal osteoma, melanoma, and retinoblastoma.

Case 394

72-year-old woman. Senile scleral plaques.

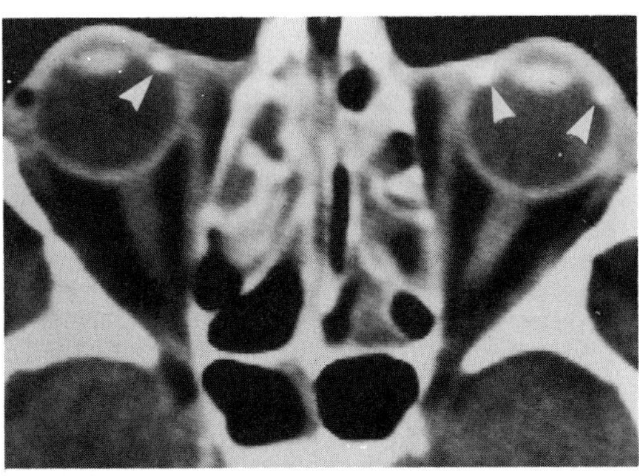

Small calcifications are commonly found near the junction of the horizontal rectus muscles and sclera in elderly patients. The calcium occurs within scleral plaques, possibly the result of chronic stress at the site of the rectus insertions. This benign phenomenon is usually bilaterally symmetric.

Case 395

1-year-old boy. Bilateral retinoblastomas.

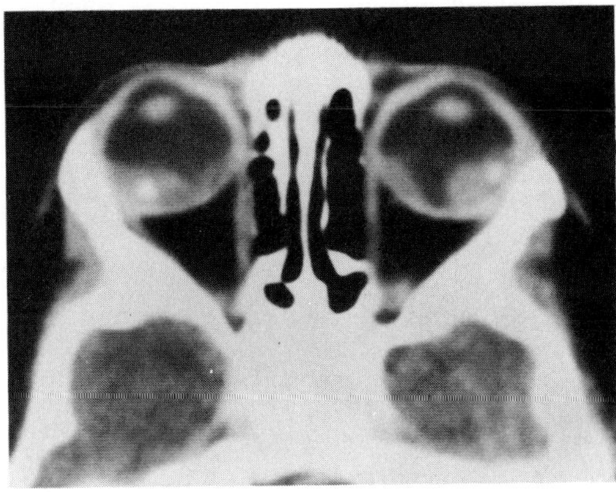

Tumors arising within the globe may be demonstrated by mass and/or calcification. In this case, the density of the tumor masses is apparent within the globes, a finding that may also be noted with orbital melanoma or metastases to the choroid.

Retinoblastomas frequently calcify and are often bilateral. CT is mainly used for assessing the retrobulbar extension of a known tumor. However, a tiny focus of calcium may be a clue to involvement of the nonpresenting eye.

Calcification of the posterior globe is also seen in choroidal osteomas, benign lesions with cancellous bone occurring in plaques along the posterior sclera.

Case 396

66-year-old man. Calcified meningioma of the optic nerve sheath.

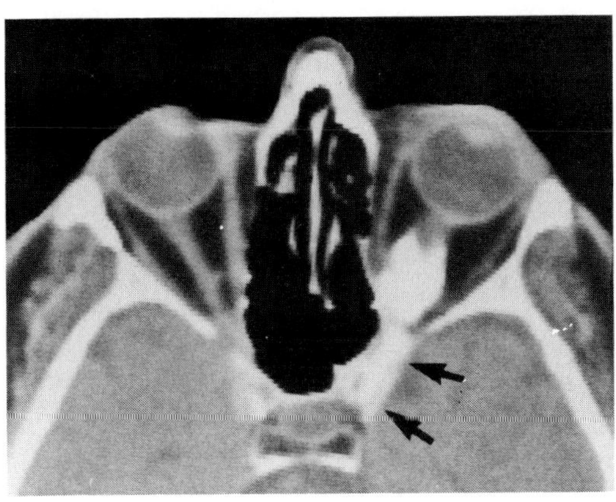

The tumor in this case has a fusiform shape that surrounds the axis of the optic nerve. Associated hyperostosis of the anterior clinoid process is present *(arrows)*.

Optic nerve gliomas may be fusiform and occasionally calcify. They do not demonstrate the central core of nerve-sparing lucency characteristic of sheath meningiomas.

Case 397

23-year-old man (coronal scan).

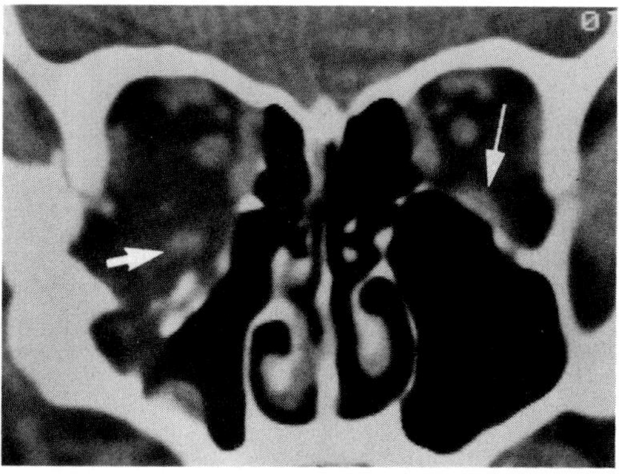

A direct blow to the eye compresses the orbital contents into the narrowing cone of the posterior orbit. The resultant increase in intraorbital pressure may cause secondary displacement of the orbital floor or medial wall.

CT scans clearly document these so-called "blow-out" fractures. Orbital fat and muscle are seen to herniate into air-containing sinuses.

The common blow-out fractures of the orbital floor are well defined on coronal scans. In this case, the floor of the right orbit is markedly depressed. The inferior rectus muscle *(short arrow)* is located far below its normal location *(arrow on the left)*.

Case 398

46-year-old man.

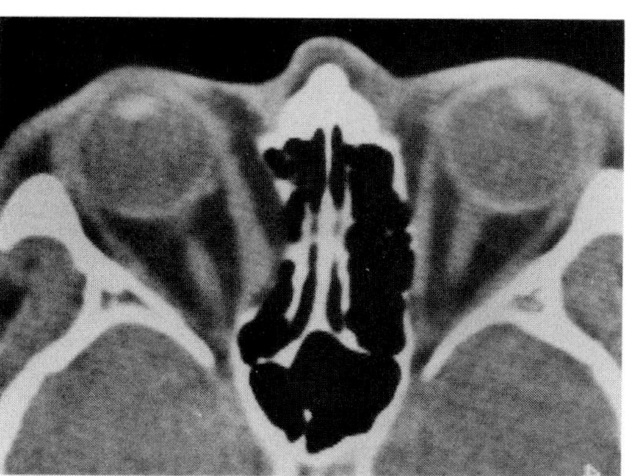

Blow-out fractures involving the medial wall of the orbit are well seen in either coronal or axial planes. This scan demonstrates orbital fat occupying the fossa formed by displacement of the lamina papyracea. The medial rectus muscle is thickened and distorted as it is drawn toward the fracture. The position of the globes is dysconjugate.

PENETRATING ORBITAL TRAUMA

Case 399

21-year-old assault victim. Lacerated globe.

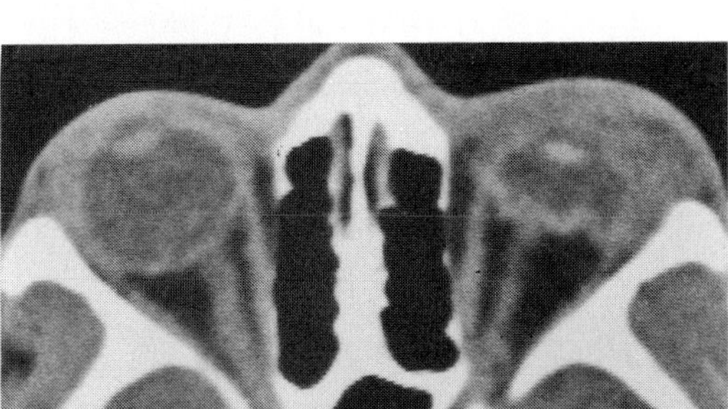
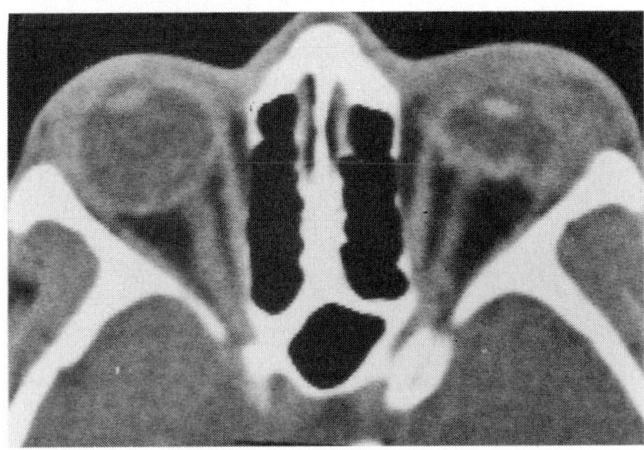

CT scans display the orbital contents in cases where facial injury may preclude ophthalmologic evaluation. In this case, a collapsed globe due to a penetrating injury is clearly demonstrated. No retrobulbar hematoma or foreign body is seen.

A small amount of head tilt may cause apparent asymmetry of normal anterior clinoid processes, as illustrated here.

Case 400

24-year-old pheasant hunter.

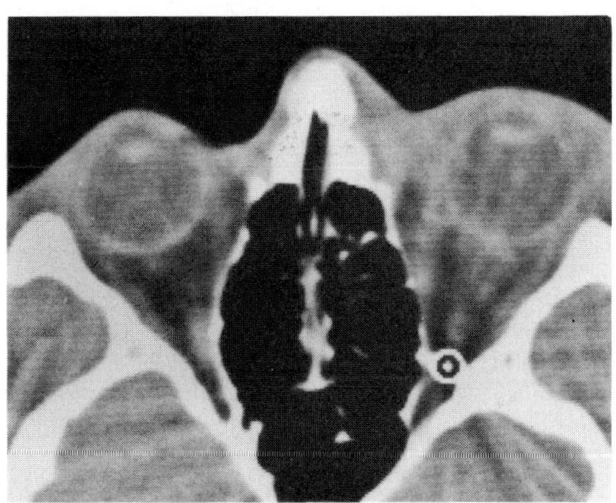

The localization of dense intraorbital foreign bodies is aided by the axial display of CT scans. A pellet is seen at the apex of the left orbit in this case.

Foreign bodies of low attenuation (e.g., wood and plastic) can sometimes be demonstrated. Associated ocular or retrobulbar injury is often apparent.

REFERENCES

1. Ahmadi J., Teal J.S., Segall H.D., et al.: Computed tomography of carotid-cavernous fistula. *A.J.N.R.* 4:131–136, 1983.
2. Balchunas W.R., Quencer R.M., Byrne S.F.: Lacrimal gland and fossa masses: Evaluation by computed tomography and A-mode echography. *Radiology* 149:751–758, 1983.
3. Berges O., Vignaud J., Aubin M.L.: Comparison of sonography and computed tomography in the study of orbital space-occupying lesions. *A.J.N.R.* 5:247–251, 1984.
4. Bilaniuk L.T., Zimmerman R.A.: Computer-assisted tomography: Sinus lesions with orbital involvement. *Head Neck Surg.* 2:293, 1980.
5. Bilaniuk L.T., Zimmerman R.A.: Computed tomography in evaluation of the paranasal sinuses. *Radiol. Clin. North Am.* 20:51–66, 1982.
6. Bryan R.N., Lewis R.A., Miller S.L.: Choroidal osteoma. *A.J.N.R.* 4:491–494, 1983.
7. Byrd S.E., Harwood-Nash D.C., Fitz C.R., et al.: Computed tomography of intraorbital optic nerve gliomas in children. *Radiology* 129:73–78, 1978.
8. Daniels D.L., Williams A.L., Syvertsen A., et al.: CT recognition of optic nerve sheath meningioma: abnormal sheath visualization. *A.J.N.R.* 3:181–183, 1982.
9. Danziger A., Price H.I.: CT findings in retinoblastoma. *A.J.R.* 133:695–697, 1979.
10. Davis K.R., Hesselink J.R., Dallow R., et al.: The role of CT and ultrasound in the diagnosis of cavernous hemangioma and lymphangioma of the orbit. *A.J.N.R.* 1:119, 1980.
11. Dresner S.C., Rothfus W.E., Slamovits T.L., et. al: Computed tomography of orbital myositis. *A.J.N.R.* 5:351–354, 1984.
12. Dubois P.J., Beardsley T., Klintworth G., et al.: Computed tomography of sarcoidosis of the optic nerve. *Neuroradiology* 24:179–182, 1983.
13. Enzmann D.R., Donaldson S.S., Kriss J.P.: Appearance of Graves' disease in orbital computed tomography. *J. Comput. Assist. Tomogr.* 3:815–819, 1979.
14. Forbes G.: Computed tomography of the orbit. *Radiol. Clin. North Am.* 20:37–49, 1982.
15. Forbes G.S., Earnest F., Waller R.R.: Computed tomography of orbital tumors, including late-generation scanning techniques. *Radiology* 142:387–394, 1982.
16. Forbes G.S., Sheedy P.F., Waller R.R.: Orbital tumors evaluated by computed tomography *Radiology* 136:101–111, 1980.
17. Gaster R., Duda E.: Localization of intraocular foreign bodies by computed tomography. *Ophthalmol. Surg.* 11:25–29, 1980.
18. Grove A.S.: Orbital trauma and computed tomography. *Ophthalmology* 87:403–411, 1980.
19. Hammerschlag S.B., Hughes S., O'Reilly G.V., et al.: Blow-out fractures of the orbit: A comparison of computed tomography and conventional radiography with anatomical correlation. *Radiology* 143:487–492, 1982.
20. Harr D.L., Quencer R.M., Abrams G.W.: Computed tomography and ultrasound in the evaluation of orbital infection and pseudotumor. *Radiology* 142:395–401, 1982.
21. Hedges T.R., Pozzi-Mucelli R., Char D.H., et al.: Computed tomographic demonstration of ocular calcification: correlation with clinical and pathological findings. *Neuroradiology* 23:15–21, 1982.
22. Hesselink, J.R., Davis K.R., Dallow R.L., et al.: Computed tomography of masses in the lacrimal gland region. *Radiology* 131:143–147, 1979.
23. Hesselink J.R., Davis K.R., Weber A.L., et al.: Radiological evaluation of orbital metastases with emphasis on computed tomography. *Radiology* 137:363–366, 1980.
24. Howard C.W., Osher R.H., Tomsack R.L.: Computed tomographic features in optic neuritis. *Am. J. Ophthalmol.* 89:699–702, 1980.
25. Lallemand P.P., Brasch R.C., Char D.H., et al.: Orbital tumors in children: Characterization by computed tomography. *Radiology* 151:85–88, 1984.
26. Leo J.S., Halpern J., Sackler J.P.: Computed tomography in the evaluation of orbital infections. *Comput. Tomogr.* 4:133–138, 1980.
27. Lloyd G.A.: Primary orbital meningioma: A review of 41 patients investigated radiologically. *Clin. Radiol.* 33:181, 1982.
28. Nugent R.A., Rootman J., Robertson W.D., et al.: Acute orbital pseudotumors: Classification and CT features. *A.J.N.R.* 2:431–436, 1981.
29. Peeters F.L., Kroger R.: Dural and direct cavernous sinus fistulas. *A.J.R.* 132:599–606, 1979.
30. Perugini S., Pasquini U., Menichelli F., et al.: Mucoceles in the paranasal sinuses involving the orbit: CT signs in 43 cases. *Neuroradiology* 23:133–139, 1982.
31. Peyster R.G., Hoover E.D., Hershey B.L., et al.: High resolution CT of lesions of the optic nerve. *A.J.N.R.* 4:169–174, 1983.
32. Peyster R.G., Savino P.J., Hoover E.D., et al.: Differential diagnosis of the emlarged superior ophthalmic vein. *J. Comput. Assist. Tomogr.* 8:103–107, 1984.
33. Ramirez H., Blatt E.S., Hibri N.: Computed tomographic identification of calcified optic nerve drusen. *Radiology* 148:137–139, 1983.
34. Rothfus W.E., Curtin H.D.: Extraocular muscle enlargement: A CT review. *Radiology* 151:677–681, 1984.
35. Rothfus W.E., Curtin H.D., Slamovits T.L., et al.: Optic nerve/sheath enlargement: A differential approach based on high resolution CT morphology. *Radiology* 150:409–415, 1984.
36. Sacher M., Lanzieri C.F., Sobel L.I., et al.: Computed tomography of bilateral lacrimal gland sarcoidosis. *J. Comput. Assist. Tomogr.* 8:213–215, 1984.
37. Sevel D., Krausz H., Ponder T., et al.: Value of computed tomography for the diagnosis of a ruptured eye. *J. Comput. Assist. Tomogr.* 7:870–875, 1983.
38. Trokel S.L., Hilal S.K.: Recognition and differential diagnosis of enlarged extraocular muscles in computed tomography. *Am. J. Ophthalmol.* 87:503–512, 1979.
39. Turner R.M., Gutman I., Hilal S.K., et al.: CT of drusen bodies and other calcific lesions of the optic nerve: case report and differential diagnosis. *A.J.N.R.* 4:175–178, 1983.
40. Unger J.M.: Orbital apex fractures: The contribution of computed tomography. *Radiology* 150:713–717, 1984.
41. Unsöld R., Degroot J., Newton T.H.: Images of the optic nerve: Anatomic-CT correlations. *A.J.N.R.* 1:317–323, 1980.
42. Weinstein G.S., Dresner S.C., Slamovits T.L., et al.: Acute and subacute orbital myositis. *Am. J. Ophthalmol.* 96:207–217, 1983.
43. Weinstein M.A., Berlin A.J., Modic M.T., et al.: Orbits, in Haaga J.R., Alfidi R.J., (eds.): *Computed Tomography of the Whole Body.* St. Louis, C.V. Mosby Co., 1983, pp. 279–311.
44. Weinstein M.A., Modic M.T., Risius B., et al.: Visualization of the arteries, veins, and nerves of the orbit by sector computed tomography. *Radiology* 138:83–87, 1981.
45. Winter J., Centeno R.S., Bentson J.R.: Maneuver to aid diagnosis of orbital varix by computed tomography. *A.J.N.R.* 3:39–40, 1982.
46. Zilkha A.: Computed tomography of blow-out fractures of the medial orbital wall. *A.J.N.R.* 2:427–429, 1981.
47. Zimmerman R.A., Bilaniuk L.T.: CT of orbital infection and its cerebral complications. *A.J.R.* 134:45–50, 1980.

CHAPTER 13

SPINAL LESIONS

LUMBAR DISC BULGE *vs.* HERNIATION

Case 401

55-year-old man. Bulging disc (L4–5).

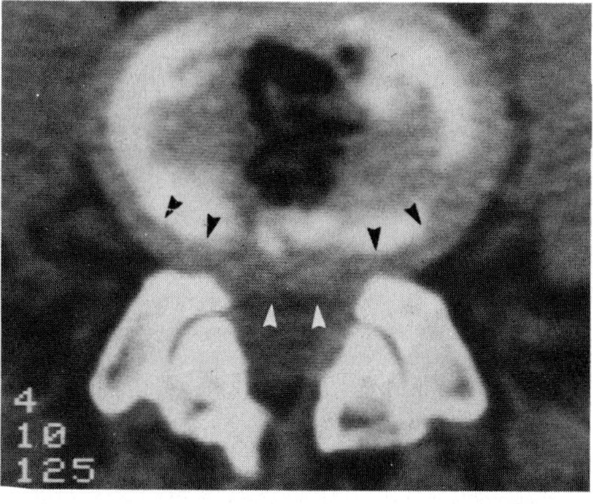

The CT definition of lumbar disc abnormalities is based on the differential attenuation of bone, disc, spinal fluid, and epidural fat. In this case, the margin of disc density *(white arrows)* bulges circumferentially beyond the dense bone of the vertebral end plate *(black arrows)*. The posterior margin of the bulging disc is defined by the slightly lower attenuation of spinal fluid within the dural sac.

The posterior margin of lumbar discs is normally slightly concave at the L-1 through L-5 levels and nearly straight at L-5–S-1. Bulging discs demonstrate a uniform, symmetric convexity. This broad curve contrasts with the focal asymmetry of disc herniation, as seen in Case 402.

The false appearance of a posterior disc bulge may be caused by oblique angulation of the scan with respect to the disc level, most commonly seen at L-5–S-1. Spondylolisthesis may also cause a prominent disc margin resembling a diffuse bulge (see Case 416).

Case 402

31-year-old man. Herniated disc (L-5–S-1).

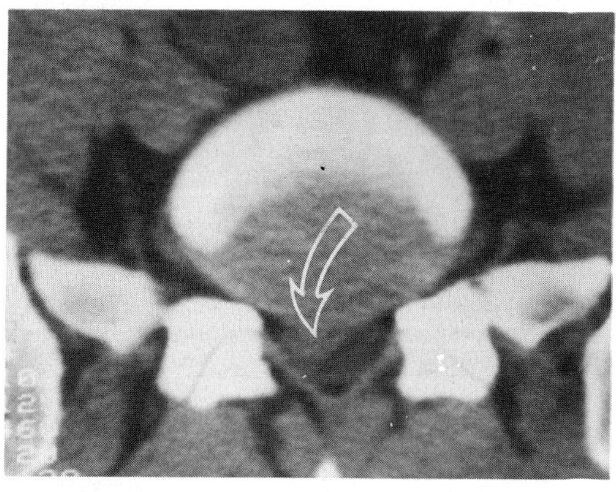

Discs herniating into the spinal canal are usually defined by the lower attenuation of spinal fluid and epidural fat.

The focal protrusion of disc density in this case *(arrow)* has a small radius of curvature that is distinct from the gently curving margin on either side. This localized change in contour contrasts with the diffuse bulge in Case 401.

Disc herniations are most common in a posterolateral direction, but midline herniations also occur. Some cases present features intermediate between Cases 401 and 402, and the distinction between an asymmetric disc bulge and a frank disc herniation is occasionally difficult.

DISC HERNIATIONS INVOLVING THE LATERAL RECESS AND INTERVERTEBRAL FORAMEN

Case 403

44-year-old man. Disc herniation (S-1).

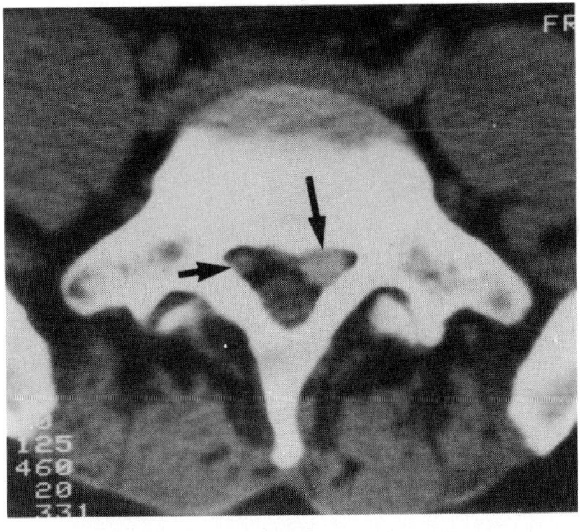

In addition to compromising the central canal, herniated discs may cause nerve compression by narrowing the lateral recess or restricting the intervertebral foramen.

The lateral recess is formed at the anterolateral corner of the spinal canal by the junction of the rostral vertebral body and pedicle. A nerve occupies this angle *(short arrow)* as it prepares to exit beneath the pedicle through the superior portion of the intervertebral foramen.

A herniated fragment extending caudally from the disc space may compromise the lateral recess and compress the exiting nerve *(long arrow)*. As seen here, the density of a herniated disc is greater than that of the root sleeve normally occupying the recess.

Compression of a nerve within the lateral recess may also be due to hypertrophic bone, as discussed in Case 413.

Case 404

53-year-old man. Disc herniation (L3–4).

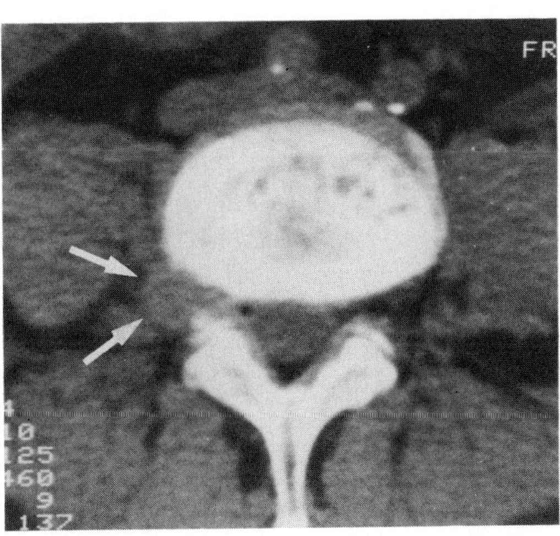

Laterally herniated discs may encroach on the intervertebral foramen. In Case 404, the dural sac is undisturbed within the central canal. However, the right intervertebral foramen is filled with disc material, obliterating the epidural fat through which the exiting nerve normally passes.

Occasional epidural masses (e.g., lymphoma or metastasis) or neuromas occupying the intervertebral foramen may present a similar appearance.

COMPOUND ROOT SLEEVES

Case 405A

50-year-old man.

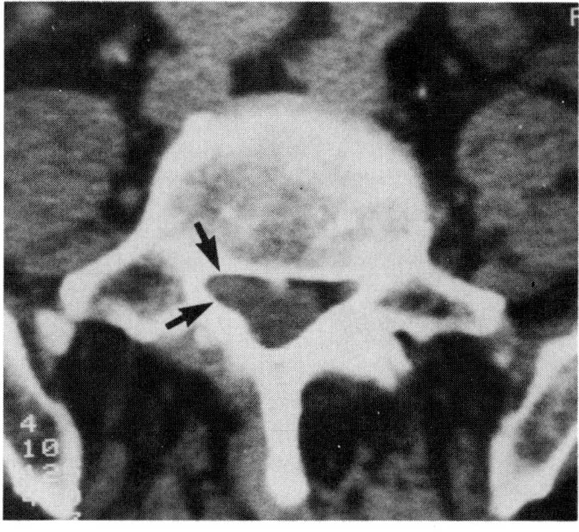

Adjacent lumbar nerves may share a common sleeve. A "conjoined" or "compound" sleeve is larger than an individual nerve and is located between the levels of the contributing roots.

This normal variant is typically discovered as an asymmetric structure occupying the lateral recess *(arrows)*. It may be misinterpreted as a herniated disc. However, the low density of spinal fluid within a compound sleeve contrasts with the increased density expected of disc material (compare this scan with Case 403). In addition, the involved lateral recess is large, favoring a congenital variation with corresponding bone morphology.

Case 405B

Same patient. Scan slightly caudal to that in Case 405A.

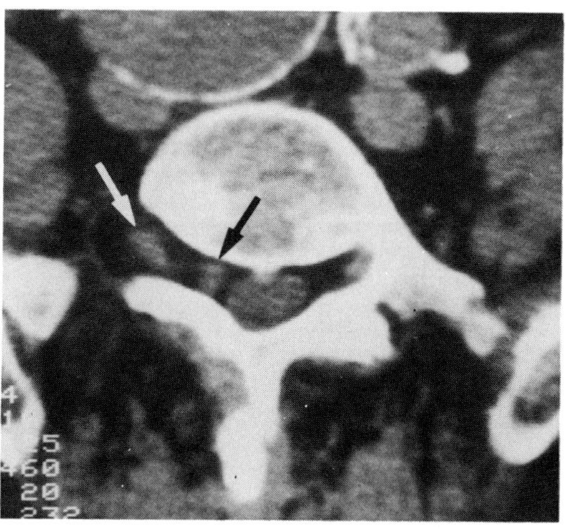

A compound sleeve may be identified by more caudal sections demonstrating the emergence of two separate roots. On this scan the compound sleeve in Case 405A is dividing, with the L-5 branch *(white arrow)* exiting laterally while the more medial S-1 root *(black arrow)* continues caudally. Myelography (CT or routine) will distinguish between compound sleeves and other lesions in ambiguous cases.

The normal left L-5 root is seen within its lateral recess, far removed from the dural sac and central canal. Calcified aneurysms of the iliac arteries are incidentally noted.

DIFFERENTIAL DIAGNOSIS: EPIDURAL DENSITY POSTERIOR TO A VERTEBRAL BODY

Case 406

45-year-old woman.

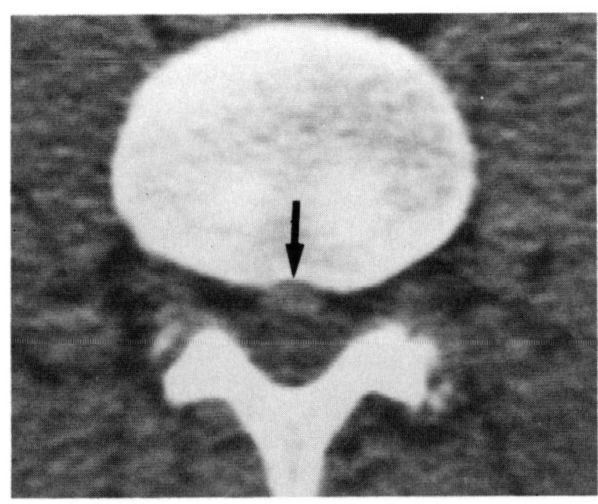

Normal Anterior Epidural Veins (L-3).

Case 407

52-year-old man.

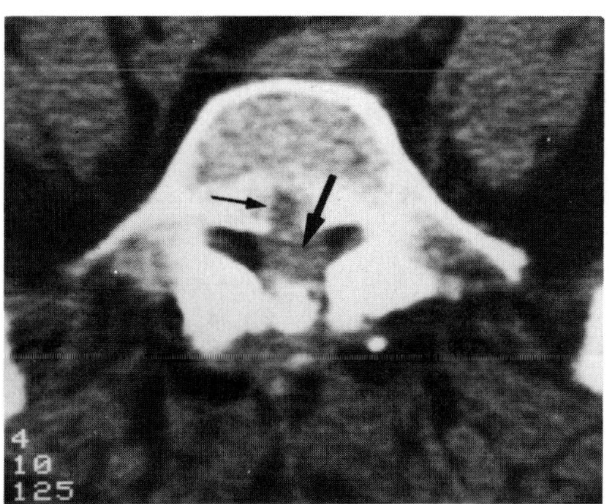

Herniated Disc Fragment (L-5; Metrizamide Scan; Prior Laminectomy).

The normal plexus of epidural veins ("retrovertebral plexus") may form a prominent structure within the anterior portion of the spinal canal. The veins are particularly noticeable at midvertebral levels near the basivertebral vein (*small arrow,* Case 407). A bone spur is sometimes seen adjacent to the vein and should not be misinterpreted as an osteophyte or calcified disc fragment.

The basivertebral vein is not seen in Case 406, and the density of anterior epidural veins *(arrow)* mimics the appearance of a midline disc fragment. The recurrent midline disc herniation in Case 407 *(large arrow)* is well defined by intrathecal contrast (see Case 419).

Adjacent sections may link a questionable midline density to vascular structures or provide confirmatory evidence of disc herniation. Scans performed after intravenous contrast infusion will define the location of epidural veins in equivocal cases.

DIFFERENTIAL DIAGNOSIS: EPIDURAL MASS WITHIN THE SPINAL CANAL

Case 408

32-year-old man.

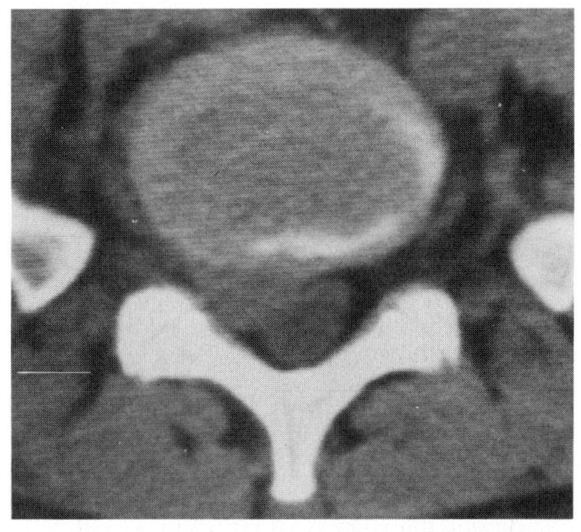

Epidural Metastasis (Seminoma).

Case 409

31-year-old man.

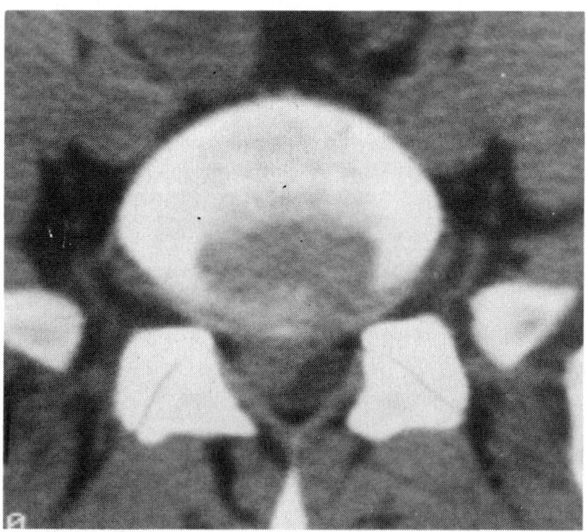

Herniated Disc.

The prevalence of lumbar disc disease does not preclude the possibility of other epidural lesions. Epidural tumors can mimic the appearance of disc herniation, as seen in Case 408. Spontaneous or post-traumatic epidural hematomas may also be confused with a herniated disc.

A clue to the nondisc nature of Case 408 is the difference in attenuation between the epidural mass and the center of the disc. Herniated fragments may appear slightly lower (or higher) in attenuation than the parent disc (as in Case 409), but a significant disparity should suggest an alternative diagnosis.

Case 410

30-year-old man complaining that his right arm "gives" when he lifts weights. Central disc herniation (C4–5; narrow window display).

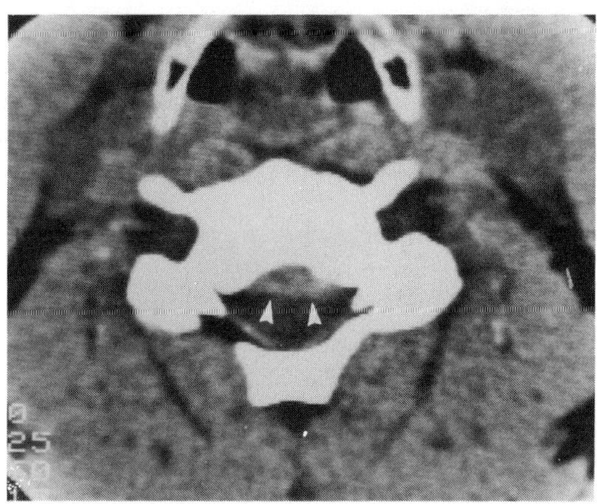

The axial perspective of CT scans is as useful in the cervical spine as in the lumbar region. However, the small size of cervical vertebrae and discs requires close placement of thin sections for adequate definition of anatomical and pathologic features. Even with good technique, the lack of epidural fat and the reduced contrast resolution of thin sections may make diagnosis difficult. Calcification is common in cervical discs and may partially offset the lack of surrounding contrast.

In this case, a large central disc herniation occupies the anterior portion of the spinal canal. The herniating disc has extended caudally from the C4–5 level to lie behind the body of C–5. The density of the disc contrasts with the low attenuation of the dural sac and epidural fat.

Case 437 demonstrates a similar central disc defined by subarachnoid contrast material.

Case 411

33-year-old man with triceps weakness and radiculopathy. Lateral disc herniation (C6–7).

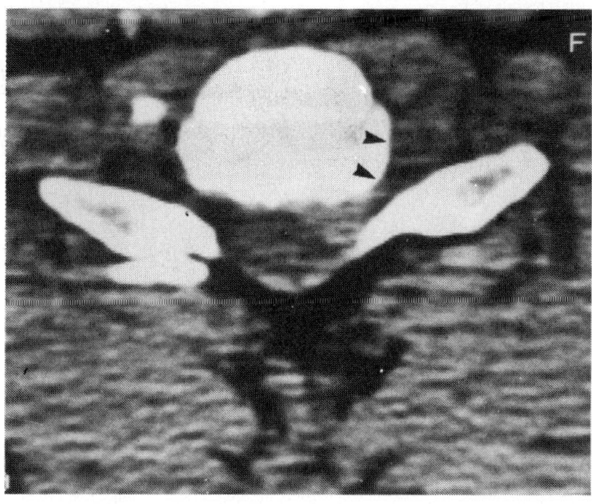

Artifact from the thick tissue and bone of the shoulders may compromise scans of the lowest cervical levels. Caudal traction on the arms may improve the quality of these images.

In this large man (300 lb), the scans at the C6–7 level (performed with arm traction) are suboptimal but do demonstrate a laterally herniated disc on the left, confirmed at surgery.

In addition to disc pathology, cervical scans may define stenosis of the central canal or intervertebral foramen caused by hypertrophy of the uncinate process *(arrows)*.

Case 412

71-year-old man. Stenosis of the central canal (L2–3).

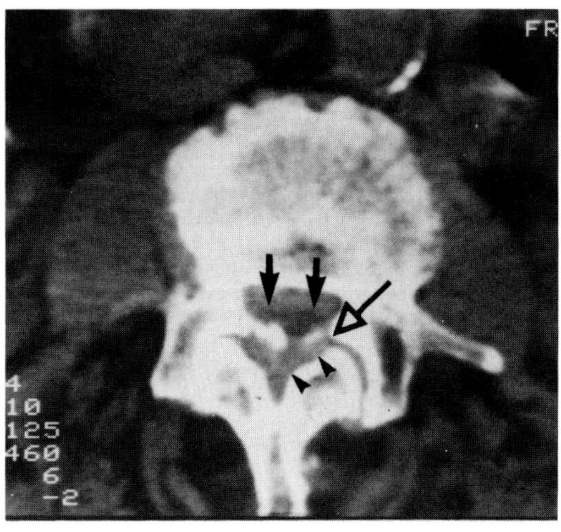

A variety of congenital and acquired factors may cause narrowing of the spinal canal. Axial scans clearly demonstrate the cross-sectional morphology and severity of such stenosis.

Congenitally stenotic canals often present a triangular or "trefoil" morphology, with short pedicles and medially bowing laminae. Congenital deformity (e.g., achondroplasia) may compress the canal sufficiently to produce symptoms of lumbar stenosis (e.g., "pseudoclaudication").

Spinal stenosis is more commonly caused by the superimposition of acquired changes on congenitally narrow dimensions. The acquired factors may be specific processes (e.g., Paget's disease, ossification of the posterior longitudinal ligament) or simple degenerative changes.

Case 412 is a typical example. The combination of disc bulge *(solid arrows),* facet hypertrophy *(open arrow),* and thickening of the ligamentum flavum *(small arrows)* causes circumferential constriction of the canal. A complete myelographic block was found at this level (see also Case 415).

Case 413

66-year-old man. Stenosis of a lateral recess (L-4).

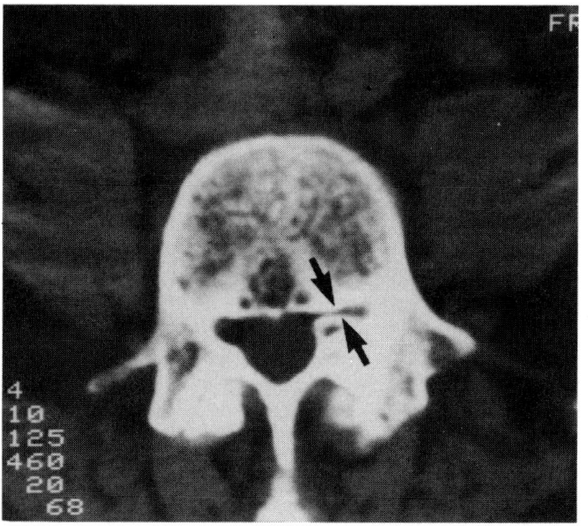

The base of the superior articular facet of a lumbar vertebra forms the posterolateral margin of the lateral recess. Hypertrophy of the facet (and/or related osteophytes) may narrow the recess and cause nerve compression, either alone or in combination with disc pathology.

In this case, the left lateral recess *(arrows)* has been almost obliterated by overgrowth of the facet joint. CT accurately demonstrates the relative contributions of disc and bone to compromise of the lateral recess or intervertebral foramen (compare this scan to that in Case 403).

LUMBAR FACET ARTHROPATHY

Case 414

74-year-old man (L-5–S-1)

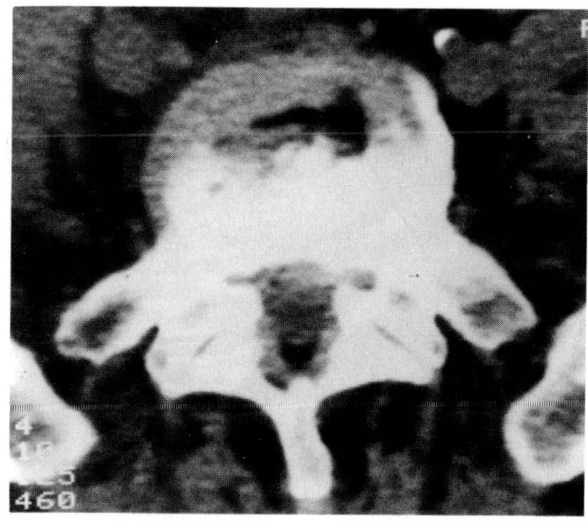

Degenerative changes of the facet joints are often seen on lumbar CT scans. Common findings include sclerosis, subchondral erosions, osteophyte formation, and narrowing of the joint space.

The capsule of the facet joint may become thickened and calcified. Rare synovial cysts arising from the joint may mimic other extradural masses.

In this case, hypertrophy and spurring of the facets has caused bilateral narrowing of the lateral recesses. Gas is present within the bulging disc, and the ligamenta flava are thickened.

Case 415

62-year-old man (L3–4).

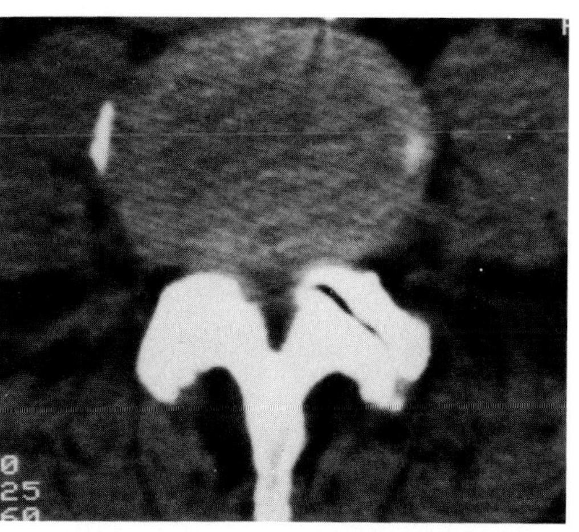

Overgrowth of the facet joint, may be a response to excessive stress caused by instability or by fusion at adjacent levels. This patient had been fused from L-4 to S-1. Facet hypertrophy has developed a "cupped" configuration, and gas is seen within the left joint. Stenosis of the central canal is present due to a combination of congenitally small dimensions and superimposed degenerative hypertrophy.

Facet arthropathy may cause back pain with radicular referral independent of canal compromise or nerve root compression.

SPONDYLOLISTHESIS

Case 416

68-year-old man (L-5–S-1).

Case 417

55-year-old man.

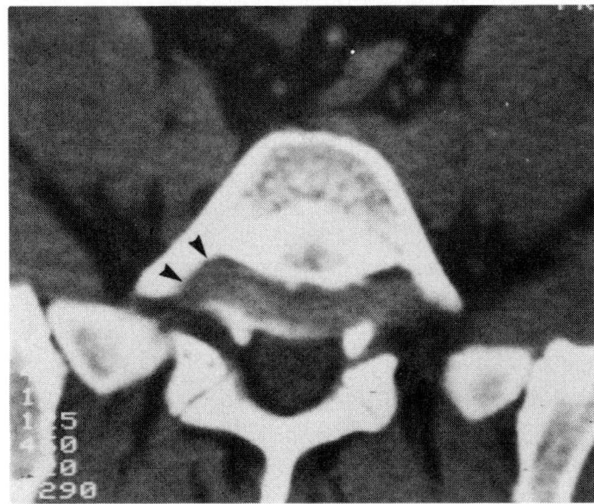

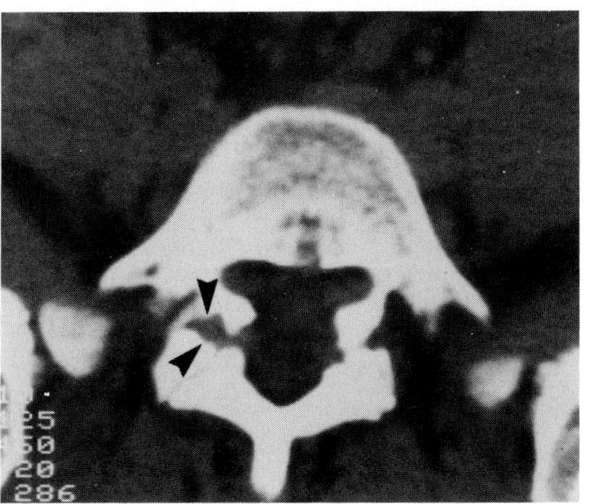

The CT features of spondylolisthesis include characteristic subluxation and visualization of associated spondylolysis.

The intervertebral disc usually maintains its relationship to the caudal vertebral body, with the rostral body slipping anteriorly. The resulting ledge or step-off from rostral body to disc may resemble a disc bulge. Anterior movement of the rostral body away from its posterior arch causes the spinal canal to become elongated in anteroposterior diameter and elliptical in configuration.

The displacement of the rostral vertebra carries the lateral recess *(small arrows)* anteriorly, so that it comes to lie above the nondisplaced disc. The associated distortion of the intervertebral foramen causes compression of the root exiting beneath the pedicle of the forward-slipping vertebra.

Degenerative spondylolisthesis may occur in the absence of spondylolysis when disc narrowing and facet laxity allow subluxation.

When present, the bone defect of spondylolysis may resemble an "extra" facet joint crossing anterior to the normal articulation *(arrows)* Spondylolysis is best seen at the midvertebral level, while the facet joint is best seen at the disc level.

Scarring and callus formation are often found adjacent to the pars defect.

POSTOPERATIVE LUMBAR SCANS

Case 418

47-year-old woman.

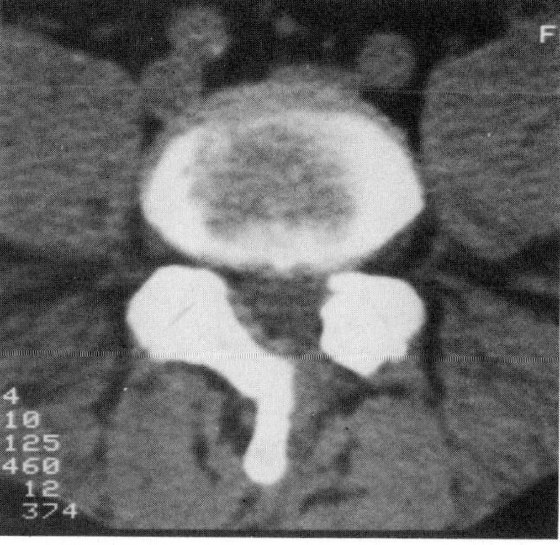

Lumbar laminectomy and discectomy lead to characteristic postoperative CT findings. A laminectomy defect is usually apparent, with well-defined margins posterior to the facet joint. (Compare this scan with the disorganized margins of spondylolysis located more anteriorly in Case 417.)

Fibrosis at the operative site replaces epidural fat and obscures the normal interface with the dural sac. The sac itself may be tethered or prolapsed toward the laminectomy defect.

Case 419

55-year-old woman (scan after metrizamide administration).

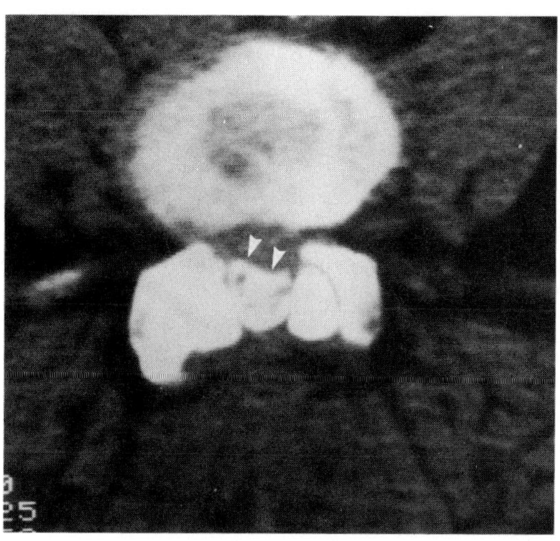

The diagnosis of residual or recurrent disc herniation may be hampered by the postoperative loss of epidural fat. Helpful clues include: (1) the mass-like margin of disc fragments, as opposed to the vague boundary of epidural fibrosis, and (2) contrast enhancement within epidural scar but not within herniated discs.

Intrathecal contrast material may be useful in difficult postoperative cases. Here distortion of the dural sac suggests a focal disc fragment *(arrows),* which was confirmed by surgery (also see Case 407).

Case 420

59-year-old woman with back and leg pain. Metastatic breast carcinoma.

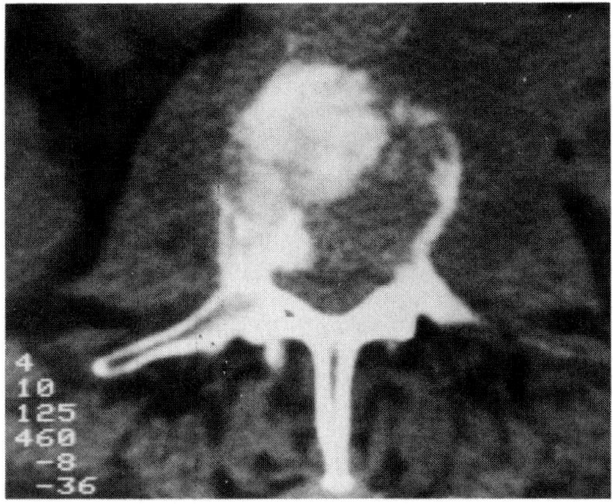

CT scans may demonstrate vertebral or paraspinal tumors that account for symptoms of local or radicular pain. In this case, a metastasis has destroyed a lumbar vertebral body and grown into the prevertebral and psoas regions. Posterior extension of a vertebral tumor may compromise the spinal canal and require emergency decompression or radiation.

Other metastases (or myeloma) may present as well-marginated lesions within a vertebral body. Reactive sclerosis may be seen in association with metastases, lymphoma, or meningiomas.

Benign vertebral lesions are also well defined on CT scans. Examples include Paget's disease, hemangiomas, and Schmorl's nodes (intravertebral disc herniations).

Case 421

55-year-old man with sacral pain. Carcinoma of the ureter.

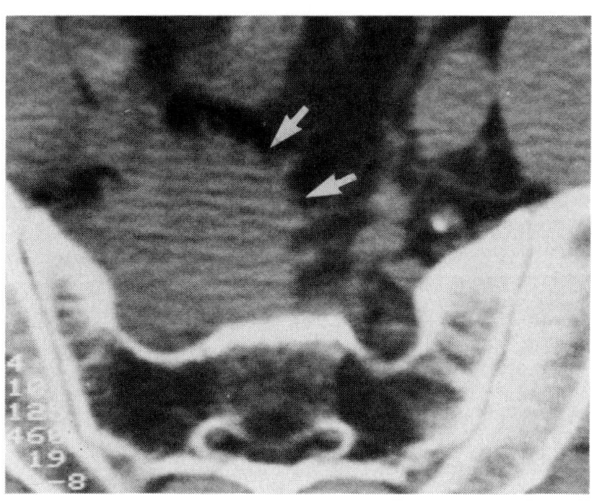

Scans through the sacrum may disclose the source of pain or dysfunction unexplained by lumbar evaluation. Here a mass *(arrows)* has grown into a sacral foramen (compare with the left side). A carcinoma of the ureter was subsequently diagnosed.

Case 422

86-year-old man. Epidermoid tumor.

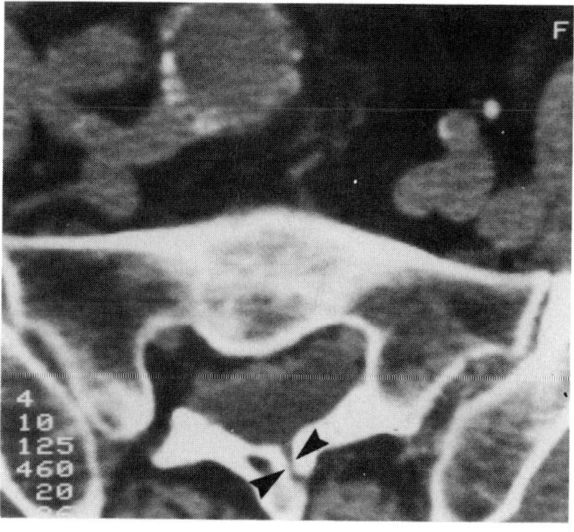

Some intraspinal tumors are apparent on routine scans, while others require subarachnoid contrast material for definition (see Cases 432 and 433).

Here a spina bifida occulta *(arrows)* is associated with a low-attenuation mass occupying much of the large spinal canal. The low attenuation of the lesion remains greater than that of epidural fat and is characteristic of an epidermoid tumor.

An aneurysm of the right iliac artery is seen at the margin of the film. Lesions of the aortoiliac vasculature and other retroperitoneal processes may be discovered incidentally when spinal scans are reviewed thoroughly.

Case 423

44-year-old woman. Cervical meningioma (postcontrast scan, C2–3 level).

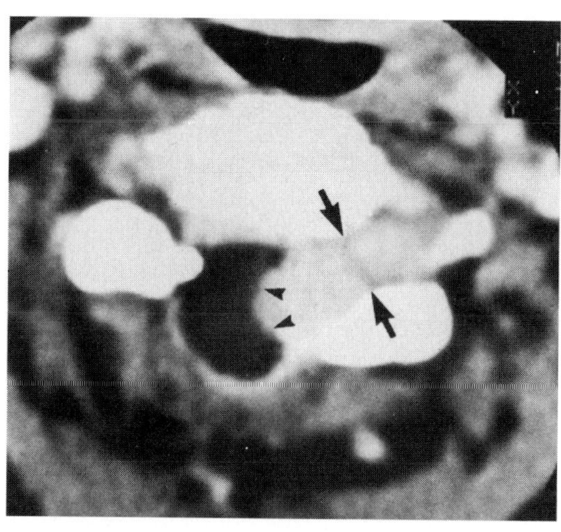

Intravenous contrast is occasionally useful in defining vascular lesions of the spinal canal. Arteriovenous malformations usually demonstrate enhancement, as do some intramedullary tumors (e.g., hemangioblastoma).

Spinal meningiomas may also be well demarcated by contrast enhancement, as seen in this case. The "dumbbell" meningioma occupies a widened intervertebral foramen *(large arrows)*. The medial margin of the tumor passes through the enhancing dura to displace the cervical spinal cord *(small arrows)*.

The spinal cord is usually visible on routine scans of the high cervical region due to contrast provided by the wide subarachnoid space at this level. This appearance should not be confused with epidural fat surrounding the dural sac at more caudal levels.

Case 424

26-year-old woman two weeks after laminectomy. Paraspinal abscess.

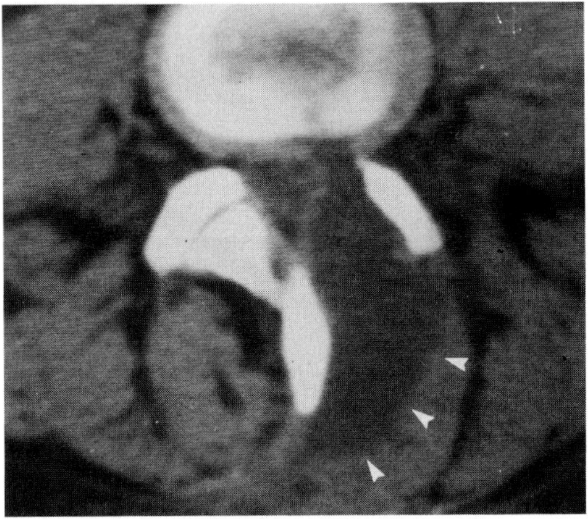

Paraspinal abscesses form homogeneous, low-attenuation collections, as seen here. The low density and sharp margins contrast with the isodensity and vague borders of cellulitis. Involvement of the psoas region is common in cases of intra-abdominal infection.

Pseudomeningoceles form another category of cystic structures that may be encountered on postoperative scans. These fluid collections expand from the dural sac into the surgical defect. In this case, the abscess cavity extends to the disc but does not communicate with the central canal.

Case 425

14-year-old girl with back pain, exaggerated lumbar lordosis, and severe limitation of lumbar flexion. Disc space infection.

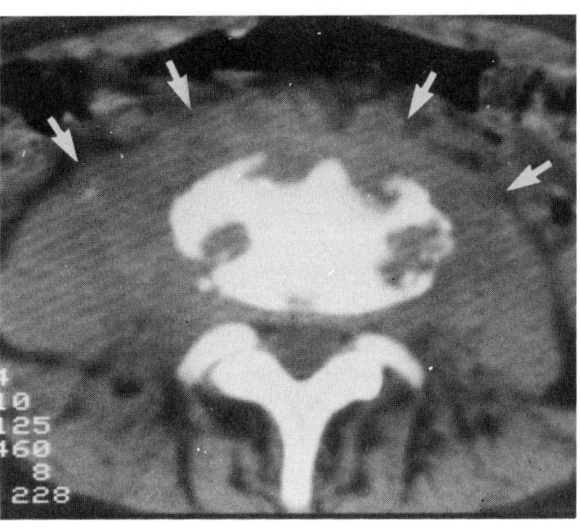

Infection of the intervertebral disc causes a ring of paraspinal edema and exudate *(arrow)* surrounding a narrowed disc space. Erosion and fragmentation of the adjacent vertebral end plates is a hallmark of discitis, as seen here.

Isolated vertebral osteomyelitis is also well demonstrated by the axial CT display. Distinction from metastasis may be difficult in the absence of associated discitis.

Case 426

52-year-old man who fell from a tree (L-1 level).

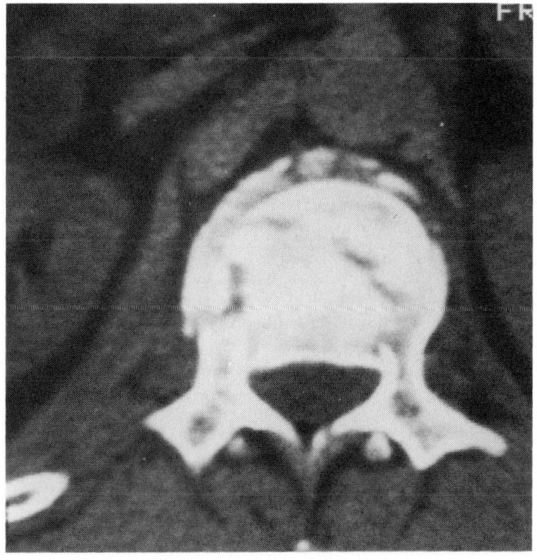

Fractures of vertebral bodies and posterior arches are well evaluated by axial scans. Despite the obvious comminution in this case, bone fragments do not significantly compress the spinal canal.

Soft-tissue injury is more difficult to judge without contrast material. Occasional epidural hematomas are imaged on high-resolution scans.

Case 427

64-year-old man injured in an automobile accident (L-2 level)

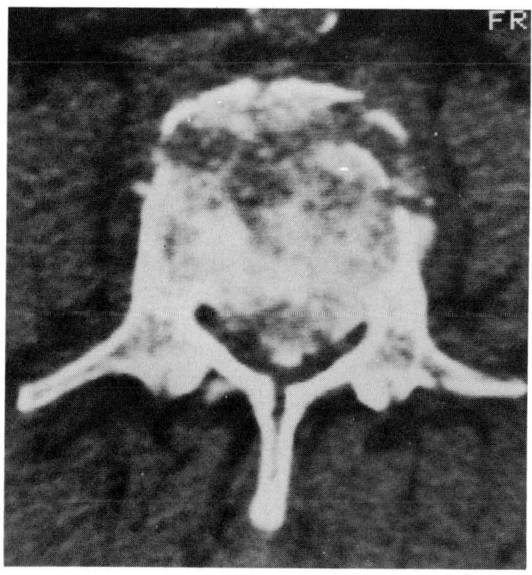

In this case, a comminuted fracture of the vertebral body is associated with displaced fragments that nearly obliterate the spinal canal. This cross-sectional display defines the need for decompression. A fracture line extends into the spinous process.

DIFFERENTIAL DIAGNOSIS: EXPANSILE LESION OF THE SACRAL CANAL

Case 428

74-year-old man.

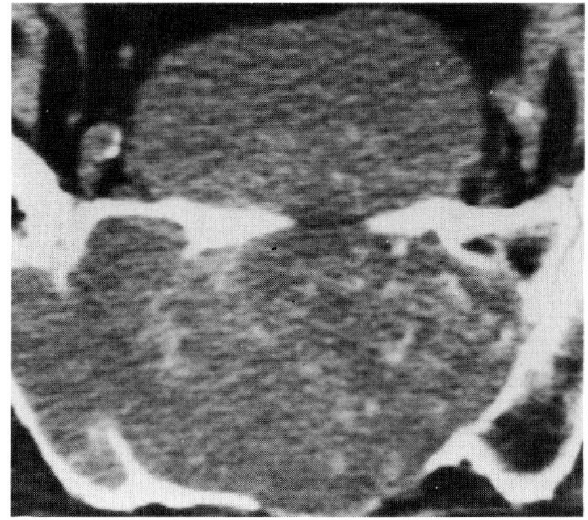

Epidermoid Cyst.

Case 429

30-year-old woman.

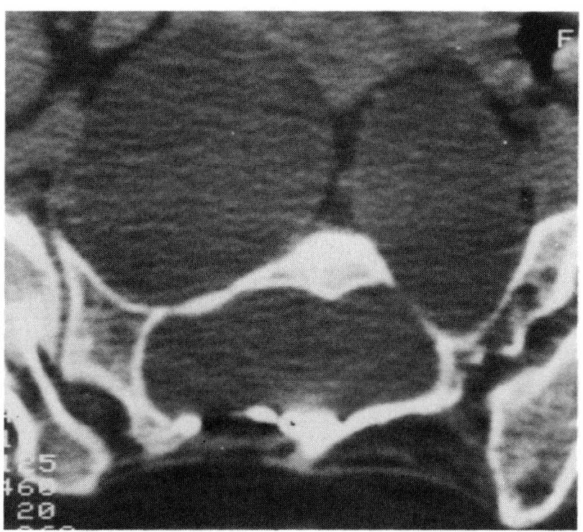

Dural Ectasia In Marfan's Syndrome.

CT is an excellent means of demonstrating the osseous and soft-tissue components of sacral lesions. The masses in these two cases have originated within the spinal canal, with expansion of bony margins and extension into the pelvis.

The patient in Case 428 had undergone subtotal removal of tumor on two prior occasions. The current mass has a bilobed configuration due to a large pelvic component and has crossed the right sacroiliac joint.

The homogeneous low attenuation of the mass in Case 429 suggests fluid content. A less dramatic but similar appearance may be seen with smaller cysts commonly found along sacral root sleeves.

Case 430

35-year-old woman. Normal foramen magnum (coronal reconstruction of axial scans with metrizamide).

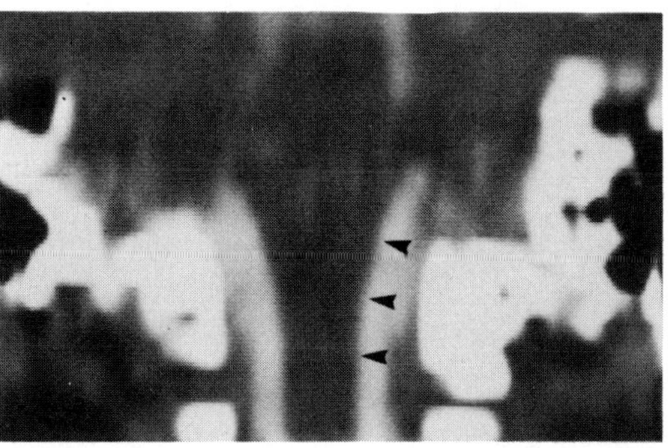

CT scanning performed with subarachnoid contrast material gives excellent definition of intradural and extradural morphology. This technique is best applied to localized regions of interest and can be supplemented by reconstruction of axial images in the coronal or sagittal planes.

Here, a coronal reformation outlines the normal cervicomedullary junction *(arrows)*. This combination of CT and subarachnoid contrast has been joined by magnetic resonance imaging as the most useful procedures for evaluating the foramen magnum region.

Case 431

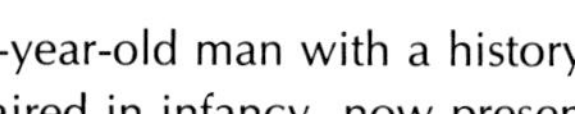

25-year-old man with a history of meningomyelocele repaired in infancy, now presenting with increasing leg weakness and sphincter dysfunction. Tethered cord (sagittal reconstruction, L-3 level, metrizamide).

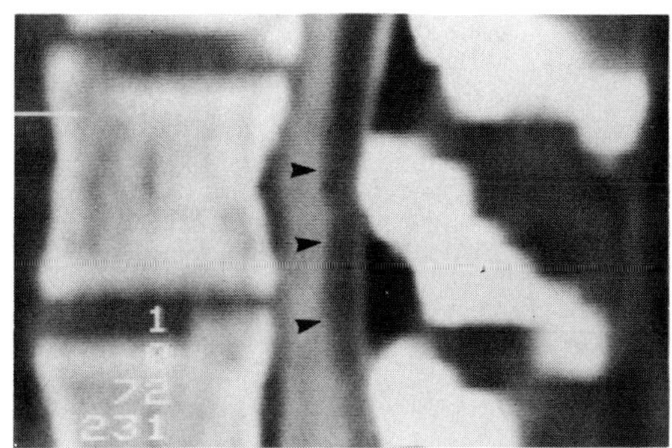

Sagittal reconstruction of axial images centered at L-3 demonstrates the low-lying spinal cord passing through the lumbar region *(arrows)*. Tethering of the cord commonly accompanies dysraphic states and is frequently associated with lipomas at the caudal end of the dural sac. The lipomas may surround and/or infiltrate the filum terminale and conus medullaris.

CT-myelography is an excellent tool for evaluating congenital malformations of the spinal canal (e.g., diastematomyelia, neurenteric cyst). The procedure may be performed as a sequel to routine myelography after a single injection of contrast material.

DIFFERENTIAL DIAGNOSIS: INTRADURAL MASS

Case 432

40-year-old man (scan with metrizamide).

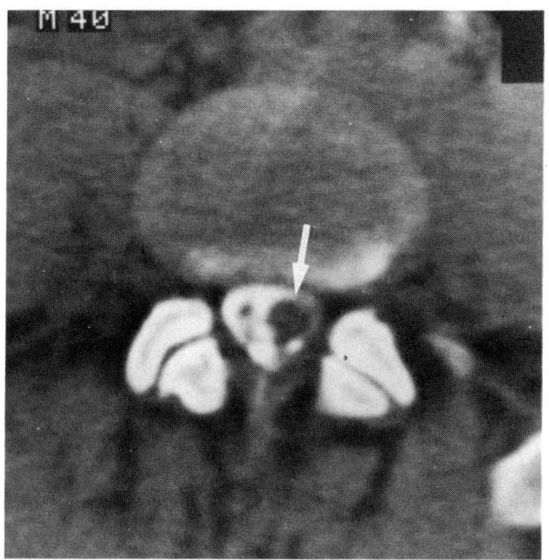

Neurofibroma.

Case 433

37-year-old woman (scan with metrizamide).

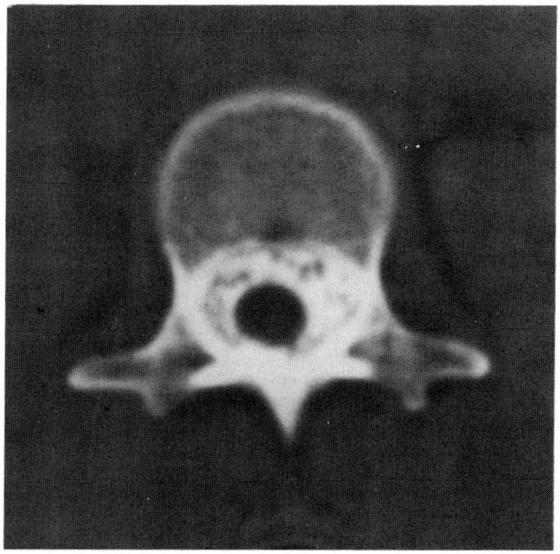

Ependymoma Of The Conus Medullaris.

CT-myelography outlines intradural masses as well-defined filling defects. The features of the lesion are rarely specific (e.g., low attenuation in a lipoma, or calcification in a meningioma).

The most common intradural tumors in the region of the conus medullaris and cauda equina are ependymomas and neurofibromas, as illustrated in Cases 432 and 433. These lesions are often indistinguishable. Both may be lobulated, and both may expand the spinal canal when large and longstanding.

Other lumbar intradural masses include metastases from systemic carcinomas (e.g., lung, breast), "drop" metastases from intracranial tumors (e.g., medulloblastoma, ependymoma, germinoma, glioma), epidermoid tumors, arachnoid or parasitic cysts, and vascular malformations. Meningiomas are common intradural, extramedullary masses in the thorax but are rare in the lumbar region.

Arachnoiditis may cause clumping of nerve roots resembling an intradural mass, usually accompanied by thickening and irregularity of the dura. A tethered spinal cord (as in Case 431) may resemble an intradural mass on a single axial scan.

Case 434

37-year-old man. Astrocytoma of the cervical cord (C6–7 level; scan with metrizamide).

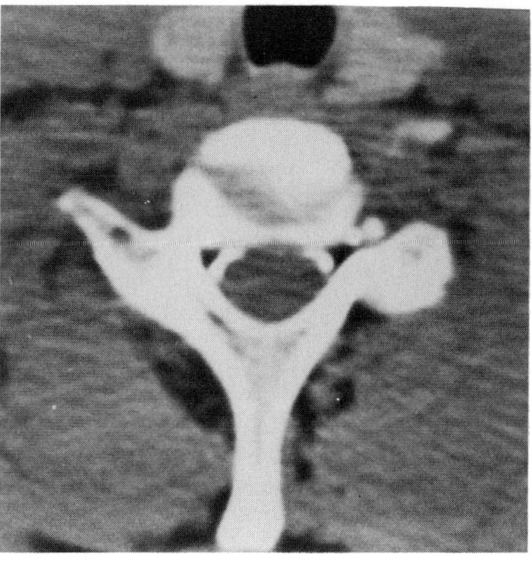

Axial scans with subarachnoid contrast material provide clear definition of the spinal cord. Partial volume effects of the dense contrast cause the apparent size of the cord to vary as the window settings are changed. However, at a given setting a pathologic expansion of the cord is easily recognized, as in this case.

The differential diagnosis of intramedullary masses includes tumors (ependymoma, astrocytoma, hemangioblastoma, lipoma, metastasis), cysts (tumor, post-traumatic, syrinx), inflammatory processes (acute myelitis, sarcoidosis, abscess), and vascular lesions (arteriovenous malformation (AVM), hematoma). When an intramedullary mass is encountered, delayed scans are useful to evaluate the possibility of syrinx (see Case 435).

Case 435

40-year-old man with a history of old trauma, now presenting with diminished sensation and atrophy of the lower extremities. Post-traumatic syrinx (T–12 level; scan with metrizamide).

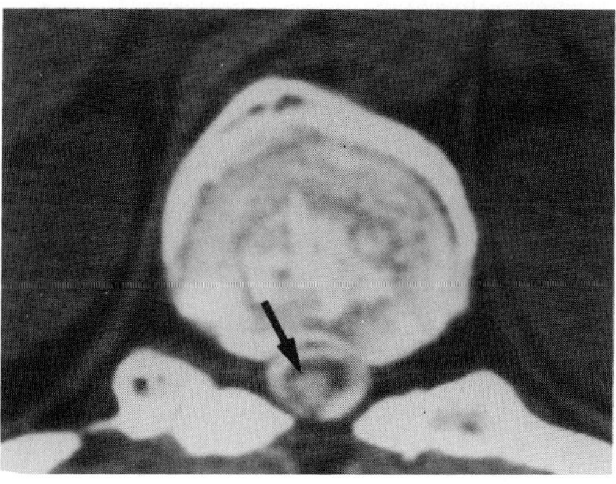

Both congenital and acquired syringomyelia may be defined by delayed scans following the injection of subarachnoid contrast material. Contrast accumulates within the cavity of the syrinx *(arrow),* creating a "target" appearance within the cord.

The syrinx cavity may be eccentric and may vary in diameter and axial extent. Cervical syringomyelia is usually a congenital abnormality, often associated with low cerebellar tonsils (Chiari I malformation). Post-traumatic syringomyelia may occur at any level.

The initial contrast scans in syringomyelia may demonstrate cord widening (comparable with that in Case 434), cord atrophy (see Case 436), or a normal cord diameter.

DIFFERENTIAL DIAGNOSIS:
FLATTENED SHAPE OF THE CERVICAL SPINAL CORD

Case 436

43-year-old man (scan with metrizamide).

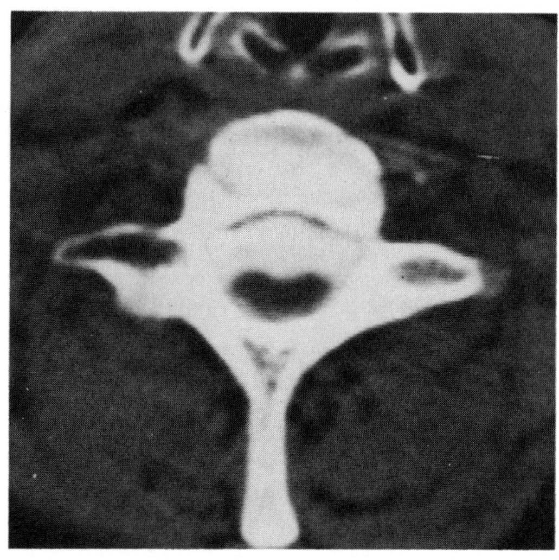

Syringomyelia.

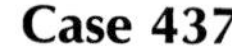

Case 437

36-year-old man (scan with metrizamide).

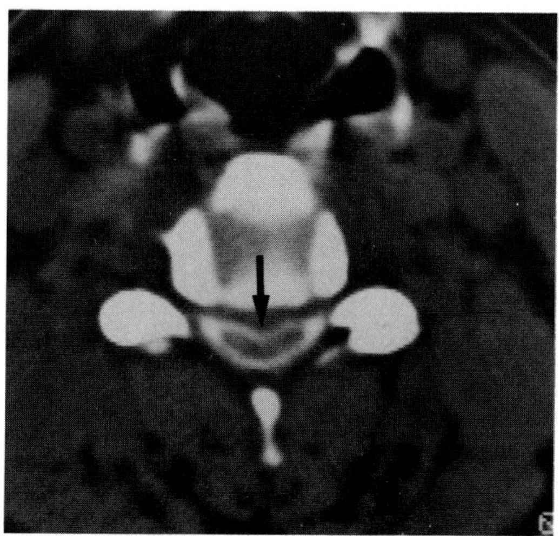

Central Disc Herniation (C4–5).

The spinal cord may become flattened in AP diameter because of atrophy or compression.

Anteroposterior narrowing is frequently seen in syringomyelia. The ventral surface of the cord may be slightly indented, while the transverse diameter is relatively preserved. Other causes of cord atrophy include trauma, multiple sclerosis, ischemia, AVM, and amyotrophic lateral sclerosis.

A similar morphology may result from compression of the cord by anterior osteophytes or cervical disc herniations, as in Case 437. Compare the spacious ventral subarachnoid space in Case 436 to the thin rim of contrast in Case 437.

REFERENCES

1. Abdullah A.F., Chambers R.W., Daut D.P.: Lumbar nerve root compression by synovial cysts of the ligamentum flavum. *J. Neurosurg.* 60:617–620, 1984.
2. Aubin M.L., Vignaud J., Jardin C., et al.: Computed tomography in 75 clinical cases of syringomyelia. *A.J.N.R.* 2:199–204, 1981.
3. Batnitzky S., Price H., Gaughan M., et al.: The radiology of syringohydromyelia. *Radiographics* 3:585–611, 1983.
4. Bonafe A., Ethier R., Melancon D., et al.: High resolution computed tomography in cervical syringomyelia. *J. Comput. Assist. Tomogr.* 4:42–47, 1980.
5. Carrera G.F., Haughton V.M., Syvertsen A., et al.: Computed tomography of the lumbar facet joints. *Radiology* 134:145–148, 1980.
6. Carrera G.F., Williams A.L., Haughton V.M.: Computed tomography in sciatica. *Radiology* 137:433–437, 1980.
7. Daniels D.L., Grogan J.P., Johansen J.G., et al.: Cervical radiculopathy: Computed tomography and myelography compared. *Radiology* 151:109–113, 1984.
8. Daniels D.L., Williams A.L., Haughton V.M.: Computed tomography of the articulations and ligaments at the occipito-atlantoaxial region. *Radiology* 146:709–716, 1983.
9. Dorwart R.H., Vogler J.B. III, Helms C.A.: Spinal stenosis. *Radiol. Clin. North Am.* 21:301–325, 1983.
10. Fitz C.R.: Midline anomalies of the brain and spine. *Radiol. Clin. North Am.* 20:95–104, 1982.
11. Fries J.W., Abodeely D.A., Vijungco J.G., et al.: Computed tomography of herniated and extruded nucleus pulposis. *J. Comput. Assist. Tomogr.* 6:874–887, 1982.
12. Gado M., Patel J., Hodges F.J.: Lateral disk herniation into the lumbar intervertebral foramen: Differential diagnosis. *A.J.N.R.* 4:598–600, 1983.
13. Grogan J.P., Daniels J.L., Williams A.L., et al.: CT criteria for recognition. *Radiology* 151:661–664, 1984.
14. Haykal H.A., Wang A.M., Zamani A.A., et al.: Computed tomography of spontaneous acute cervical epidural hematoma. *J. Comput. Assist. Tomogr.* 8:229–231, 1984.
15. Heinz E.R., Rosenbaum A.E., Scarff T., et al.: Tethered spinal cord following myelomeningocele repair. *Radiology* 131:153–160, 1979.
16. Helms C.A., Dorwart R.H., Gray M.: The CT appearance of conjoined nerve roots and differentiation from a herniated nucleus pulposis. *Radiology* 144:803–807, 1982.
17. Hemminghytt S., Daniels D.L., Williams A.L., et al.: Intraspinal synovial cysts: natural history and diagnosis by CT. *Radiology* 145:375–376, 1982.
18. Hermann G., Mendelson D.S., Cohen B.A., et al.: Role of computed tomography in the diagnosis of infectious spondylitis. *J. Comput. Assist. Tomogr.* 7:961–968, 1983.
19. Kaplan J.O., Quencer R.M.: The occult tethered conus syndrome in the adult. *Radiology* 137:387–391, 1980.
20. LaMasters D.L., Watanabe T.J., Chambers E.F., et al.: Multiplanar metrizamide-enhanced CT imaging of the foramen magnum. *A.J.N.R.* 3:485–494, 1982.
21. Landman J.A., Hoffman J.C., Braun I.F., et al.: Value of computed tomographic myelography in the recognition of cervical herniated disc. *A.J.N.R.* 5:391–394, 1984.
22. Lanzieri C.F., Hilal S.K.: Computed tomography of the sacral plexus and sciatic nerve in the greater sciatic foramen. *A.J.N.R.* 5:315–318, 1984.
23. Mawad M.E., Hilal S.K., Fetell M.R., et al.: Patterns of spinal cord atrophy by metrizamide CT. *A.J.N.R.* 4:611–613, 1983.
24. Meyer J.D., Latchaw R.E., Roppolo H.M., et al.: Computed tomography and myelographyy of the postoperative lumbar spine. *A.J.N.R.* 2:223–228, 1982.
25. Mikhael M.A., Ciris I., Tarkington J.A., et al.: Neuroradiological evaluation of the lateral recess syndrome. *Radiology* 140:97–107, 1981.
26. Miyasaka K., Isu T., Iwasaki Y., et al.: High resolution computed tomography in the diagnosis of cervical disc disease. *Neuroradiology* 24:253–257, 1983.
27. Naidich T.P., McLone D.G., Mutluer S.: A new understanding of dorsal dysraphism with lipoma (lipomyeloschisis): Radiologic evaluation and surgical correlation. *A.J.N.R.* 4:103–116, 1983.
28. Nakagawa H., Okumura T., Sugiyama T., et al.: Discrepancy between metrizamide CT and myelography in diagnosis of cervical disk protrusions. *A.J.N.R.* 4:604–606, 1983.
29. Neave V.C., Wycoff R.R.: Computed tomography of cystic nerve root sleeve dilatation. *J. Comput. Assist. Tomogr.* 7:881–885, 1983.
30. Post M.J.D., Green B.A.: The use of computed tomography in spinal trauma. *Radiol. Clin. North Am.* 21:327–375, 1983.
31. Price A.C., Allen J.H., Eggers F.M., et al.: Intervertebral disk-space infection: CT changes. *Radiology* 149:725–729, 1983.
32. Price H.I., Batnitzky S., Levine E., et al.: The computed tomographic findings in benign disease of the vertebral column. *Radiographics* 4:283–313, 1984.
33. Quencer R.M., Green B.A., Eismont F.J.: Posttraumatic spinal cord cysts: Clinical features and characterization with metrizamide computed tomography. *Radiology* 146:415–423, 1983.
34. Risius B., Modic M.T., Hardy R.W., et al.: Sector computed tomographic spine scanning in the diagnosis of lumbar nerve root entrapment. *Radiology* 143:109–114, 1982.
35. Schubiger O., Valavanis A.: CT differentiation between recurrent disc herniation and postoperative scar formation: The value of contrast enhancement. *Neuroradiology* 22:251–254, 1982.
36. Schubiger O., Valavanis A.: Postoperative lumbar CT: Technique, results, and indications. *A.J.N.R.* 4:595–597, 1983.
37. Scotti G., Musgrave M.A., Harwood-Nash D.C., et al.: Diastematomyelia in children: Metrizamide and CT metrizamide myelography. *A.J.N.R.* 1:403–410, 1980.
38. Scotti G., Scialfa G., Pieralli S., et al.: Myelopathy and radiculopathy due to cervical spondylosis: myelographic-CT correlates. *A.J.N.R.* 4:601–603, 1983.
39. Sobel D.F., Barkovich A.J., Munderloh S.H.: Metrizamide myelography and post myelographic computed tomography: Comparative adequacy in the cervical spine. *A.J.N.R.* 5:385–390, 1984.
40. Soye I., Levine E., Batnitzky S., et al.: Computed tomography of sacral and presacral lesions. *Neuroradiology* 24:71–76, 1982.
41. Teplick J.G., Haskin M.E.: Computed tomography of the postoperative lumbar spine. *A.J.N.R.* 4:1053–1072, 1983.
42. Teplick J.G., Haskin M.E.: CT and lumbar disc herniation. *Radiol. Clin. North Am.* 21:259–288, 1983.
43. Teplick J.G., Haskin M.E.: Intravenous contrast-enhanced CT of the post operative lumbar spine. *A.J.N.R.* 5:373–383, 1984.
44. Teplick J.G., Peyster R.G., Teplick S.K., et al.: CT identification of postlaminectomy pseudomeningocele. *A.J.N.R.* 4:179–182, 1983.
45. Wane A.M., Lewis M.L., Rumbaugh C.L., et al.: Spinal Cord or nerve root compression in patients with malignant disease: CT evaluation. *J.C.A.T.* 8:420–428, 1984.
46. Whelan M.A., Hilal S.K., Gold R.P., et al.: Computed tomography of the sacrum: II. Pathology. *A.J.N.R.* 3:555–559, 1982.
47. Williams A.L.: CT diagnosis of degenerative disc disease. *Radiol. Clin. North Am.* 21:289–300, 1983.
48. Williams A.L., Haughton V.M., Daniels D.L., et al.: Differential CT diagnosis of extruded nucleus pulposis. *Radiology* 148:141–148, 1983.
49. Williams A.L., Haughton V.M., Daniels D.L., et al.: CT recognition of lateral lumbar disc herniation. *A.J.N.R.* 3:211–213, 1982.
50. Williams A.L., Haughton V.M., Meyer G.A., et al.: Computed tomographic appearance of the bulging annulus. *Radiology* 142:403–408, 1982.
51. Williams A.L., Haughton V.M., Syvertsen A.: Computed tomography in the diagnosis of herniated nucleus pulposis. *Radiology* 135:95–99, 1980.
52. Yu Y.L., Stevens J.M., Kendall B., et al.: Cord shape and measurements in cervical spondylotic myelopathy and radiculopathy. *A.J.N.R.* 4:839–842, 1983.
53. Zilkha A., Irwin G.A., Fagelman D.: Computed tomography of spinal epidural hematoma. *A.J.N.R.* 4:1073–1076, 1983.

INDEX

B

D

E

F

H

I

M

N

O

P

Q

R

S

W